EXCEPTIONAL INFANT

Psychosocial Risks in Infant-Environment Transactions

Exceptional Infant

Infant Volume 4

PSYCHOSOCIAL RISKS IN INFANT-ENVIRONMENT TRANSACTIONS

Edited by Douglas B. Sawin, Ph. D.,
Raymond C. Hawkins, II, Ph. D.,
Lorraine Olszewski Walker, R.N., Ph.D., &
Joy Hinson Penticuff, R.N., Ph.D.

BRUNNER/MAZEL New York

Library of Congress Catalog Card Number 68-517
ISBN 0-87630-222-3
ISSN 0071-3295

FOREWORD

When Graham Sterritt and Girvin Kirk joined me in the early 1970s editing *EXCEPTIONAL INFANT, VOLUME 3: Assessment and Intervention,* the emphasis in selecting articles for the book was on identifying and disseminating reports of action and innovation.

The spirit of the times stressed program building. Even though the Great Society of the 1960s was already becoming a relic of the past, developmental disabilities had just been discovered as a previously neglected frontier for social reconstruction. In many communities across the United States there was a gathering wave of new concern, new energy, new techniques and new funds to seek to improve the lives of disabled babies and young children.

In order to fulfill its intended function as a guide to further action, that book was organized to let one group of program builders help other program builders find useful answers to the specific question: "What shall we *do?"*

This new book, *EXCEPTIONAL INFANT, VOLUME 4,* reflects a different fundamental spirit. This new spirit may be summed up by the two questions: "What shall we *think about?"* and "What shall we *seek to understand?"*

The 15 major chapters and the associated commentary collected here examine a pervasive set of interconnected questions that have not received adequate recognition in the past. These questions deal with subtle interactions between child and environment when either or both are characterized by inherent obstacles to optimum development of children's growth potential.

The professions that deal with childhood disability have known for years that infancy is the period of maximum dependency and vulnerability. We have known that this is the period when disabled babies have most to gain and most to lose from environmental forces that shape their fate. Yet we have not focused concentrated attention on the full complexity of infant-environment relationships. We have not devoted sufficient analysis to understanding the lines of positive and negative force

v

between the constitutional disorders babies bring with them into the world and the environmental disorders these babies find awaiting them when they get here.

The editors and authors whose work this volume represents have pursued a major undertaking in repairing conceptual deficits in the field. These studies of psychosocial risks in infant-environment transactions embody a new spirit of intellectual depth in what in the past have often been excessively mechanistic and simplistic patterns of explanation and implementation.

As we move forward in the 1980s it is essential that we come to terms with another point we often overlook.

Understandably, we often fixate our attention upon pre-emptive life tragedies that are the daily work of the community of professions that deal with infant disabilities. We often fail to recognize that society's concern for victims of medical and social disadvantage is a topic on the public agenda that must jostle for a place in the public mind with other issues of major public concern. Funding levels are determined by political decisions that reflect public awareness and public commitment.

We know and care about babies whose lives are tragic right from the start. We are prepared to pay part of the costs of giving these babies the help they need. We frequently assume everybody cares, or that they would care if they knew what we know, and that they would pay, too.

It is often a shock to us to discover that this isn't true. Many don't know. Many don't want to know. And many others, whether they know or not, put their priorities elsewhere.

In this period when public attention increasingly is directed elsewhere, budgetary pressures constantly constrain us from *doing more* about problems we think deserve top priority. Within this constraint, perhaps it is right for us to be concerned now with *learning more*—and doing better.

In this respect, *EXCEPTIONAL INFANT, VOLUME 4* is a major step in the right direction. The rich collection of articles assembled here gives impressive evidence of enriched understandings of the life plight of those who must grapple with the heavy burden of infant disability. Progress is evident on virtually every page. This volume demonstrates that our professional community has the capacity to renew itself continually, to broaden the scope of relevant issues, to mobilize fresh knowledge, and to reexamine old ideas in terms of new values.

BERNARD Z. FRIEDLANDER, PH.D.

West Hartford, Connecticut
April, 1980

PREFACE

A better understanding of fetal and infant development has been the goal of recent extensive research conducted by investigators from diversity of disciplines including medicine, psychology, nursing, and social work. As our knowledge of normative developmental patterns has emerged, attention has been increasingly directed toward the factors which place some infants at risk for abnormal, or at least sub-optimal, development.

This volume is the fourth in the *Exceptional Infant* series. The editors and contributors to this volume address a range of topics pertaining to psychosocial risks in infant-environment transactions. We have defined psychosocial risks in infancy as the psychological (intellectual/cognitive, personality/temperamental, and social/behavioral) characteristics of infants *and* the social, environmental factors that place infants at a disadvantage for current adaptation and functioning ("competence"), as well as for future psychological and physical development.

The aim of this volume, which represents the product of a year-long symposia series held at the University of Texas at Austin and funded by a grant from the National Institute of Child Health and Human Development, was to explore theoretical and methodological perspectives that will facilitate systematic research of the nature of psychosocial risks. A second goal of the editors was to prepare a comprehensive "taxonomy" of psychosocial risk factors as a means of organizing the literature to facilitate its use by other researchers. The concluding section of this volume comprises the taxonomy of citations and an accompanying, cross-referenced bibliography.

Our operational definition of psychosocial risks in infancy reflects two assumptions regarding the unit of analysis. First, we believe that the prime focus should be upon the psychological characteristics of the infant that are predictive of current adaptation and future competence. Second, these infant characteristics shape, and are shaped by, social environmental factors such as the development-fostering qualities of families, in a complex, ongoing transactional process.

vii

FIGURE 1

Psychosocial Risks in Pregnancy and Early Infancy

PARENT   INFANT

BIOPHYSICAL RISKS
  Personality genetics
    (e.g. temperaments)
  Constitutional factors
    (intactness of sensory-motor,
    perceptual, and cognitive ap-
    paratus; physical illness; age;
    physique, hormones; nutrition-
    al status; pregnancy-birth com-
    plications, toxic effects of drugs,
    alcohol, tobacco;)

PSYCHOSOCIAL RISKS
  Age; educational level;
  SES and other demographics;
  Marital status, quality of marital
    relationship;
  Parenting models
    (attitudes about parental roles
    and infant care, preferences for
    certain infant characteristics,
    e.g. sex, due to familial educa-
    tional, and sociocultural influ-
    ences;)
  Life stress

Genetic-

$\longrightarrow$

Congenital
Influences

BIOPHYSICAL RISKS
  Personality genetics
    (e.g. temperaments, sex)
  Constitutional factors
    (intactness of sensory-motor,
    perceptual, and cognitive ap-
    paratus, physical illness; phys-
    ical characteristics; prematur-
    ity; PBC's; congenital impair-
    ments and neurodevelopmental
    lags; atypical birth weight;
    medication side effects;)

PSYCHOSOCIAL RISKS
  Learning influences
    (cognitive competencies & per-
    formance)
  Adoptee status;
  Birth order

⌐↓   CAREGIVER-INFANT TRANSACTION   ↗↙

(Rearing Process)

RECIPROCITY
shaping

P ————————→
←———————— I

feedback

1. Synchronous
2. Asynchronous
   a. Parent's violation of infant's limits
   b. Infant's violation of parent's limits
   c. Mutual violations
3. Early separation effects
4. "Optimally stimulating environment"
5. Invulnerable parents and families

↓
OUTCOMES

FIGURE 2

DEVELOPMENTAL OUTCOMES

INFANT AND YOUNG CHILD

1. "Normal" child
2. Developmental disabilities and mental retardation
3. Emotional and psychophysiological disorders
4. Hyperactivity and conduct disorders
5. Depression
6. Physical growth problems (obesity, failure to thrive)
7. Abuse
8. Psychosis (including Early Infantile Autism)
9. "Invulnerable child"

PARENTS AND FAMILIES

1. Normal parents and families
2. Parental reactive disorders
3. Marital discord
4. Disturbed family relations
5. Invulnerable parents and familes

PSYCHOSOCIAL INTERVENTION

What form? For whom?
When? How effective?

A framework for conceptualizing the major features of psychosocial risks is presented in Figure 1. Distinguished in this flow chart are the *types* of risks (i.e., biophysical vs. psychosocial) and the hypothesized *direction of influence* of these risk factors.

Biophysical risks (i.e., medical, genetic, and constitutional factors) are distinguished from psychosocial risks, which are the focus of this edited volume. Whereas biophysical risks are hypothesized to exhibit a unidirectional influence upon the infant, chiefly operative through genetic and congenital mechanisms, psychosocial risks are manifested *bidirectionally* through asynchronous caregiver-infant transactions, in which biophysical characteristics may, or may not, play a predisposing, mediating role. Some hypothesized developmental outcomes of psychosocial risks for the infant and young child (e.g., developmental disorders, physical growth problems, abuse, "invulnerableness") are presented in

Figure 2. The impact of an infant at psychosocial risk upon the family is implicit in these outcomes. Finally, four questions are raised regarding psychosocial intervention: What form should it take? For whom (i.e., for the infant and/or parents)? When? How effective? While the answers to these questions are not in this volume, we hope that the ideas and research presented herein will move us closer to answers and will stimulate and guide research toward even more informed answers than are possible from the literature to date.

The editors of this volume would like to acknowledge the substantial support and help that we have received in organizing the symposia series and in preparing this volume. We gratefully acknowledge the help of Dr. Martin Manosevitz in the preparation of the grant proposal for funds to sponsor the project. The idea to do so and the selection of the project members were his. Dr. Carol Deets was extremely helpful in sensible, instrumental ways during the preparation of the grant proposal.

We thank Rachael Daum for applying her excellent organizational skills to the day-to-day progress of the symposia series and the preliminary bibliographic work for the taxonomy. Bonny Keeler, Susanne Doell, and Pam Cobb contributed substantially to the final preparation of the taxonomy for which we are indebted to them.

The Center for Research for Mothers and Children, NICHD, NIH made the project possible with their generous support. We thank them not only for their support but for their willing cooperation at every stage of the project.

Our greatest debt is to the contributors to this volume who have made our task a reasonable one and who have made each of us better informed researchers of psychosocial development in infancy. Each of the contributors has been responsive to our purpose and most cooperative in facilitating the prompt completion of this volume. We thank them each sincerely.

DOUGLAS B. SAWIN, PH.D.
RAYMOND C. HAWKINS, II, PH.D.
LORRAINE OLSZEWSKI WALKER, R.N., PH.D.
JOY HINSON PENTICUFF, R.N., PH.D.

Austin, Texas
April, 1980

CONTENTS

Foreword v
> By Bernard Z. Friedlander

Preface vii

I. THEORETICAL PERSPECTIVES AND DEVELOPMENTAL MODELS OF
PSYCHOSOCIAL RISKS IN INFANCY 3

   1. Implications of Plasticity and Hierarchical Achievements
for the Assessment of Development and Risk of
Mental Retardation 7
> By J. McVicker Hunt

   2. Genetics of Psychosocial Risk 55
> By Lee Willerman

   3. A Diathesis-Stress Model for the Study of Psychosocial
Risks: The Prediction of Infantile Obesity 70
> By Raymond C. Hawkins, II

II. DEVELOPMENT OF EARLY PATTERNS OF PARENT-INFANT
INTERACTION: THE ROLE OF THE PARENT AND OF THE INFANT ... 87

   4. Disruption and Asynchrony in Early Parent-Infant
Interaction 91
> By Evelyn B. Thoman

   5. Interactions of High-Risk Infants: Quantitative and
Qualitative Differences 120
> By Tiffany Martini Field

   6. The Primacy of Social Skills in Infancy 144
> By Edward Tronick

III. ISSUES IN PSYCHOSOCIAL RISK: PARENT-INFANT SEPARATION,
EARLY INTERVENTION, AND BIO-ETHICAL CONSIDERATIONS 159

7. Disruption of Attachment Formation Due to Reproductive
Casualty and Early Separation 161
By Joy Hinson Penticuff

8. Fathers and Risk: A Hospital-Based Model of Intervention 174
*By Ross D. Park, Shelley Hymel, Thomas G. Power, and
Barbara R. Tinsley*

9. Pain-Filled Fruit of the Tree of Knowledge: Problems
and Paradoxes in the Sanctity of Life 190
By Bernard Z. Friedlander

Commentaries on Chapter 9:

Infanticide, Parental Crisis, and the Double-Edged Sword:
A Commentary 197
By Larry A. Bugen

A Physician's Perspective on the Problems and Paradoxes
in the Sanctity of Life 200
By Anne B. Fletcher

Perspectives on Decisions for Nontreatment of Damaged
Newborns 204
By James M. Diamond

Alternatives to Passive Euthanasia for Ameliorating the
Psychosocial Burdens of Parents Giving Birth to
Severely Damaged Infants 208
By Raymond C. Hawkins, II

IV. PARENTAL ATTITUDES ABOUT INFANTS: ISSUES IN ASSESSMENT
AND IMPLICATIONS FOR PARENTING BEHAVIOR 213

10. Parental Models: A Means for Evaluating Different
Prenatal Contexts 215
By Mary E. Pharis and Martin Manosevitz

11. Early Parental Attitudes and the Parent-Infant Relationship 234
By Lorraine Olszewski Walker

V. METHODOLOGICAL ISSUES IN ASSESSING INFANT CHARACTERISTICS
AND THE QUALITY OF PARENTS-INFANT INTERACTIONS 251

12. Dimensional Analyses of Newborn Behavior and Their
    Significance for Later Behavior: The Example of
    the Bethesda Longitudinal Study 255
    By Raymond K. Yang

13. Analyzing Behavioral Sequences: Differences Between
    Preterm and Full-term Infant-Mother Dyads
    During the First Months of Life 271
    Roger Bakeman and Josephine V. Brown

14. Lag Sequential Analysis as a Data Reduction Technique in
    Social Interaction Research 300
    By Gene P. Sackett

VI. OVERVIEW AND INTEGRATION OF CURRENT PERSPECTIVES ON
PSYCHOSOCIAL RISK AND INFANT DEVELOPMENT 341

15. Issues in Early Reproductive and Caretaking Risk:
    Review and Current Status 343
    By Arnold J. Sameroff

VII. A TAXONOMY OF PSYCHOSOCIAL RISK FACTORS IN
INFANCY: A GUIDE TO RECENT RESEARCH 361

Comprehensive Bibliography 397

Name Index 447

Subject Index 455

EXCEPTIONAL INFANT

Psychosocial Risks in Infant-Environment Transactions

Part I

THEORETICAL PERSPECTIVES AND DEVELOPMENTAL MODELS OF PSYCHOSOCIAL RISKS IN INFANCY

The papers comprising the first section of the volume represent initial attempts to formulate developmental models for psychosocial risk in infancy. These models should be helpful for determining the more important questions that researchers might address.

There are three basic theoretical paradigms implicit in our definition of psychosocial risks in infancy. The first paradigm is an *individual differences perspective* on characteristics of the developing infant in which the phenotype psychological characteristics of the infant are derived from underlying genotypic, genetic and congenital mechanisms. Implicit in this paradigm is a "continuity" assumption, in which characteristics of atypical infants, present at birth or shortly thereafter, provide a template shaping both the subsequent cognitive and behavioral competencies of the infant and also the infant's social environment. The second theoretical paradigm emphasizes the *development fostering qualities of the social environment* which promote infant adaptive modifications. This second paradigm assigns more importance to the quality of the infant's social environment in influencing subsequent development. The third model incorporates the infant and environmental variables within a diathesis stress, transactional context, where biophysical characteristics of the infant increase susceptibility to psychosocial stressors.

The paper by J. McVicker Hunt, entitled "Implications of Plasticity and Hierarchical Achievements for the Assessment of Development and Risk of Mental Retardation," provides a broad historical and conceptual overview of infant development and cultural-familial retardation, stressing the importance of the development-fostering qualities of the social environmental context. Dr. Hunt defines the concept of "plasticity" in

3

psychological development. Plasticity refers to an organism's capacity to make adaptive modifications to novel experiences. He summarizes the new evidence for plasticity, including his recent work concerning the effects of perceptual-cognitive and language training upon the developmental level of Iranian infant and preschool orphans. He next considers the implications of plasticity for theories of development in infants and children, contrasting the notions of heritability and educability. Hunt makes the contention, utilizing the range of reaction concept, that every child born without gross pathology or retardation has the genotypic potential to achieve all the abilities required for participation in the mainstream of any culture of the world. For, as a given heritability index holds only for a particular sample of life histories and for the particular sample of genotypes that are involved, educability is by definition the outcome of potential. The education process is limited only by the ingenuity of humankind to create development-fostering experiences from birth on and perhaps even earlier. Hunt comments on the implications of plasticity for the assessment and measurement of development as well, summarizing again the advantages of his criterion-referenced approach over the more traditional norm-referenced procedure. Finally, he examines the implications of plasticity for the assessment of infants and young children at psychosocial risk and for intervention strategies, speculating on how infant development researchers and practitioners may use the concept of plasticity to guide them in designing more ingenious programs to cope with what Hunt refers to as "the challenge of incompetence in poverty."

In his paper, entitled "Genetics of Psychosocial Risk," Lee Willerman provides us with a good example of the individual differences perspective toward characteristics of the developing infant, emphasizing genetic and congenital mechanisms. Dr. Willerman summarizes the evidence for the substantial genetic heritability of certain important infant psychological characteristics (e.g., capacity for cognitive growth). He cautions environmental enrichment proponents, such as Dr. Hunt, to demonstrate that observed improvements in infant or childhood cognitive level are due to what he calls "fertilizer effects" as opposed to "hothouse effects." Willerman analogizes that, in the hothouse, growth can be more rapid, but final attainment may not differ from expectation. Environmental enrichment programs exhibiting fertilizer effects, in contrast, increase ultimate attainment in addition to speeding up development. Most importantly, Willerman emphasizes the important consequences of taking a genetic perspective on psychosocial risks. He contends that multiple pathways exist to mental retardation; some are largely environmental but others are genetic in origin. He advises researchers to use more powerful research designs (e.g., adoptee methods) to permit separation of gene and environmental effects, thus encouraging efforts to dissect the heterogeneity of psychosocial risk outcomes.

Dr. Ray Hawkins outlines yet a third theoretical paradigm for the study of psychosocial risks—a *diathesis-stress model* illustrated for the prediction of infantile obesity. According to this model, specific biological/genetic characteristics of the infant (i.e., the "diathesis") may predispose heightened susceptibility to environmental stressors, leading to developmental disorders such as the onset of childhood obesity. Thus a genetic predisposition toward excess adipose tissue formation or underactive temperament may interact with infant overnutrition due to asynchronous caregiver-infant feeding transactions with the result being obesity.

This diathesis-stress model incorporates the features of the other two paradigms such that the reciprocal influences of infant characteristics and the development fostering qualities of the social environment reflect a *transactional process* yielding a continuity in the quality of infant individual adaptation to successive developmental tasks. Prediction of psychosocial risk outcomes for the infant and parents may be made from such a model (i.e., there is a developmental continuity), but these predictions must be based upon measures of both individual infant characteristics and characteristics of the social environment in transactions across development (Matas, Arend, & Sroufe, 1978; Sameroff, this volume).

1

Implications of Plasticity and Hierarchical Achievements for the Assessment of Development and Risk of Mental Retardation

J. McVICKER HUNT

University of Illinois

What I wish to do first is to show how the evidences of plasticity in psychological development led to recognition of social-class inequities of opportunity for early learning, how this led, in turn, to the mounting of Project Head Start, and how disappointment with the results led both psychologists and politicians to revisit the belief that heredity is the reason for the prevalence of school failures among children of poor uneducated parents. Second, I wish to examine the relevance of indices of heritability to educability, and to summarize some of the new evidences of plasticity, or the effects of experience on psychological development. Third, I wish to indicate the implications of this evidence for our conception of the nature of psychological development. Fourth, I wish to indicate the implications of the evidences of plasticity for assessing psychological development and educational achievement. Fifth, I wish to suggest their implications for assessing risk of mental retardation. Finally, I would like to indicate what now appears to be the nature of our hope of coping with the "challenge of incompetence and poverty."

The preparation of this paper has been supported by a grant from the Waters Foundation of Framingham, Mass. I wish to acknowledge this support with gratitude.

PLASTICITY AND SOCIAL-CLASS INEQUITIES

As long as the social Darwinism of Herbert Spencer and other 19th century sociobiological thinkers prevailed, it supported the beliefs in fixed intelligence and predetermined development (Cremin, 1962). As long as these beliefs prevailed, our traditional value of equality of opportunity had no apparent relevance to social class variations of opportunities during the preschool years.

In his book, *The Children's Cause*, Gilbert Y. Steiner (1976) credits two books that came out in the early sixties with changing this state of affairs. These books were my own *Intelligence and Experience* (Hunt, 1961) and one entitled *Stability and Change in Human Characteristics* by Benjamin Bloom (1964). These books assembled the accumulated evidence of the role of early experience in psychological development. In doing so, they made our traditional value of equality of opportunity relevant to the variations of opportunities during the preschool period which are associated with education, poverty, and social class. Yet, Steiner contends, these books would probably have had only academic significance had not President John F. Kennedy had a mentally deficient sister. Kennedy made the "war on poverty" the center of attention in his administration. Furthermore, he appointed his brother-in-law, R. Sargent Shriver, as Director of the Office of Economic Opportunity, newly organized to conduct this "war." Shriver's wife, Eunice Kennedy Shriver, had chosen as their pediatrician Dr. Robert Cooke. The Cookes, like the Kennedys, had a child who was mentally deficient.* Cooke was thereby attuned to the scientific literature in this domain. He knew of these books and other literature. When, in 1963-64, Cooke was chairman of a White House task force concerned with formulating the role that the federal government might play in fostering early child development, his task force made two recommendations that the Congress accepted and voted into operation. One was to increase support for scientific investigation of child health and development with the formation of the National Institute of Child Health and Human Development. Dr. Cooke's task force

---

* I use the words "mentally deficient" when there is a detectable pathology to account for observed retardation in behavioral development. I distinguish "mental retardation," which is merely descriptive, from "mental deficiency" which is based on some kind of pathology. A mentally deficient individual will be observed to be mentally retarded, but individuals may become mentally retarded also as a consequence of experience of poor development-fostering quality.

also contended that the state of the art was already such that it would justify a massive intervention in early education for children of the poor designed to prevent what I have called the "incompetence" that often results from an early life in the poverty sector. This second recommendation was the basis for the launching of Project Head Start.

Why the Results of Project Head Start Were Limited

Project Head Start, however, had other as well as educational aims. One of these concerned health gains to be assessed in medical terms; in this respect, it is significant that the person selected to direct Project Head Start was Dr. Julius Richmond, a child psychiatrist. Another aim of the program was to give the people from the poverty sector more control over their own lives and the lives of their children. This aim falls in the domain of community action, and it is significant that social workers figured heavily in shaping the operation of Project Head Start. When it came time to evaluate the project, however, the evaluation focused on the educational aims. Perhaps this was because failure in school is the most obvious deficiency of children from the poverty sector. Perhaps it was also because psychologists have developed tests of intelligence and of educational achievement, and these made it appear to be relatively easy to objectify the degree to which the educational aims of the project were achieved. So, the first evaluative studies, which appeared in the first volume of *Racial Isolation in the Public Schools* (U. S. Commission on Civil Rights, 1967) and in *The Impact of Head Start* (Cicirelli et al., 1969) conducted by the Westinghouse Learning Corporation, reported only a comparison of the test gains and the permanence of those gains in the children of uneducated parents of poverty who had and had not participated in Head Start programs. The upshot of these evaluative reports was that, yes, the children who participated in Head Start for at least a year gained more in academic achievement than did children with comparable levels of risk who did not participate. The gains from a single summer of participation, however, were miniscule. Moreover, those gains from a full year of participation were insufficient to enable participating children to become equals in academic achievement of children from middle-class backgrounds. Furthermore, by the time they entered the second grade, those who had participated in Head Start were no longer ahead of those who had not participated. In other words, the gains lacked permanence. This was the general picture because the evaluative studies had focused entirely on the achievement of the academic aims.*

One can properly ask why the impact of Project Head Start fell so far short of the hopes for it. If one accepts as valid the evidence of plasticity or the effects of experience in early psychological development, there are a variety of factors in the answer. First, the hopes were unrealistic. The very idea that it would be possible to overcome within a summer or even a year the effects of the experience of poor development and learning opportunities so common in the homes of poor uneducated parents was preposterous. Many of us most concerned with the effects of early experience and education (e.g., Cynthia and Martin Deutsch, Susan Gray, and myself), questioned the wisdom of launching such a large-scale program without a tested educational technology. When I wrote Julius Richmond in this vein, he responded that the medical consequences alone would justify launching the project. Unfortunately, the achievements in the medical domain received little attention. Not until Edward Zigler became the Director of the Office of Child Development were these and the effects in other domains assembled for Congress in order to show them the wisdom of continuing support for Project Head Start. Zigler then refocused the goals of the project on "social competence" which, at least by implication, he defined as ability to cope with the exigencies of living in the most general sense (see Zigler & Trickett, 1978). Our concerns were more limited, namely, to educational competence, and the doubts of such people as Martin and Cynthia Deutsch, Susan Gray, and myself were based upon our recognition that a large-scale project was being launched before a tested technology for compensatory education had been developed.

Project Head Start actually deployed the nursery schooling then prevalent in America. At least two of the early examples of nursery schooling did start with compensatory goals in view (Maria Montessori, 1909; Margaret McMillan, 1919), but most nursery schooling stemmed from Froebel's (1826) emphasis on play, based on his religious faith that the exercise of natural, God-given inclinations would optimize development, and from the laissez-faire emphasis of G. Stanley Hall, based on his faith

---

* Since this was written, evidence of delayed effects of compensatory education has come to my attention from the follow-up studies of consortium of pioneers in the use of preschool education to prevent school failure by children of poorly educated parents of poverty (Lazar & Darlington, 1978; Lazar, Hubble, Murray, Roache, & Royce, 1977). Moreover, an economic analysis of at least one of these preschool projects has found these delayed, or "sleeper," effects to make it cost effective (Weber, Foster, & Weikart, 1978).

in the notion of recapitulation (see Pruette, 1926). Hall had an appreciation of the epigenetic nature of development. He conceived exercise of the behavior characteristic of each stage of development to be essential for the appearance of the behavioral patterns to come. This justified laissez-faire permissiveness for him. These early roots of laissez-faire permissiveness were greatly bolstered in the 1920s and 1930s by the influence of psychoanalysis as it was understood in the child guidance movement (Healy, Bronner & Bowers, 1930). At this time, neurotic inhibition and compulsiveness were commonly viewed as a consequence of the influence of over-controlling mothers. From this view, the purpose of nursery schooling was to keep children out of the reach of over-controlling mothers for about half of each day so that they would be less likely to develop superegos so strong as to produce neurotic inhibitions and compulsive characters. Because of this history, the prevailing kind of nursery schooling that we disseminated in Project Head Start was poorly suited for the compensatory task of teaching the symbolic and motivational achievements so commonly weak in the children of poor, uneducated parents.

Another reason for the limited and transient gains from Project Head Start is the confusion of our community-action goals with our educational goals. Community action meant getting the parents to participate in the educational process. This was a laudable aim, but bringing parents into the management and educational operations without adequate training led to confusion and compromised the compensatory educational efficiency of many of the programs (Payne, Mercer, Payne & Davidson, 1973).

Yet another factor limiting gains resulted from the fact that only a few people had any inkling of the specific nature of the developmental deficiencies in children of these poor and uneducated parents, and those who did have at least a limited understanding of these deficiencies had little influence on the planning of the curricula disseminated. Neither did any of the people concerned understand what Piaget (1945) has termed the "equilibrium" or "equilibration" (Piaget, 1977). This concept concerns the role of the discrepancy between cognitive achievements and cognitive demands of situations in functioning and education that I have attempted to encapsulate in what I like to call "the problem of the match" with emphasis on the emotional and motivational aspects (see p. 00). As long as the concept of predetermined development prevailed and age was considered to be the essential consideration in the choice of learning experiences, however, little progress in understanding the role of this discrepancy in the educational process could be made.

There is also at least one hypothesis which suggests that perhaps the worst possible age was chosen for compensatory education. This is the hypothesis of *phrenoblysis* put forth by Herman P. Epstein (1974a, 1974b). He contends that there are periods of rapid growth of the brain relative to the soma which alternate with periods of relatively slow brain growth. Epstein, a biophysicist, got interested in this problem after coming to feel that the educational experience of his daughter was highly unfortunate. He undertook to examine the annual increments in head size and discovered that substantial changes occurred during certain periods but not during others. The periods of rapid growth in human children were from age 2-4, 6-8, 10-12, and from 14-16. There is also a sex difference in the ages of the last period of rapid growth indicated. Next, he asked whether these periods meant anything intellectually, and he began to look for evidences of changes in the IQ in longitudinal testing. He discovered that these same periods are associated with significant increases in IQ. Since the IQ was designed to be constant in groups, the existence of significant increases associated with various ages is of interest. From these relationships he derived the hypothesis that, due to the endogenous processes of brain growth, there are periods when experience can make a lot more difference in children's achievement levels than they would in other periods.

I have taken Epstein's hypothesis seriously enough to look at the results of Head Start in this manner. To make a long story short, the gains that occur during the fourth year (when compensatory education is introduced at age three rather than four) are definitely larger than those obtained during the fifth and sixth years. Also, those gains which are being reported in the Follow Through Program are substantially larger than those that occur during the fifth year. These data are nicely consonant with Epstein's hypothesis, *but* they do not necessarily constitute evidence for it because the proportion of the total achievement at three is considerably less than that at four and five, and the duration of compensatory education is substantially greater for those children in the Follow Through Program than for those in Head Start. Nevertheless, it is not inconceivable that the fifth year in the lives of children may have been a poor time to institute a program with a compensatory purpose.

Revisiting the Hypothesis of Heritability

Presenting here all these reasons why Head Start failed to achieve more than it actually did is based upon the presumption that these children from uneducated poor families have the necessary genotypic potential to learn what the schools attempt to teach and to acquire the knowledge, the skills, the motivations, and the values required for a productive role in the mainstream of society. Despite these various factors limiting the results from Project Head Start, the so-called "failure" of the Project has prompted a revisiting in those traditional beliefs in intelligence being essentially fixed and development being predetermined by heredity.

In his widely read paper entitled, "How Much Can We Boost IQ and Scholastic Achievement?", Arthur Jensen (1969) opened with this sentence: "Compensatory education has been tried and it apparently has failed" (p. 1). The remainder of his paper aims to answer the question, "Why?" It presents a long discourse on the measurement and meaning of heritability which adds up to the proposition traditional in textbooks of psychology before World War II, namely, that approximately 80% of the variance in the IQ, but somewhat less of the variance in the scores on tests of achievement, is attributable to heredity. Since only 20% of the total variance remains, he argues that neither compensatory education, nor even life experience in general, can be expected to have much influence on those social-class and racial differences in performance on tests of intelligence and academic achievement.

This argument from Jensen (1969, 1972, 1973) has received support from the authority of Nobel prize physicist, William Bradford Shockley, partial support from Richard Herrnstein (1971, 1973), and others. Moreover, it has rearoused the emotionality of the old harangues on the relative influence of heredity and environment which I had hoped would by now be "by the boards." This paper of Jensen's, however, was discussed by the Nixon cabinet in some detail (Hirsch, 1976), and it seems to have had some importance in reducing the enthusiasm of the Nixon Administration for both the Office of Economic Opportunity and Project Head Start.

RELEVANCE TO EDUCATION: HERITABILITY OR THE RANGE OF REACTION

In view of what is in essence a revisiting of the beliefs in fixed intelligence and predetermined development backed with evidence from measures of heritability, let me counter with the proposition that measures of heritability are irrelevant to educability (see Hunt, 1977).

At best, indices of heritability constitute an indirect approach to the assessment of educability. They are indirect because they involve statistical assessments of heritability, or the percentage of variance in measures of such a trait as the IQ, which must then be subtracted from 100%, the total variance, to obtain an estimate of the variance in the trait attributable to experience. In the argument of Jensen, the proportion of the variance in the IQ attributed to heredity is 80%. His argument and his percentage was traditional in textbooks of psychology before World War II. Since heritability is 80%, so the argument goes, this leaves only 20% of the variance in the IQ attributable to variations in life experiences. Thus, little effect from a program such as Head Start is possible.

Actually, indices of heritability are irrelevant to educability for two main reasons. First, *educability* is, by definition, a matter of *potential*. It is a matter of what characteristics and competencies an individual might develop with differing life experiences. *Heritability* indices are only *properties of* the *particular populations* on which they are based. This means that each index of heritability applies only to that particular variation of genotypes and that particular variation in life histories from which it is derived. No matter how many samplings under existing social conditions result in indices of heritability approximating 80%, they are not applicable to any new population for which new child-rearing practices have been devised. The ultimate level of competence attainable is clearly a matter of human ingenuity in the domains of child-rearing and education (see also Hirsch, 1972).

A second reason for this irrelevance derives from the fact that measures of heritability concern individual differences in the measures of various competencies whereas educability is concerned with achieving those competencies demanded by the standards of the culture for a productive role. One of the great misfortunes in the history of the influence of psychology on education has been this emphasis on individual differences. This emphasis may reflect the idea of the struggle for existence which emerged from the first studies of human population in relation to the food supply made during the 18th century in the stormy society of pre-revolutionary France. It was formulated most clearly in the famous *Essay on the Principles of Population* by Parson Thomas Malthus in 1978. Charles Darwin acknowledged this as the guiding idea for his *Origin of the Species* in 1859. The idea was also central to Francis Galton's study of *Hereditary Genius* in 1869. It was this work which launched the study of individual differences and emphasized the role of heredity in their causation. Moreover, in his first study, where he followed Galton in the use of twins for determining the relative importance of heredity and environment, E. L. Thorndike (1905) contended that: "In the actual race of life, which is not to get ahead, but to get ahead of somebody, the chief determining factor is heredity" (p. 553). While competition clearly plays a useful role in various aspects of life, the goal of education is much less "to get ahead of somebody" than it is for individuals to attain sets of competencies required by the culture for productive participation somewhere in the mainstream of their society. Thus, the goal of *educability* is not to be defined competitively in terms of the individual's position in some sample of the population, but rather by the attainment of abilities, attitudes, kinds of knowledge, kinds of skills, and values required for productive and respected participation somewhere in the mainstream of the society. What is important for education, therefore, is not individual differences in achievement reflected in the measures of the variance, but rather the achievement of a standard of excellence in performance required by a mainstream position within the society. Since measures of heritability aim to account for variance in potential or ability, this constitutes a second reason for their irrelevance to educability.

There are empirical aspects of this second reason for the irrelevance of indices of heritability to educability. One consists of the fact that the more similar the rearing conditions of individuals are, the smaller is the variance among individuals in the ages of attaining developmental landmarks and in measures of development or educational achievement. For instance, the standard deviation of the ages of the children of Metera Center who are at the upper three levels in the development of object permanence was only a third that of home-reared children from working-class families at the same level even though the former averaged substantially older than the latter (Paraskevopoulos & Hunt, 1971). In the same study, similar but less prominent trends in the standard deviations and means of ages were found for those at the upper levels of vocal imitation. Another example may be found in connection with a series of interventions in child-rearing practices at the Orphanage of the Queen Farah Pahlavi Charity Society in Tehran. There, those interventions which tended to reduce the variation in the life experiences of the children resulted in very substantially reduced standard deviations of the ages at which they achieved the top steps on the ordinal scales of Uzgiris and Hunt (1975).

Such a finding has also been reported by Smilansky (1979)* for the children of Oriental Jews of professional status and of marginal working-

---

* Recalled by Hunt and others from Smilansky's oral presentation, but omitted from this publication.

class status who have migrated to Israel. For those settling in cities, where the life experiences of the children from birth on are controlled by the parents and involve the differences in their tutelage, the difference in mean IQ is between 30 and 40 points. On the other hand, when these two classes of parents have settled in kibbutzim, where children from both classes of parents share daily life with their caretakers in the baby houses, the difference between the mean IQs of the children of parents from these differing social classes is reduced to between five and 10 points. At this writing, relatively few of such data appear to exist. Those which exist indicate that the more alike the life histories of individuals are, the less the variance among them in rates of development and in such measures of ability as the IQ. We should have many more of such data.

The Range of Reaction

A second empirical aspect of this second reason for the irrelevance of heritability to educability comes from evidence deriving from a strategy of investigation suggested by the *range of reaction*. The range of reaction is a concept of geneticists authored by Richard Woltereck in 1909 (see Dunn, 1965, p. 95ff). Woltereck was a zoologist who worked with variations in measurable characteristics of pure lines of daphnia reared under differing conditions of nutrition and temperature. Whereas an index of heritability is the property of a population, the range of reaction is the property of an individual genotype. For this reason, a major share of the work on the range of reaction has been done by botanists because they have had the methodological advantage of plants that clone. Cloning permits an investigator to have numerous individuals with the same genotype. Samples of cloning plants can therefore be reared under differing conditions, and the variation in the phenotypic characteristics can be observed and measured. Woltereck's work, even though it appears to have stemmed from that of Johannsen (1903, 1909), the Danish botanist who first distinguished observable, measurable *phenotypes* from *genotypes*, concerned the phenotypic modifications produced in pure lines of daphnia, a species of crustacia, by development under diverse conditions. These modifications in phenotypic characteristics led him to the concept of the *range of reaction*.

Variations in competencies, semantic mastery of various kinds of information, and motivations in identical twin human beings reared under diverse conditions fit perfectly the definition of the range of reaction, and they would have the essence of relevance to educability. Unfortunately, there is a paucity of such data. Studies of identical twins reared apart have been done, but they have usually been done to obtain the correlation between the IQs of such twins for comparison with the correlation between the IQs of fraternal twins to obtain indices of heritability (see Jensen, 1967), or with the correlation between identical twins reared together to determine how much rearing apart lowers the correlation (see Burt, 1966). In either case, the concern is with individual differences rather than with how much measures of competence can be modified. Moreover, the variations in the development-fostering quality of rearing conditions for those reared apart have not been large, have often failed to involve the first months or even years of life, and certainly have not involved specific treatments designed especially to foster various aspects of development.

The maximal observed difference between the IQs of a pair of identical twins reared apart to the best of my knowledge is 17 points and this difference was reported in a study by Holzinger (1929). Moreover, only Holzinger, again to the best of my knowledge, has also reported a correlation of pair differences in IQ with assessments of the amounts of difference in the development-fostering quality of the rearing conditions in the homes in which the twins were reared apart. This correlation was reported to be +.70. In the logic of correlation coefficients, such a finding would suggest that approximately half of the variance in the IQs of Holzinger's sample of identical twins should be attributed to their differing life experiences. Even for that pair in Holzinger's sample with a difference in IQ of 17 points, however, only a moderate difference is evident in the development-fostering quality of their life experiences.

In order to determine the potential size of the range of reaction for educability by rearing identical twins apart, it would be necessary to rear one of each pair under such conditions as those in the Tehran Orphanage when Dennis (1960) visited there to find 50% of those infants in their second year not yet sitting up and more than 80% of those in their fourth year not yet walking. It would be necessary to rear the other twin in each pair from birth through at least toddlerhood by caretakers taught how to foster initiative, trust, vocal imitation, and language such as we employed with our fifth sample of foundlings at the Orphanage of the Queen Farah Pahlavi Charity Society in Tehran (see below, and Hunt et al., 1976). Thereafter, the former twin would have to continue his/her life in an understaffed orphanage with no continuing relationships with any adult person while the latter should have a continuing affectionate relationship with one or more adults who would provide understandable answers to his/her "why?" questions, and such educational experiences as James Mill and his wife provided for their son, John Stuart. Who knows how much the IQs of pairs of identical twins with such widely different life histories might differ? For both ethical and humanitarian reasons, of course, no such studies will ever deliberately be made. In passing, it is worth noting, however, that I would expect heredity to figure in the amount of difference obtained. For instance, I would expect greater differences between the IQs of pairs of twins without detectable pathology at birth than for pairs of twins with Down's syndrome if both were reared under such contrasting conditions (see Hunt, 1961, p. 323ff).

There is, however, an alternative version of this strategy suggested by the concept of the range of reaction which is entirely feasible. It consists of comparing the means and standard deviations of such measures of phenotypic competence as the IQ in groups of children from the same population who have been reared under differing circumstances. Since the range of reaction is the property of a given genotype, an alternative stretches the definition of both the genotype and the norm or range of reaction. The alternative strategy suggested substitutes samples for individuals and a population, defined as a group of males and females with equal opportunities for mating, for a genotype. When samples of infants from a given population are reared under differing conditions, the difference between the resulting means of the measure of the phenotypic characteristic is an average of the ranges of reaction for the population to the differing sets of rearing conditions. Such differences have the essence of relevance to educability. Moreover, it is from the differences between the mean measures of achievement for samples, as nearly random as feasible, from the same population reared under radically different conditions, that the new evidences of plasticity have come.

NEW EVIDENCES OF PLASTICITY

Since 1966, I have had underway such a program of research at the Orphanage of the Queen Farah Pahlavi Charity Society in Tehran (see Hunt et al., 1976). The findings from this program have been supplemented by those from the studies conducted in a variety of places. At the Tehran Orphanage, the independent variable has consisted of a series of interventions into the child-rearing practices of the institution. Each kind of intervention has been followed longitudinally. Consequently, the dependent variables have consisted of the means and standard deviations of the ages at which infants achieved the steps on each of seven ordinal scales inspired by the observations of Jean Piaget (Uzgiris & Hunt, 1975). For both ethical and investigative reasons, we chose not to have simultaneous treatment and control groups (see Hunt et al., 1976). We chose, rather, to base our comparisons of the means and standard deviations of the ages of achieving the steps on our ordinal scales between successive samples, or waves, of infants for which each successive intervention was intended to improve the development-fostering quality of the life experience.

The infants in each of the groups, which we have termed "waves," have been foundlings. This is to say that the infants were without known parents or relatives. They had typically been left in a mosque or on the steps of a police station, often wrapped in swaddling clothes and placed in a paper sack. From these places, they were taken to the Municipal Orphanage of Tehran. Whenever the program called for a new wave of foundlings, one collaborator, Mehri Ghodssi, the director of the Orphanage of the Queen Farah Pahlavi Charity Society, and her attending pediatrician obtained them from those available in the Municipal Orphanage. Aside from their being foundlings, the only criteria for selection as our subjects were being less than a month old and an absence of detectable pathology. Thus, these successive waves of infants in our program approximate samples from a single population as nearly as one is likely to achieve in human society.

For the first, control wave of 15 foundlings, the only intervention in the child-rearing practices of the orphanage consisted of examining each infant individually with our Piaget-inspired ordinal scales every other week during their first year and every fourth week thereafter until they were transferred to another orphanage at some time around three years of age. This same scheme of assessing the dependent variables was employed with each successive wave.

The second wave of 10 foundlings got what was intended to be auditory-visual enrichment consisting of tape-recorded music and mother-talk, which the infant could obtain at will by pulling on a cord attached to a plastic bracelet around his/her wrist, or of movement in a mobile hung over the crib which the infant could obtain by body shaking. The auditory and visual inputs were thus intended to be made responsive to the infant's spontaneous actions. Unfortunately, this intent was aborted for this second wave because the resident director at the time failed to keep the apparatus in order. We appear actually to have done some damage to the infants in this wave even though their caretakers were instructed to care for them in the same fashion they cared for those without the apparatus. The caretakers may perhaps have failed to follow this instruction because they felt that these infants, with this apparatus on their cribs, who were housed in the same ward along with between 20 and 30 others, were getting something extra.

The third wave of 10 foundlings got what we called "untutored human enrichment." For this group, the infant-caretaker ratio was reduced from 10:1 to 10:3. The caretakers, however, were free to do whatever came naturally, and each was equally responsible for all 10 infants.

The fourth wave, this time of 20 foundlings, got the auditory-visual enrichment that had been planned for the second wave, and this time the apparatus was kept in repair and the details of the plan were followed reasonably well.

The fifth wave of 11 foundlings also got "human enrichment," but this time we taught the caretakers what to do to foster development. We taught them by means of a translation of Badger's Teaching Guides for Infants (1971a) and Toddlers (1971b). These guides were also revised to include instructions concerning how to foster vocal imitation, upon which the phonological aspect of language is based, and semantic mastery for those experiences intimately involved in the caretaking operation such as the parts of the body, the pieces of clothing worn, and the verbs for the various operations. Also, unlike the case for Wave III, each caretaker was put in charge of specified infants. It was intended that each should be in charge of three of the foundlings, a reduction in the infant-caretaker ratio from 10:1 to 3:1 approximately matching that for the third wave. The director of the orphanage, however, had visited Metera Center in Athens. There, she had observed a program with an infant-caretaker ratio of 3:1 upon which she chose to improve despite methodological objections. Consequently, four of the caretakers had but two infants in their care and only the fifth had three. These were our five waves. Each wave was more than a year old before the next wave was assembled, and sometimes nearly two years separated successive waves.

The seven ordinal scales inspired by Piaget's observations that were used to assess the effects of the successive interventions were: (1) object permanence, (2) development of means, (3) vocal imitation, (3b) gestural imitation, (5) operational causality, (6) object relations in space, and (7) schemes for relating to objects (for descriptions of these scales, see Uzgiris & Hunt, 1975).

For a full account of the results, I must refer you to the monograph already mentioned (Hunt et al., 1976). There it will be seen, first, that except for the abortive attempt at auditory-visual enrichment for Wave

II, each intervention served, at least ultimately, to hasten development. This is to say that each intervention reduced the mean ages at which the successive waves attained the top steps on all these scales. Second, it will be seen that the untutored human enrichment provided for Wave III hastened only the development of posture and locomotion. This is to say that it reduced the mean age of achieving a sitting posture and of cruising while holding on to the sides of the crib, and it failed completely during the first year to influence the rate of development on any of our Piaget-inspired scales. During the second year, however, this untutored human enrichment did serve to hasten the achievement of the top steps on all of the Piaget-inspired scales. Third, it will also be seen that the audiovisual enrichments provided for Wave IV served to hasten the early development of the infants as measured by the mean ages at which they acquired the lower steps on these scales. After they were approximately 40 weeks of age, however, the infants of Wave V, who received the tutored human enrichment, pulled well ahead of those of Wave IV. Here I must limit further presentation of the results to the differences between the mean ages at which the 25 infants in Waves I and II, combined, and the 11 infants of Wave V achieved the top steps on the seven scales. These appear in Table I.

TABLE 1

Mean Ages in Weeks of Achieving the Top Steps on the Several
Uzgiris-Hunt Scales by the Combined[a] Control Group and by the
Group Reared by Tutored Caretakers with the Differences
Between Them and Between Mean Ages of Achievement
Transformed to IQ-Ratios

Scales	Nb	I & II Estimated[c] Mean Age	Nb	V Mean Age	Difference in Mean Age	in IQ-Ratios
I. Object Permanence	15	127	11	93	34	32
II. Development of Means	12	148	11	94	54	41
III-A. Vocal Imitation	10	156	11	93	63	49
III-B. Gestural Imitation	8	158	11	71	87	83
IV. Operational Causality	14	138	11	85	53	40
V. Object Relations in Space	12	141	11	88	53	35
VI. Schemes for Relating to Objects	2	169	11	90	79	45

a. The combination included the 15 controls for which the only intervention consisted of examinations every other week during the first year and every fourth week thereafter till they were transferred to another orphanage.
b. The numbers of children who demonstrated the critical behavior for the top step of each scale. The number of controls (Waves I & II) was 25, that of the group reared by tutored caretakers (Wave V) was 11.
c. In estimating the mean age of achieving the top step on each scale, the mean age of transfer (169 weeks) has been used for those who failed. This yields very conservative estimates of the lags among the controls.

Table 1 shows that the differences in mean ages of achieving the top steps on the several scales varied considerably. The largest difference, 87 weeks, occurs for the scale of Gestural Imitation. The next largest, 79 weeks, occurs for Schemes for Relating to objects. Here the top step consists of spontaneously naming the objects presented to the infants by the examiner. Of the 25 infants in Waves I and II, only two ever spontaneously named an object before they departed the orphanage at about three years of age. These two exceptions had been pets of caretakers.* On the other hand, of the 11 foundlings in Wave V whose caretakers were taught how to foster vocal imitation and semantic mastery, all spontaneously named objects before they were 22 months old.

The smallest difference in Table 1, that of 34 weeks, is to be found for the mean ages of attaining the top step of object permanence. This is much smaller than the largest difference obtained in our research between mean ages of achieving the top step on the scale of object permanence. The largest difference has been that between the mean age (182.3 weeks) at which the top step on this scale was achieved by infants reared from birth at the Municipal Orphanage of Athens and the mean age (73.02 weeks) at which it was attained by eight consecutive infants born to the uneducated parents of poverty served by the Parent and Child Center of Mt. Carmel, Illinois. These eight Mt. Carmel infants, however, had the experiences provided in a program of educational day-care based on the already-mentioned teaching guides of Earladeen Badger. These guides emphasized the importance, according to the theory behind what I call "the problem of the match" (Hunt, 1961, pp. 267ff; 1966, p. 131), of providing materials to keep infants interested. It so happened, however, that the toy which most attracted the interest of these infants from their seventh to their 17th month of life was a shape box. This box was about six inches in each of three dimensions, had a hinged top with holes of five shapes, and blocks shaped to match these holes. Once a block dropped through the hole of the same shape, it disappeared while making a distinct sound from landing on the bottom of the box. The block could then be retrieved by lifting the top. Although we have not yet reproduced this effect, this experience with the shape box appears

---

* According to the account that I got, these two infants who became pets in Waves I and II had been ill when very young. Those who gave special care to these infants appeared through this care to become attached to them, thereby exemplifying Festinger's (1957) theory of cognitive dissonance. The examiners who reported this seemed to feel that becoming attached to infants through special care given during an illness was "perfectly natural."

serendipitously to have had a marked hastening effect on the rate of advancement on this branch Piaget (1936) has called object construction.

This largest obtained difference of 109 weeks is not readily interpretable, however, because we have no ready frame of reference for such data. This difference can readily be transformed into one between means of the IQ-ratio for object permanence, and for the purpose of communication, it may be worthwhile. Once the transformation is made, the difference becomes one of the order of 90 points between the mean IQ-ratio for children at the Municipal Orphanage in Athens and the mean IQ-ratio for those who got the educational day-care at Mt. Carmel. This maximal obtained difference in the mean ages of attaining the top step on the scale of object permanence cannot be properly taken as a range of reaction because the men and women served by the Parent and Child Center of Mt. Carmel did not have equal opportunities for mating with those of Athens. Yet, it is reasonable to attribute the difference in rates of object construction to life experiences because there is no reason whatever to believe that the children of poor, uneducated parents in Mt. Carmel, Illinois, had greater genotypic potential for object construction than the illegitimate children born to largely working-class parents in Athens. The credibility of this interpretation becomes even greater when one considers that these eight consecutive infants born to parents served by the Parent and Child Center of Mt. Carmel achieved the top step on the scale of Object Permanence at a mean age (73 weeks) which is 25 weeks younger than that (98 weeks) at which a sample of 12 home-reared infants from predominantly professional families in Worcester, Massachusetts, attained it (see Hunt et al., 1975). Transformed into points of the IQ-ratio for object permanence, this advance is of the order of 34 points. Since it directly contradicts the hypothesis that social class differences are hereditary, this advance must be attributable to the experiences in the educational day-care.

Thus far, I have been discussing the effects of experience on the rate at which specific branches of development occur. The mean of these differences in mean ages of achieving the top steps on all seven of the ordinal scales is 65.43 weeks. When this difference is transformed into a mean IQ-ratio for all seven scales combined, the result is a difference of 46.7 points. Since standard IQs are based upon a substitutive average across branches to obtain the mental age, this difference in mean IQ-ratio for all seven branches represents a good approximation of the difference of the mean IQ for the 25 foundlings in Waves I and II from the mean IQ for the 11 foundlings in Wave V. Perhaps you should know that

Humphrey (personal communication) has found scores based on performances on a composite of Piaget's tasks showing a correlation of +.87 with the Stanford-Binet IQs. And the 11 foundlings of Wave V achieved the top steps on five of these seven scales at younger average ages than did a sample of 12 home-reared infants from predominantly professional families in Worcester, Massachusetts (see Hunt et al., 1976).

Non-Metrical Effects of the Interventions

These effects on the mean ages of attaining the top steps on these ordinal scales are representative of those psychological performances for which we have a metric. We had no good metric for their achievement of early learning, or for social attractiveness, or for such personality characteristics as mood, initiative, and trust. Yet, the contrast between the children of Wave V and those of Waves I and II in such characteristics appears to be every bit as marked as that on those variables for which we did use measures with a metric.

Consider first language achievement (see Hunt, 1979a). As noted above, only two of the 25 controls in Waves I and II ever spontaneously named an object during their first three years. One can safely say that the remaining 23 had achieved neither expressive nor even receptive language by that age. One can justify the statement that they lacked expressive language without difficulty for their only vocalizations consisted of crying and of yelling in anger. Moreover, these vocalizations seemed to be directed at no one in particular, but rather at the world at large.

It is more difficult to justify the statement that they lacked receptive language. The justification I have is based on what I like to call "horseback research." During my visit to Tehran, when the children in Wave I were approximately 30 months old, I would stand near several of them and request either one of their caretakers or an examiner to tell a specified one of them to "Go to the man," namely, me. Only the two pets ever responded to such verbal directions. Yet, if I looked directly at the child concerned, smiled and thrust out my arms in a gesture of invitation, I regularly got one of two reactions. Under half of the children would come directly to me, but the faces of the others would cloud up in distress as they withdrew further from me. Either reaction indicated an appreciation of the meaning of my gesture, but there had been no such sign of such appreciation of the meaning of the verbal directions. Other such tests of receptive language were also improvised, but this was the least complex of them. Thus, even at 30 months of age, all but two of the 15 controls in Wave I appeared to be without either expressive or receptive language. There were similar findings for the 10 infants of Wave II on a later visit.

Of the 11 infants in Wave V whose caretakers got instruction in the fostering of vocal imitation and semantic mastery, on the other hand, all had not only spontaneously named objects well before they were two years old, but, by age two, they also had vocabularies of at least 50 words. This was ascertained by touching features of their faces, parts of their bodies, various of their garments, and pieces of furniture while asking, in Persian, "What's that?" Moreover, the quality of their imitative pronunciation of strange words was judged by one of the Persian examiners to be better than that of four children from Wave III still available in the orphanage who were then over four years old. These four children had also received human enrichment, but without a specific caretaker

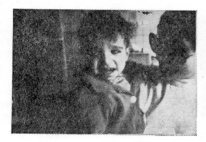
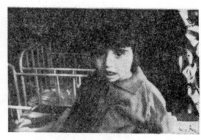
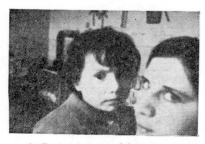
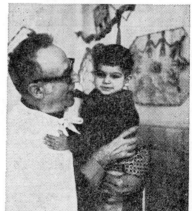

FIGURE 1. Four of the foundlings from the control wave were reared according to the usual child-rearing practices of the orphanage except for the repeated examining. The infant-caretaker ratio was about 30 to 3. The infants were about 20 months of age when these snapshots were taken.

knowledgeable in how to foster vocal imitation and semantic mastery. This contrast in language achievement was obviously exceedingly sharp and deep in a qualitative sense even though we have no nice metric for it.

Consider next the contrast in appearance. In Figure 1, first, we have snapshots of four of the controls. Note their glum expressions with an absence of any sign of enthusiasm, interest, or initiative. The appearance of the child pictured in my arms was taken while I was uttering my imitation of infant vocalizations in order to elicit a pseudo-imitative response from him. His expression hints at a mild degree of interest, but there was no pseudo-imitative response even though he was then at least 18 months of age. He has the most attractive and interested expression on any of the controls for which snapshots were made.

Parenthetically, these snapshots were originally taken only for me to have a means of identifying the subjects. There was no plan to use them as evidence. In fact, it was only after I had assembled the pictures to

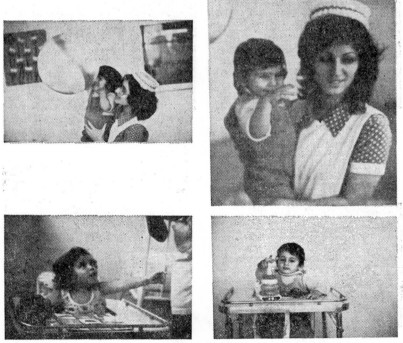

FIGURE 2. Four of the foundlings reared by caretakers, who were taught how to foster psychological development including vocal imitation and semantic mastery, were 18 to 22 months of age when these snapshots were taken.

accompany my acount of our success in fostering language achievement that I realized how they could also illustrate the contrast in appearance and social attractiveness so obvious when one saw the children in action.

In Figure 2, for contrast, are snapshots of four of the infants from Wave V who received the tutored human enrichment. On the left in the top pair is Cambiz. Note the enthusiasm with which he is striking the ball that hangs by a string from the ceiling. If one did not hold him firmly, the force of his efforts would throw him from one's arms to the floor. The picture on your right of the top pair is of Shabnam. Note her interested expression and her waving. She was the youngest of Wave V. Even though she was somewhat less than 18 months of age when this snapshot was made, she already had a vocabulary of over 50 words. The third picture, lower left, is of Monee. Note how his arm is outstretched presumably in a request for attention or perhaps for help from a caretaker. When this snapshot was taken, Monee was about 22 months of age. Not only could he name correctly some 50 things, but he also showed semantic mastery for the elementary abstraction of colors by correctly naming reds, yellows, greens, and blues when they were pointed to in pictures along the walls. When one realizes that somewhat less than a fourth of the children in Head Start show such mastery of colors, this demonstrated no small achievement for a foundling of less than two years who had been reared in an orphanage. The picture on the lower right is of Parviz, busy with his stacking toy. He had a vocabulary of about 50 words, and he would usually correctly name any of the four primary colors when they were pointed to, as would Cambiz. Unfortunately, I did not personally try all children of Wave V on color naming.

I believe you will agree that these four children of Wave V appear more attractive socially than do the controls. Their attractiveness, I believe, derives from their interested facial expressions and the evidence of either enthusiasm or initiative in their postures or gestures.

As further evidence of their social attractiveness, it is interesting to note that seven of these 11 children in Wave V were adopted by childless couples in Tehran while only two of the preceding 55 infants in the first four waves were ever adopted. Moreover, those two were adopted when they were less than six months old because they were pretty babies. These seven were adopted as two-year-olds because they were alert, interested, socially responsive, full of initiative and trust, and therefore socially attractive.

It is worth calling attention to this contrast in appearance because one often hears, even from psychologists, the contention that the difference of children in educated families of the middle class from those of poor, uneducated parents must be hereditary because they "look so different." In these studies, as already noted, each wave has consisted of foundlings taken from the Municipal Orphanage of Tehran when they were no more than a month old and were without detectable pathology. In other words, each wave came from the same basic population. Thus, these differences in age of achieving the top steps on the ordinal scales, in language achievement, and in appearance must have arisen out of their rearing conditions.

Other Such Data

These data on the effects of experience from our own research are limited to the first two or three years of life. Although such data are limited, there are some which extend assessment of the effects of experience to older ages.

First, there is the evidence of the damage from orphanage rearing. It appears to be of the order of 50 IQ points. This statement is based upon the evidence in Dennis' (1973) *Children of the Creche* and in the study by Skeels and Dye (1939) on the effects of transferring infants from an Iowa orphanage to a ward of moron women in an institution for the mentally deficient, where they were later adopted. In this study by Dennis, the Lebanese foundlings who remained in the Creche until they were seven or 12 years of age had IQs averaging 53 and 54 respectively, whereas groups of foundlings who were adopted before they were two years of age had average IQs of slightly above 100.

In the study of Skeels and Dye, which began with a clinical surprise, the "contrast" group, who had an average IQ of 86 when first examined, showed progressive retardation during the two ensuing years of life in the orphanage, lost an average of 26.2 IQ points, and averaged in IQ slightly under 60. The transferred group had an average IQ of only 64 at the time of transfer. With the experience provided by the attentions of the moron women in the institution for the mentally deficient, the members of this transferred group made an average gain of 28.5 IQ points, and averaged at the final testing 92.46. What is probably most important is that 11 of the 13 children in the transferred group became sufficiently attractive to be placed in adoptive homes where they increased further their earlier gains in IQ points.

After a lapse of 21 years, Skeels (1966) ascertained the adult status of these 25 individuals in a follow-up. In education, those in the contrast group completed a median of less than the third grade; those transferred completed a median of the twelfth grade and four went on to college. One of those four, who had an IQ of only 72 at the time of transfer when he was a little over 23 months of age, later earned a doctorate in counseling psychology at the University of Minnesota. He was on hand to speak at the ceremonies for the Kennedy Awards for Harold Skeels and Marie Skodak. There was a similar contrast in occupational levels. Of the 12 in the contrast group, one had died in adolescence following continued residence in a state institution for the mentally deficient and four were still wards of institutions. Of the remaining seven, only one had attained more than marginal employment. Of the 13 who were transferred, the range of occupations extended from domestic service for two girls who had never been placed in adoptive homes, to business and professional occupations. Only two of the subjects from the contrast group ever married. One had one child, mentally retarded, and was subsequently divorced. The other was the exception to marginal employment for this group; he had "a nice home and a family of four children, all of average intelligence" (Skeels, 1966, p. 55). Of the 13 transferred, 11 married, and nine of the 11 had a total of 28 children whose IQs ranged from 86 to 125, with a mean of 104, and all of these second-generation children were in appropriate grades for their age.

The study by Skeels and Dye (1939) illustrates how the depth of retardation in early development increases with continuing experience of poor development-fostering quality typical of understaffed orphanages. The advances shown by the infants in the transferred group illustrate how retardation can be reversed through improvements in the development-fostering quality of experience when those improvements come early enough with people responding to the spontaneous actions of children. This occurs even though the responding people may be moron women in an institution for the mentally deficient. The findings of Skeels' follow-up study illustrate how both the retardation and hastening of development become greater with the prolongation of experiences of, respectively, poor and good development-fostering quality.

The Milwaukee study has demonstrated that favorable rearing conditions can foster the psychological development of infants of poor uneducated black mothers bringing their average IQ at 66 months of age to 124, or 24 points above the norm of 100 (see Heber, 1978; Heber et al., 1972). The 40 black mothers of the subjects of this study had IQs of 75 or below. The 20 infants in the treated group got home visits during their first six months, and thereafter were taken five days a week to a center where each child had a tutor. The tutors were provided with curricula designed to foster cognitive development and language skills. The infants of the other 20 mothers were reared at home. Home visitors kept contact with the untreated families, counseled the mothers in home management, but not in child-rearing. Both the treated and the untreated children got the same schedule of repeated testings. At 66 months of age, IQs of the treated group averaged 124 while those of the untreated group averaged 94. Heber (1978) has now followed the school progress of these children through the third grade to their 108th month of age. Once their development became entirely dependent upon the development-fostering quality of experience afforded by their homes and the public schools, the average IQ of the treated group dropped from 124 to 109. At the same time, the IQs of the untreated group also continued to drop to the upper 70s. Thus, while both groups lost IQ points, the treated group maintained their 39 points of superiority over those in the untreated group. Clearly, the combination of the gains associated with educational day-care in the treated group, followed by the evidences of retardation once the children in this group were dependent entirely upon their own homes and the schools to sustain their development, indicates that plasticity can cut both ways. The fact that the treated group retained the superiority gained during their early educational day-care combined with the evidences of how difficult it is to overcome through compensatory education the effects of three or four years of experience of poor development-fostering quality indicates that, in the domain of psychological development, the old adages apply, "A stitch in time saves nine," or "An ounce of prevention is worth a pound of the cure."

In combination, these findings of 50 IQ points of retardation from orphanage rearing combined with the 24 points of advance of the treated group over the norm of 100 in the Milwaukee study suggest that the range of reaction in individuals without pathology must extend on the average to about 75 points.

Another source of evidence that the mean values of the IQ for groups can be substantially raised through improving the development-fostering quality of their experience has come from adoption studies. One such study by Scarr and Weinberg (1976) indicates that most, if not all, of the inferiority of black and interracial children in IQ is a function of rearing conditions. Their study compared the IQs of black and interracial children adopted by white parents into 101 Minnesota families with IQs of black children reared in their biological families within the same region of the country. By virtue of the history of slavery and economic discrimination against black people, a major share of the parents in the biological families are from the uneducated lower-class. In the Scarr-Weinberg study, the distribution of educational levels for the biological parents of their subjects corresponded to the distribution "for that age consort of the population." On the other hand, the educational level of the adoptive parents was much above the average as was their occupational status and income. Where the mean of the IQs of black children reared in their own homes within the North Central region is only 90, the mean IQ of all black adoptees was 106. Thus, the mean IQ for the black children adopted into white homes was a full standard deviation above the mean IQ of black children reared by their biological parents from within the North Central region. Moreover, those black children adopted during their first year had a mean IQ of 111 as compared with a mean of 97.5 for those who were adopted later. Thus, for those adopted early, the gain was of the order of 20 IQ points or 1.33 standard deviations. Such gains were obtained with the customary rearing practices of the educated, middle-class white parents and without any of that special pedagogic expertise for infants and young children that appears to be developing (see Hunt, 1979b). This study shows again that a major share of the gain obtainable early will be sustained if the development-fostering quality of children's experience is continued beyond the sensorimotor phase.

Another adoption study by Schiff et al. (1978) indicates that at least the predominant share of the observed inferiority of the IQ and of school failure found in the children of working-class parents is a function of their life experiences. This study examined the files of all of the children who had been abandoned at birth between 1962 and 1968 in the files of six public agencies from various parts of France. The investigators focused attention on cases where the *absence* of professional qualification was known for *both parents*. In a fifth of these cases (i.e., 32), the children had been adopted before the age of six months into a family of high socio-professional status. Both the IQ scores and the school records for all 32 of these children were obtained. Moreover, the investigators were able to find the biological mothers of 28 of these 32 children, and 20 turned out to have children of school age whom they had reared. IQ scores and school records for all 39 of these biological children of these 20 mothers were obtained. The IQs of the adopted children averaged 108.7 (S.D. = 10.7), as compared with an average of 94.9 (S.D. = 11.3) for the biological children. This is a difference in mean IQs of approximately one norm-based standard deviation of 15 points. When Schiff et al. compared the observed rate of school failure for the adopted children (18%), they found it to be compatible with the rate expected solely from the social status of the adoptive parents (23%), but very much below the rate expected from the social status of the biological parents (69%). Schiff and his collaborators conclude that "our results bring no information about estimates of the 'heritability' of IQ scores, but they do underline the fallacy of using such estimates to 'explain' scholastic and intellectual failures of working-class children" (p. 1504).

Despite the paucity of data from this research strategy suggested by the range of reaction, those available demonstrate clearly that variations in the development-fostering quality of experience over time can produce very substantial modifications in the mean levels of developmental and educational achievement. In the familiar terms of the IQ, such modifications have ranged from one to at least three norm-based standard deviations, and if one combined the evidence from studies of the retardation from orphanage-rearing with studies of the advancements from educational day-care, it would appear that the range of reaction for means of the IQ for groups of children without pathology must extend to the order of five standard deviations. Clearly, such effects of experience on the average level of competence achieved is infinitely more relevant to the issue of educability than indices of heritability can possibly be.

IMPLICATIONS FOR THE THEORY OF PSYCHOLOGICAL DEVELOPMENT

In our traditional theory of psychological development, we psychologists have thought it to consist of two separate processes: maturation and learning. Maturation has been conceived to consist of a growth process dictated by the genes (see e.g., Carmichael, 1954, Chap. 2-6). As Arnold Gesell wrote, "From the moment of fertilization, intrinsic and extrinsic factors cooperate in a unitary manner; but the original impulse of growth and the matrix of morphogenesis are endogenous rather than exogenous. The so-called environment, whether internal or external, does not generate the progressions of development. Environmental factors support, inflect, and specify; but they do not engender the basic forms and sequences of ontogenesis" (1954, p. 354). An element of truth resides in these propositions for it is indeed impossible to flutter a limb until that limb has developed, or to change through experience the behavioral structure involving the peculiar anatomy of one species into that of another. Genetically based individual differences certainly exist. On the other hand, learning, defined broadly to include all of the experiences that foster development, appears to play a much larger role than Gesell envisaged for it.

It is not the environment, however, that is itself important in development. Rather, it is the effects of experience, where experience is defined as the use of sensorimotor and all other kinds of behavioral organizations as well as the adaptive modifications in them elicited by the environmental circumstances encountered in the course of development. Thus, the sequence of movements shaped by the growth of the embryonic chick within the egg has been shown to be important for the repertoire of the behavior in chicks present at the time of hatching (see Kuo, 1932). Moreover, recent evidence has demonstrated that early experience plays a very substantial role in the maturation of microstructures in the brain (see Greenough, 1976). The marked retardation in the behavioral development associated with being reared in an understaffed orphanage where the environmental circumstances remain essentially constant indicates that for development to occur, there must be changes in the environmental circumstances encountered which are appropriate for the developmental achievements of the infant. Such evidence further suggests that psychological development comes about through the exercise of maturing systems and through the adaptive modification of these systems which are elicited by the environmental circumstances encountered. But it is what the infant does in the course of interacting with the situations he/she encounters that influences his/her psychological development.

It is also important in this connection to understand that the development-fostering quality of the situations encountered is a function of how well the demands they create match the structures of organizational behavior that the infant or child has already achieved. Even though the concept of "readiness" has been widely used among educators for years, its psychological nature has been vague. In general, it has simply meant that the child has not matured sufficiently to have the abilities needed. Piaget, therefore, must be credited with recognizing the psychological and developmental nature of this readiness, and it is through this recognition that the inadequacy of those key behavioristic concepts, *stimulus* and *response,* becomes clear. He has discussed this relationship under the terms *equilibrium* (Piaget, 1936, 1947) and *equilibration* (Piaget, 1977). Cognitive appreciation of such a matter as the transitivity of perceived differences (taller, heavier, etc.) does not exist unless a child has developed through his maturation and past experience the operational structure which Piaget (1947, 1977) terms "serial ordering." Without cognitive appreciation of the meaning of a situation, the situation exerts no demands. It is like the proverbial business of "talking to a pig about Sunday." Piaget has extended his conception from the cognitive appreciation of meanings, principles, and relationships to physical reactions to objects by saying that "A subject is sensitive to a stimulus only when he possesses the scheme that permits the capacity for response" (Piaget, 1977, p. 5).

Some of Piaget's (1936) most penetrating discernments of the nature of development came from observing his own three children. In those observations he illustrated over and over how developmental advancements came about through the assimilation of new perceptions and information into existing sensorimotor organizations and through adaptive modification of existing sensorimotor organizations to cope with new situations, yet he made no mention of the emotional and motivational aspects of this process or of the relationship between situational demands and the structures of the behavioral organizations already achieved.

What I have discussed as "the problem of the match" in my theorizing about both intrinsic motivation and psychological development, which involves this ubiquitous relationship, has emphasized the emotional and motivational aspects of it (Hunt, 1965, 1966, 1971). I recognize that cognitive appreciation of the situation is essential. Otherwise, the situation exerts no demands for adaptive modifications. An infant's cognitive grasp of a situation may be sufficient for it to create demand, and also to create demands beyond the infant's capacity for the required adaptive modification of his relevant sensorimotor systems. When this is the nature of the relationship between situational demands and an infant's achievements, distress is invariably the consequence. Although one can find illustrations of distress from such a source in Piaget's (1936) illustrative descriptions of concrete behavior in specified situations, Piaget has made nothing of it theoretically. Perhaps it was being engrossed with recent evidences of the emotional and motivational aspects of information processing (Hunt, 1963) that prompted me to note numerous instances of such distress in my "horseback" research on the matter. For instance, whenever I have attempted to get an infant to match pictures when that infant was still showing motor trial-and-error when attempting to place blocks in the holes of the shape-box, my attempts have always produced withdrawal and distress, and often tears. All too often my attempts have spoiled budding friendships. On the other hand, if an infant has already achieved the scheme of inspection and can look at a block and, from his perception of its shape, put it directly into the hole of that shape, the game of matching pictures evokes interest and joyful excitement. All too often I have had to leave the game before the infant was ready to stop.

Serious damage can and is all too often done when adults demand repeated encounters with such overmatches. It makes little difference whether the method of preventing withdrawal is punishment or extrinsic reward for persisting. Unless the adult is able to provide a help that enables the infant to make the necessary adaptive modifications in his/her behavioral organizations, the child tends to lose confidence in his competence. The damage to development from such overmatches is illustrated by the finding in a study. Correlating the errors in mothers' reports of what their four-year-olds would do in coping with each test in a graded series of 96 items with the numbers of these tests passed by their children, the resulting coefficient of correlation was −.80. Most of it, as would be expected, however, was based upon errors in which the mothers overestimated the aptness of their children's performances. This is to say that the correlation of the numbers of overestimations of their children's performances with the numbers of the tests they passed was −.77 (Hunt & Paraskevopoulos, 1980). The counsel to parents to avoid "pushing" their children gets empirical justification from this finding.

On the other hand, the retardation associated with rearing in understaffed orphanages appears to result from the continued sameness and unresponsiveness of the situations that infants encounter there. Situations must be responsive to avoid habituation, or extinction, of the orienting and attentional responses to repeated encounters with perceptual events unrelated to the infant's spontaneous actions. From such considerations, it would appear that psychological development occurs at approximately an optimum rate when the situations that infants encounter provide a graded sequence of demands which the child can appreciate and which are sufficiently discrepant from those that gave rise to his/her existing achievements to attract his/her interest and perhaps be a little surprising. This interest motivates the use of their sensorimotor organizations and the additional demands will call forth adaptive modifications in existing behavioral organizations. For parents, caretakers, and teachers arranging and maintaining a sequence of situations that interest children and with which they can cope is a problem. I like to call it "the problem of the match."

In the course of his/her early development, each infant must construct from his interactions with his circumstances both his schemes for processing information and his understanding of his world, physical and social.

There are two major aspects of this process which must be credited largely to Piaget. First, the interactions of the newborn human infant with situations are already far more organized than would be indicated by John Locke's contention that the mind of a newborn is a blank page on which perception writes, or by the early behaviorists' concept of a multiplicity of reflexes which can, through association or conditioning, come to be elicited and organized in an infinite variety of ways. The infant comes with a set of behavioral systems ready-made, but these must be shaped and adapted through functioning to meet the demands of each culture. Second, such conceptual components of reality as objects, space, time, and causality—the givens of epistemological philosophers from Plato to Kant—do not exist at birth, and Piaget (1937) must be credited with the discovery of this fact. Some of these constructs are so much alike across cultures that the words representing them can be directly translated from one language to another. Others show considerable variation. Moreover, in their creation, the schemes for processing information and these structures of knowledge go through an epigenesis. Although evidence exists calling various aspects of Piaget's (1936, 1937) description of the stages of the sensorimotor period into question, the overall nature of the epigenesis seems generally correct. What is still missing is the nature of the constructions and of the experiences which are required to bring them about. For instance, is the nature of development along all branches alike? Or is that for object construction a matter of growing something akin to Hebb's (1949) "cell assemblies," that for imitation a matter of acquiring motivational habits, and that for language a matter of learning sets? Until we know more both about the nature of the constructions and about the kinds of experience which foster their development, we shall have a limited understanding of psychological development and a weak technology of early education.

My major point here is to provide a conception of how experience plays the major role in the rate of psychological development that the evidences on plasticity indicate that it can play. I am fairly confident that it also plays an equally major role in the level of competence ultimately achieved, but except for that from comparing the evidences of competence across the centuries, the only evidence directly relevant to this issue of which I know is that in the follow-up study of Skeels (1966).

It should be noted that this conception of psychological development and of its dynamics does not deny the existence of genetic variation among individuals within the human species. It does suggest, however, that for traits such as intelligence, or competence, which come about through an epigenetic accumulation of achievements built one upon another, there is a tremendous amount of plasticity. From the evidence that I know well, I am inclined to believe that every child born without pathology has the genetic potential necessary to achieve all the abilities, information, and values required for productive participation in the mainstream of any society on this earth. I do not believe, on the other hand, that life histories can be arranged to make such intellectual giants as Aristotle, Thomas Aquinas, Galileo, Newton, Shakespeare, Milton, or Einstein of every child born. I no more believe this than I believe that the life history can be arranged to make an outstanding pianist, pugelist or professional basketball player out of every child born. It should be noted, however, that participating productively in no society requires such outstanding abilities or characteristics. It also should be noted that pathological handicaps are another story. I suspect that such handicaps account for that small cluster regularly found on the lower tail of the distribution of IQs from large samples. Pathological handicaps clearly limit development and educability.

IMPLICATIONS FOR THE ASSESSMENT OF PSYCHOLOGICAL DEVELOPMENT

These evidences of plasticity and those of hierarchical organization in the work of Piaget have implications for the assessment of psychological development and especially as such assessment is involved in the educational enterprise.

First, Use of Tests for Prediction

The use of intelligence tests to predict the performance of students in school has been highly unfortunate for educational purposes. Such a use confuses prediction with explanation and understanding. In at least three ways, it has frustrated Binet's (1909) hopes that tests of intelligence would enable educators, following Pestalozzi's metaphor of education as farming, to modify the method of cultivation to increase intelligence defined as "capacity to learn with instruction" (Binet, 1909, pp. 54-55). First, the very idea that the IQ provides a measure of future potential as well as past achievement has tended to produce in teachers expectations for their pupils that damp their ingenuity in instruction. The saddest answer a teacher can give to "How is X doing?" is "As well as can be expected." Actually, IQs show little relationship with how much pupils learn with instruction; they merely correlate with performance on tests that follow instruction (Woodrow, 1938, 1939). In other words, those pupils who are ahead in academic achievement before instruction begins tend to remain ahead following exposure to the curricular experience falsely considered to be instruction (see Hunt, 1975c; Hunt & Kirk, 1971).

Second, tests of intelligence were created to reflect individual differences. For such a purpose, the norm-referenced model was appropriate. Unfortunately, this same model was extended to the testing of educational achievement, so the emphasis in achievement tests has been placed on interpersonal comparisons in the form of rank in norming groups. This tends to distract both pupil and teacher from the specific and concrete goals of teaching-learning tasks. Moreover, it creates for pupils a frustrating double bind. If excellence is defined as producing test performance within the top 10% of the class, 90% of the individuals in that class must inevitably fail to achieve excellence. It is chiefly for this reason, as I see it, that our norm-referenced approach to testing is in trouble. It is in trouble with minority groups, a majority of whom are largely uneducated and poorly employed, because they have become resentful about receiving evidence interpreted to mean that they are inherently inferior because of their biological nature. If accepted, such a verdict would leave them without hope of improving their status with effort. They question the validity of the evidence, and quite properly, I believe. They see this so-called test evidence as an unfair obstacle in the way of their access to equality of opportunity. Moreover, this norm-referenced approach to assessment is also in trouble with the law, and precisely because judges and juries discern the dissonance between the evidences of plasticity in psychological development and this use of norm-referenced tests to assess genotypic potential, and therefore the individual's worth in the future rather than merely his past achievement (see Hunt, 1975d).

This idea that non-referenced tests of intelligence measure potential gets encouragement from the conception of intelligence as a power that matures with age at a constant rate. Empirically, considerable constancy exists in the IQ. Constancy of the average IQ for groups of individuals is, however, completely irrelevant to the proposition that intelligence is a power which matures at a constant rate. It is irrelevant because choosing test items to represent a given mental age when from two-thirds to three-fourths of the children of that age passed the items insures the constancy of the average IQ for any group.

Seemingly more relevant is the evidence of constancy in the IQs of individual children. Here, however, individual curves of mental growth have shown marked inconstancy of the IQ, especially during the first three years of life (see Jones, 1954). In view of the evidences of such marked plasticity as I have summarized, moreover, I suspect that a very large share of this empirical constancy in individual IQs is a function of the relative constancy in the development-fostering quality of the rearing conditions in most homes, neighborhoods, and social classes. This suspicion was brought home to me by the findings of Yarrow, Rubenstein, and Pedersen (1975). In their study, measures of such things as the responsiveness of caretakers and of the inanimate materials available to the infants in their homes (measures based on only two three-hour periods of observation), showed correlations approaching +.6 with measures of the persistence of the infants in striving for the goals which they themselves had chosen. This fact that measures based on only two three-hour periods of observation could have such a high correlation with measures of performance at age six months suggested that the consistency of the development-fostering quality of such experience must be far greater than has been realized.

Here I wish not to be misunderstood. I do not mean that IQs are without validity for predicting the performances of children on tests of academic achievement which are given after only a few weeks, or even months, following the testing that yielded the IQ (see Hunt, 1961, p. 311ff). Moreover, insofar as such an omnibus measure of intellectual development as the mental age yields information about the average level of a child's existing achievements, it may properly be helpful in academic placement. On the other hand, an average level of developmental achievement cannot show the detail of individual achievements along separate branches of development required for effective educational diagnosis.

Second, Use of Tests for Diagnosis

The existence of the problem of the match makes it important to create instruments for assessing the existing achievements of young children. Such a diagnostic use of tests beyond that rough assessment of the average level of development from the mental age remains only potential because our ignorance of the nature and the order of attainments in the hierarchy of achievements, especially beyond the sensorimotor phase, is tremendous. This ignorance exists, I fear, because only in the past two decades have an appreciable number of investigators entertained even the concept of such a hierarchy of achievements as that introduced by Jean Piaget (1936) only 42 years ago. Another reason for this ignorance may reside in the nature of our traditional tests of intelligence (see Hunt, 1975, 1976). When Binet and Simon (1905) hit upon their substitutive averaging to obtain the mental age, their procedures served to obscure the independent rates of advances along the several branches of development. It failed to hide them completely, for the discovery of "scatter" on the IQ scales clearly implied their existence (e.g., see Harris & Shakow, 1938; Wallin, 1922). Hiding the independent rates of development along the several branches also obscured the relationship between kinds of experience and kinds of development such as are now being uncovered serendipitously with the aid of ordinal scales for several branches of sensorimotor development (see Hunt, 1977). Recall, for instance, that the educational intervention which advanced the progeny of poor, uneducated parents six months ahead of home-reared children from predominantly professional families in the age of attaining top level object permanence left the former five months behind the latter in the age of attaining the top-level of vocal imitation. Vocal imitation appears to underlie the attainment of the phonological component of language (see Hunt, 1979a; Hunt et al., 1976). Thus, the finding that the Mt. Carmel children earned low scores on tests of intelligence at age three despite their advancement in object construction is hardly surprising.

When in 1912, Wilhelm Stern adopted the IQ-ratio of mental age to chronological age, he devised another metric which further obscures the independent rates of development along separate branches and the hierarchical nature of developing abilities as well as providing an operation within the instrument for assessing development perfectly attuned to Galton's assumption of a rate predetermined by heredity. So long as our ignorance remains, the use of tests for effective educational diagnosis will continue to be largely potential, and the behavioral signs of the interest of children in materials arranged to foster their development will be the best means available for solving the problem of the match. Hopefully, serendipitous discoveries of new relationships between kinds of experience and kinds of developmental advance will ultimately lead to an identification of separate branches in the development beyond the sensorimotor phase for which instruments of assessment can be devised.

Third, Tests to Assess the Attainment of Learning-Teaching Goals

Until about half a century ago, the tests most commonly used to determine whether children were learning in school consisted of questions or problems illustrative of what the teacher intended for her pupils to learn. Grading was based upon the percentage of questions correctly answered or problems correctly done. Although variations in accomplishment were recognized, no one thought of measuring the learning accomplishment of a student from his/her rank within the class or with some unfamiliar norming group. When the tradition of individual differences entered the domain of education, the norm-referenced tests of intelligence became the models for norm-referenced tests of achievement. These seldom matched well the emphases of individual teachers. The result was a separation of testing from teaching. The emphasis on individual differences yielded meaning to test performances chiefly in terms of the individual student's rank within a norming group or perhaps within his own class. I have myself been guilty of setting up tests for which the scores could tell a student nothing about how well he had mastered the material taught because the only meaning from them came from the student's percentile rank in the class. Moreover, I have said and heard many other professors say something equivalent to: "Every class has its top quarter, its bottom quarter, and its middle 50% with their C's." Such an attitude, however, tends to distract both student and teacher from the specific educational goal. More important, it fails to provide a concrete standard of educational achievement. I suspect that this separation of testing from teaching has had no small part in the deterioration of educational achievement during these past two decades, when, among other things, youth turned against the business of competing for educational status.

With the advent of instructional research with teaching machines and programming concepts (see Lumsdaine & Glaser, 1960), it was quickly discovered that norm-referenced tests are poorly adapted for evaluating the results of instruction. They were poorly adapted for this purpose precisely because they were designed to bring out individual differences in ability or achievement rather than to determine how well individual students were achieving the goal of each specific learning task. The consequence was the development of "criterion-referenced" tests.

It was Robert Glaser (1936) who first differentiated "criterion-referenced" tests from "norm-referenced" tests, coined these terms, and elaborated the requirements of the former for measuring the outcomes of instruction. The purpose of "criterion-referenced" tests is to discover whether and to what degree the individual student has achieved the learning goal. Such tests are "criterion-referenced" because it is the goal of the learning task which provides the criterion of success. While norm-referenced tests provide no concretely specific standard of excellence, criterion-referenced tests do. Moreover, that standard is independent of how well or poorly others do. Instead of separating the focus of teacher from that of student, criterion-referenced tests help to focus the attention and ingenuity of both student and teacher on the learning task. Such an approach to educational testing permits and even encourages classmates to become collaborators rather than contestants in the learning process. Such tests tend to focus the attention of students and parents from minority groups on the learning task without facing them with numbers that are made to indicate their inherent inferiority. They enable any student willing to make the necessary effort to escape the Catch-22 predicament which results from defining excellence in terms of performances above the 90th percentile. It is my guess that no single change in the educational enterprise would do more to counteract the recent drift away from academic excellence than a general institution of criterion-referenced testing in the place of norm-referenced testing in our schools.

There are two problems of educational assessment that criterion-referenced tests cannot solve. One of these is the diagnostic task involved in the problem of the match. The second is the problem concerning whether a given set of teaching-learning goals can lead to the proficiencies which the culture in general demands and which are required for success in various occupations and professions. Norm-referenced tests can be useful in assessing the success of educational programs, but most of them are too general to assess the fit between an individual's skills and the requirements for successful performance in specific categories of jobs.

IMPLICATIONS FOR THE ASSESSMENT OF RISK
OF MENTAL RETARDATION

All but one of the existing attempts to assess the risk of mental retardation of which I know are based upon evidences of already existing retardation in the performances of infants or young children on various kinds of norm-referenced tests. If one takes seriously the evidences of plasticity and hierarchy in the behavioral achievements which constitute early psychological development, evidences of already existing retardation indicate that it is already likely to be late for educational intervention. Behavioral retardation results inevitably from pathological mental deficiency. Moreover, it is very difficult to distinguish from evidence in test behavior the retardation of a pathological mental deficiency from the retardation resulting from experience of poor development-fostering quality. From such considerations, it follows that the assessment of risk should include obtaining evidences of the quality of the development-fostering experience a given infant is likely to have. Although educational intervention can have only limited success with pathological mental deficiency, the earlier that educational intervention begins, the greater will be its effect. Although effective compensatory education may be feasible even in early adolescence (Reuven Feuerstein of Israel, 1979, 1980), it is far more effective and less expensive to prevent that retardation resulting from experience of poor development-fostering quality than it is to compensate for it later. This is one of the main lessons to be learned from our efforts with compensatory education.

The only existing instrument that takes into account the unlikelihood of opportunities for development-fostering experience of high quality is that of Earladeen Badger (1979, 1980a) of the Department of Pediatrics in the Medical School, University of Cincinnati. The indicators employed in this instrument involve only the distal, social conditions which indicate that the development-fostering quality of an infant's experience is likely to be poor.

One category of these distal indicators is the "maturity of the mother." The criteria of "maturity" include the mother's age, her education (was she a regular student or does she have a history of special education?), evidence of the mother's commitment to plans, evidence of behavioral deviance (e.g., records of criminal behavior or child abuse), and mental health. Especially important under this rubric is freedom to be concerned with the welfare of another, or the absence of narcissistic self-centeredness.

The second category of such indicators in the Badger instrument is called the "quality of the mother's planning." The instigators in this category include whether the mother has used birth control and how consistent her use has been, whether abortions and miscarriages are part of her history, whether she has other children and what the temporal spacing between them has been, and how regular the mother was in making the prescribed visits to the clinic for prenatal care.

A third category of indicators is called the "family support system." This category includes the living arrangements (whether the mother lives alone, with her parents, with the father of the child, or with whom?), and what and how definite are the mother's plans for the care of her child. These plans may include herself as a caretaker, a relative as caretaker, a friend, an institution, or no plans at all.

A fourth and final category of indicators is called "economic status." This category includes the census tract of the mother's domicile, the mother's income, the number of people living under one roof in the mother's domicile, the mother's welfare status (including how many generations of family have been on welfare, whether only the mother is on welfare, whether the mother is dependent but working), whether the mother has a telephone in her domicile, and the number of children under five in the mother's domicile. In addition, the Badger instrument includes evidence of the infant's development as shown by performance on easily-administered screening tests. The scoring of this instrument and its predictive validity are still under investigation.

This Badger instrument is very likely, in my judgment, to be a distinct advance over any of the other instruments for the assessment of risk of mental retardation that I know about. It is an advance precisely because it attempts to take into account indicators of the likelihood that the development-fostering quality of the infant's experience will be poor. Insofar as it is possible to recruit those mothers for whom there are high indications of this risk, such an instrument affords at least the possibility of preventing retardation by teaching the mother how to provide the experiences that will foster early psychological development. Unfortunately, the indicators employed in the Badger instrument are largely of the distal variety. Only indirectly do they indicate the intimate, proximal transactions between the infant and his inanimate and social circumstances which provide the experiences that foster or hamper development.

The ultimate approach needed for the assessment of risk should be based upon the nature of the more intimate, proximal transactions between the infant and his circumstances both physical and social. At the present writing, no such instruments exist. Moreover, neither is there much dependable information about the nature of the proximal experiences that hamper and foster development. Yet, research which points to the possibility of such instruments does exist. Their importance as well as hints of the nature of the achievements that comprise competence and of the nature of some of those experiences which promote development are indicated by evidence from the Harvard Preschool Project (see White, 1975, 1978; White, Kaban, Shapiro & Attanucci, 1977; White & Watts, 1973). Where nearly most attempts at compensatory education have involved children already four years of age, with a few beginning at age three, the evidence from this project has indicated that the achievements which make a child outstanding for competence are already largely established by age three. Competence for White and his collaborators includes not only what intelligence tests measure, but the ability to anticipate the consequences of actions and events, ability to sense dissonance or to note discrepancies between observations and expectations, ability

to take the perspective of another person, ability to deal with such abstractions as positions, numbers, and rules, and ability to make interesting associations. Other aspects of such early competence include language
skills (mastery of the phonology of the language or good pronunciation
of the phonemes of the language, semantic mastery of commonly experienced objects and events, and at least the beginnings of an appreciation
of syntax in understanding statements and in making them),* attentional
competence (e.g., ability to listen to what is said by others and to keep
track of two or more things simultaneously or in rapid alternation),
and in executive competence demonstrated by creating and carrying out
complex plans of a number of steps. The already-outlined evidence of
great plasticity in the rate of general development as well as in the rate
of specific branches also imply that the development-fostering quality of
the experience afforded by homes is indeed exceedingly important. The
importance of the early home experience may well account for the fact
that higher proportions of the variance in intelligence, social status, and
income are associated with the variations among homes than with that
among schools (Jencks, 1972). This Harvard Preschool Project has also
correlated measures of the quality of various kinds of intimate, proximal
experiences with measures of various kinds of competence. Thus, White's
project is one source of the kinds of home experience that foster development and thereby reduce the risk of mental retardation.

At least two strategies of research are yielding evidence of the kinds
of experiences that reduce the risk of mental retardation. One of these
consists of correlating assessments of home conditions with measures of
psychological development. This strategy has been employed in a variety
of studies (see Hunt, 1979b). Several of these have shown unexpectedly
high correlations of the responsiveness of both the inanimate and social
environments to the spontaneous actions of infants with the development
of intentionality. This intentionality, when it is reinforced by responses
from the environment that match the achievements of the child, leads
to that self-winding initiative which appears to be so fundamental later
to a child's ability to modify his own environment in order to satisfy his
own developmental need. It was the supposed importance of the responsiveness of the environment that dictated making the tape-recorded music
and mother talk responsive to the efforts of the infant foundlings at the
orphanage in Tehran. Yet, some of the most convincing evidence for this

---

* Not all of these components of language skill are made explicit in the books and
papers of White and his collaborators (see also Hunt, 1979a).

principle is to be found in a study by Yarrow, Rubenstein, and Pedersen (1975). In their study, it will be remembered, measures of such things as the responsiveness of caretakers and of the inanimate materials available to the infants in their homes showed correlations approaching $+.6$ with measures of the persistence of the child in striving for goals they themselves had chosen. During the past few years, various pediatric investigators have reported that leaving neonates with their mothers continuously during those first days following birth in a lying-in hospital appears to result in a mutual relationship termed bonding. This appears to result in a relationship which quickly takes on that quality of reciprocal interaction characteristic of conversation (Brazelton, Tronick, Adamson, Als & Wise, 1975; Trevarthen, 1974). I suspect that the experiences of importance for the infant in this situation come from the tendency of a mother totally absorbed in her new baby to respond imitatively to its actions, especially facial expressions and vocalizations. In the epigenesis of intrinsic motivation, such imitative feedback is familiar because it is like the infant's spontaneous action, and the familiarity of the feedback makes it especially reinforcing (see Hunt, 1965, 1971, 1979c). In this reciprocal interaction between mother and infant, the mutual expectancies developed comprise shared information, or knowledge, and the beginnings of the rules for social communication. It is thus that the Papouseks (1977) speak of such early infant-mother interaction as the basis for a "cognitive head start." I suspect that this is also the experiential source of that sense of "trust" as well as of the self-winding initiative that Erikson (1950) emphasized as essential achievements of the first two years.

A serendipitous finding from our own deliberate interventions in child-rearing at the Tehran Orphanage, which is another source of evidence of the nature of early experiences that reduce the risk of mental retardation, has corroborated the importance of the responsiveness of the social environment for the development of intentions and the traits of initiative, interest, and trust that underlie both social attractiveness and judged competence at ages two and three. When the caretakers of the foundlings in our fifth wave at the Tehran Orphanage were instructed to imitate their cooings and babblings, we originally expected to foster only the development of the inclination for pseudo-imitation and vocal games. We expected to lead the infant gradually to the game of "follow-the-leader" and to an inclination to imitate strange and unfamiliar vocal patterns. This was expected to facilitate the acquisition of the phonological aspect of language. The serendipitous finding was the marked effect on social attractiveness which appears to have its basis in the outgoing interest and initiative of the foundlings in Wave V late in their second year. Caretaker imitation of the infants' cooings and babblings is a special form of situational responsiveness which is specified to an infant's spontaneous vocal actions. The effects, however, appear to extend well beyond imitation and language behavior to a generalized interest in others, and to initiative in establishing relationships and in obtaining wants (see Hunt, 1980).

There is also a reverse side of this picture coming from those studies which employ the strategy of correlating assessment of home conditions with measures of development. Unresponsive environments clearly hamper and retard early development. For instance, the greater the prevalence of noise that is irrelevant to the spontaneous actions of infants, the less advanced they are on several of our Piaget-inspired scales (Wachs, 1976, 1978; Wachs, Uzgiris & Hunt, 1971). These negative correlations are high, even above —.70, they have appeared as early as seven months of age, and they are evident throughout the first two years. Their explanation appears to reside in the fact that the adaptive response of an infant to repetitive stimulation of any kind that is irrelevant to an infant's actions consists of habituation, or extinction of the orienting attentional response (see Hunt, 1963, pp. 62-63; John & Schwarz, 1978, pp. 17-18). Moreover, it has been demonstrated that sense impressions of any kind to which this orienting or attending response has been extinguished served poorly, or not at all, as conditional stimuli or cues in learning (Maltzman & Raskin, 1965). Inasmuch as the noise of such irrelevant speech from either unconcerned adults or televisions tends to be more common in the homes of the uneducated poor than in those of the educated middle-class, it is hardly surprising that the children of the uneducated parents of poverty are less attentive to teacher talk than are children from better educated families and also do a poorer job of discriminating and pronouncing vocal sounds and words than the latter (for references, see Hunt, 1969, pp. 202-214). Moreover, very recent evidence from a cross-lagged panel analysis of a battery of measures taken at four different grade levels suggests that the hampering effects of such early extinction of attention to adult speech persists throughout the school years. In this analysis, the only high correlation (+.73) was that between measures of listening and comprehension at grade five and an intellectual composite measure at grade 11 (Atkin, Bray, Davison, Herzberger, Humphreys, & Selzer, 1977).

Now let us turn back to development-fostering experiences. When an interest in novelty appears in the development of intrinsic motivation, it is typically accompanied by the emergence of the locomotor abilities of creeping and scooting and the manipulative abilities to drop or even to throw objects (Piaget, 1936). Such newfound abilities produce problems for mothers, or caretakers, but they are especially difficult for mothers living in the crowded quarters of poor people. The locomotor abilities enable infants to get into situations dangerous to their welfare, and their manipulative abilities enable them to damage things valued by the mothers. Moreover, vocal interaction between the infant and the mother is especially important during this phase because one aspect of the interest in novelty motivates genuine imitation through which the phonological repertoire of the mother's language is achieved. As White and Watts (1973) have noted, the demands on mothers during this phase of infant development are a major source of stress. Yet, the skill of mothers in arranging for their infants situations that will enable them to use their newfound capacities successfully and that will demand adaptive modifications in them is apparently one of the major sources of positive correlation between the development-fostering quality of experiences and the development of competence. For purposes of the assessment of risk, therefore, indicators of the likelihood of an infant's having experiences which show a high correlation with measures of developmental advance is important for inclusion in instruments designed to measure risk of mental retardation.

To sum up, the chief implication of the evidences of plasticity and hierarchical achievement in early psychological development for the assessment of risk for mental retardation is that the likelihood of opportunities for those intimate, proximal experiences which have been found to foster development should be included in the instruments to assess this risk. So far, however, the only instrument which attempts this, as far as I know, deals only with the distal, social circumstances presumably correlated with such likelihood. The possibility for developing instruments based more directly on opportunities for intimate, proximal experiences that foster development exist in the published research concerned with relationships between kinds of rearing conditions and measures of developmental advance. At this point, the best I can do is to point out how the implications of plasticity and hierarchy indicate what might be done to develop better instruments for the assessment of risk for mental retardation.

HOPES OF COPING WITH THE CHALLENGE
OF INCOMPETENCE AND POVERTY

During the early 1960s, the accumulated evidences of plasticity in psychological development were taken to imply that children in their fifth year could be compensated for the lack of opportunities for experiences of high development-fostering quality by giving them a summer or a year of nursery-school through Project Head Start. When such nursery schooling failed to achieve the gains hoped for, some people revisited the old beliefs in development predetermined and intelligence fixed by heredity while others attempted to improve the technology of compensatory education. So far, however, it has been exceedingly difficult to achieve large developmental gains in children whose experiences during the first four years of life have failed to foster the competencies essential for success in school and life in general. This difficulty may be as great, or perhaps even greater, for the motivational domain than for the cognitive domain. Such appears to me to be the implication of the fact that both the largest gains during, and the largest losses following termination are to be found for the direct, "pressure cooker" teaching of Bereiter and Engelmann (1966). Evidence for both is to be found in studies by Karnes, Teska, and Hodgins (1969) and by Weikart et al., (1978).*

The deficit in the motivational domain may be epitomized by the inattention to adult talk so common among children from uneducated, poor families. It is conceivable that such attentional deficits might be corrected with reinforcement of attending behaviors, but, to my knowledge, no such attempts have yet been made. What is clear, on the other hand, is that attempts at compensatory education beginning early in the fourth year produce more substantial gains than those attained from beginning in the fifth year (see Weikart et al., 1978). Moreover, the gains obtained with Phyllis Levenstein's (1976) Mother-Child Home Program when children are between 15 and 18 months of age are still greater than those obtained with compensatory education begun early in the fourth year. Levenstein's Mother-Child Home Program also has the advantage of using mothers as teachers of their own children. Her program provides toys for mother-child dyads. These are brought to the homes by paraprofessional interveners. These interveners have been instructed, through

---

* The newer evidence of "sleeper" effects of compensatory preschool calls this inference into question because it looks as if these more enduring effects belong in the domain of motivation. Perhaps such effects result from increasing trust of those outside the family, perhaps from increases in the strength of the internal locus of control acquired in compensatory education. So far, the reasons are unclear.

the *Toy Demonstrators Visit Handbook,* to show the mothers how to interact with their children in the course of play with the toys in order to teach them such things as the labels for colors, forms, and sizes, how to manipulate toys according to verbalized instructions, and how to elicit from the children questions about the toys and verbal responses to them. The toys later give way to books, and the interveners demonstrate how to use the books to interest and to elicit active involvement and questions from the children. Moreover, since the mothers do the actual teaching, the annual cost per child tends to be less than that for compensatory education where the student-teacher ratio must be held close to five to one. Such evidence, along with that already described above, clearly suggests that where there is risk for mental retardation in infants without pathology, the strategy of choice is to teach parents how to prevent the retardation before it occurs. Perhaps it is worth repeating that the old adage appears to apply: "An ounce of prevention is worth a pound of the cure."

Until recently, however, the problem of recruiting parents for training in parenting has constituted a serious problem. It was a serious problem in the attempt at educational intervention with mothers in their homes by Karnes, Teska, Hodgins and Badger (1970). Although Levenstein has contended that recruitment is not a problem for her program, it is highly doubtful that she has enticed into her Mother-Child Program an appreciable percentage of those mothers whose circumstances and personalities put their children under the greatest risk for mental retardation. This recruitment problem has been especially vexing for pediatricians serving the teenage mothers who choose to keep and raise their illegitimate children. Fortunately, this highly vexing state of affairs has instigated the finding of a solution to the recruitment problem.

When the Department of Pediatrics in the Medical School of the University of Cincinnati invited Earladeen Badger to try her Infant and Toddler Learning Programs with the teenage mothers from the poverty sector, most of them with illegitimate offspring, she immediately recognized the recruitment problem. After examining her own experience as a mother, she recalled that her emotional concerns for her own babies had been subjectively strongest during the days immediately following their births while she was in the lying-in hospital. From this experience of her own, she decided to approach the teenage mothers with whom she was asked to work by visiting them in the lying-in hospital during the first or second day following that on which they had given birth. She discovered that none of those 36 approached on these days refused recruitment. Moreover, she was able to hold all but two of the 36 for more than a year of weekly meetings to which they usually brought their infants. Moreover, there was about 90% attendance at these meetings. The infants of these mothers did substantially better than those of mothers in a contrast group who got help only through a home visitor.

Since this pilot study was done, Badger and her staff have turned this pilot program into a service program. In the pilot, Badger herself conducted all aspects of the work: recruitment, all the classes, etc. In the service program, it has been necessary to divide the responsibility. Thus, personal continuity between recruitment and the conduct of the classes no longer exists. Nevertheless, the staff has now approached over 1,000 teenage women from poorly educated families of poverty on the first or second day following the birth of their first child to invite them to participate in classes for parenting. Few have directly refused the invitations. Existing reports cover only 771, of whom 673 were black and 98 were white. Even though they did not decline the invitation to participate, 25% of the black women and 66% of the white failed to attend the classes. Of the whole group, 55% attended 15 of the 20 classes and thereby obtained the high school credit for which Badger had arranged. Not only have the progeny of those attending the classes in the service program continued to fare substantially better than those of control mothers in the pilot study during their first year, but the mothers themselves have gained from their participation (Badger, 1980b; Badger & Burns, 1980). One kind of gain consists of an increased sense of their own worth. This shows as increased ambition in returning to school and in improving skills that will lead to better employment and is a kind of effect of training for parenting first discovered by Gray and Klaus (1965). It has since been reported by Miller (1968), Karnes, Teska, Hodgins, and Badger (1970), and Weikart and Lambie (1967). Another gain consisted of "getting on the pill" to prevent further pregnancies.

Since plasticity cuts both ways, when these teenage mothers return to school, their infants tend to lose their gains toward the norms of the first year. When their care is left to their untrained grandmothers or to other poorly educated caretakers, the development-fostering quality of their experience declines. They do not truly lose developmental ground. Rather, when the development-fostering quality of their experience declines, the infants from more privileged circumstances, who constitute the majority of those on whom test norms were based, gain more rapidly than these whose young mothers have had to leave them to the care of others, both less well trained for parenting and less concerned for their infant's welfare (see Badger, 1977, 1980b).

The availability of care with a strong educational component is highly important for these infants of mothers who return to school. Moreover, the mothers themselves are likely to need continued counsel and help if their infants are to escape the crippling deficits so common among children of the poorly educated parents of poverty. These deficits show not only on tests of intelligence but in deficiencies of language skill in their fifth year (Kirk & Hunt, 1975; Kirk, Hunt, & Volkmar, 1979). Recognizing this need, Badger has enticed a number of social agencies, which include those concerned with child welfare and child protection, the family societies, and the schools, to commit members of their own staffs to continue the training for parenting of these women who have participated during the first year of their infants' lives in the program of the Department of Pediatrics of the University of Cincinnati and of other women like them. Her work has led to the formation of a non-profit corporation entitled United Services for Effective Parenting (USEP) for the city of Cincinnati, and about 20 chapters of this organization have now been established in the State of Ohio (Badger, 1980c). To me such a program looks promising because it calls for an adaptive modification in the policies and functioning of these social agencies. I call the change an adaptive modification of their policies and functioning because it consists of a shift of priority from their various forms of treatment to one of prevention.

During the last six years, I have been asking people in a position to observe whether they have ever found a case of child abuse on the part of a mother or a father who had participated in these and other classes in parenting. This constitutes an informal use of the method of critical incidence. It is of interest, and perhaps of great significance, that thus far I have been unable to uncover a single such instance. This suggests that child protection agencies and also family agencies may advisedly shift a portion of their regular staff effort in treatment to one of prevention. Moreover, in view of the expense and relative ineffectiveness of special education with children of uneducated parents of poverty, I believe our school systems would profit by shifting a substantial portion of their effort in special education to such prevention.

SUMMARY AND CONCLUSIONS

This paper has indicated how the evidences of plasticity in psychological development, which had accumulated through the sixth decade of this century, led, once they were assembled, to a recognition that the inequities in opportunities for the experiences that foster early development across the social classes are inconsistent with our traditional value of equality of opportunity, and this recognition prompted the mounting of Project Head Start.

Although the so-called failure of Head Start has prompted some to revisit the traditional beliefs in the development of competence predetermined and intelligence fixed by heredity, there is new and better evidence for plasticity and hierarchy in the achievements comprising the early development of competence in infants and young children than we have ever had before.

In fact, heritability indices based on the differences of correlations of intelligence and achievement in pairs of individuals with differing degrees of genetic relationship are completely irrelevant to educability. What is relevant to educability are the great modifications in the mean rates and levels of developmental and educational achievement associated with differing life histories. Despite a paucity of studies employing a strategy of investigation suggested by the concept of the range of reaction, the size of largest obtained differences between the means of measures of the rates of development in samples of individuals from the same population being reared under radically differing conditions suggests that the range in the mean of reaction must be of the order of three standard deviations of the IQ.

In view of such evidences of plasticity and the evidences of hierarchy, we need to modify our conception of development from that of a unitary process that comes about at a genetically predetermined rate to one of several branches which develop only as the activities elicited by the circumstances encountered lead to adaptive modifications in the structures of behavioral organization that an infant or child brings to each encounter.

In view of the evidences of plasticity, we need to modify our methods of assessing psychological development and educational achievement. In order to learn more about the specific relationship between kinds of experience and kinds of developmental advance, we need to determine what branches exist and to assess them separately. Within the educational enterprise, we need to shift our focus of concern from measuring individual differences to determining the achievement of the specific, concrete goals of learning tasks. This means a shift for most purposes from norm-referenced tests to criterion-referenced tests.

In view of the evidence for the importance of experience in early development, we need to modify our method of assessing risk of mental retardation from early normative testing for signs of already-existing retardation to the development of instruments which will show the likelihood of infants getting experiences of a development-fostering quality which will prevent mental retardation.

Since compensatory education is both difficult and expensive socially, and since parents are inevitably in the best position to foster the development of their young during the first three years of their lives, we should be exploring more accurately the various means of teaching parents to be better educators of their progeny, and we should be taking care to recruit those parents most likely to provide experiences of poor development-fostering quality into classes for parenting. Finally, if we can get existing agencies to devote part of their existing effort to prevention instead of persisting in devoting it all to repairing developmental damage already done, there would be a hope of coping with the challenge of incompetence and poverty.

2

Genetics of Psychosocial Risk

LEE WILLERMAN
University of Texas at Austin

Let us start our discussion of the genetics of psychosocial risk with the plant that was present at the creation of genetic science—the common garden pea. Mendel found that seeds from one inbred strain produced only tall plants while seeds from another inbred strain produced only dwarf plants. If conditions of soil and weather were unfavorable, however, the growth of each plant could be reduced considerably while still preserving the rank ordering of their heights.

It would be meaningless to assign greater responsibility to either the genes or the environment in producing the ultimate height of each individual plant, for both are inextricably entwined. This is not to say, however, that it is meaningless to assess the relative contribution of *variations* in genes or *variations* in environments to the differences in height among the plants. Thus, one could determine the proportion of variance in height due to different genotypes and the proportion of variance in height due to different environmental conditions. As a prerequisite, however, independent estimates of genotypes and environments must be obtained. To the extent that both are confounded, it is virtually impossible to disentangle the independent effects of either or to determine whether there are interactions between certain genotypes and certain environments which are not readily predictable from knowledge of either genotypes or environments alone.

Much of the unproductive conflict between hereditarians and environmentalists rests on the confusion of *differences* among individuals with *absolute* levels of performance. This distinction, which is plain in the garden pea example, namely, that unfavorable environmental conditions can stunt the growth of plants while still preserving genetic differences in height, when applied to an emotionally charged concept like intelligence, suddenly becomes incomprehensible.

To take but one example of this confusion, consider the classic study of Skodak and Skeels (1949). They obtained IQs and educational data on biological mothers who had given up their children for adoption. As much as 13 years later the adopted away children were tested and educational data were obtained on the adoptive parents. The correlation between the IQs of the biological mothers, who had had no contact with their children after adoption, and their adopted away children was .44. Furthermore, the biological mothers' education correlated .38 with their children's IQ while the adoptive parents' education correlated only .04. These results were interpreted as consistent with a strong genetic influence, because when genes are the only factors responsible for familial resemblance on a trait, the expected correlation between one parent and a child is about .5. (The reason that it is only .5 and not 1.0 is that a single parent contributes only half the genetic complement to the child; the spouse contributes the other half.)

Were these the only important findings in the study, there would have been little conceptual turmoil. But, there was a finding that appeared to be in conflict with the genetic conclusion; the biological mothers averaged only an IQ of 86 while their children averaged 107 on the most comparable test. How could genes be important if IQs could be raised by 21 points with exposure to the different (and presumably superior) environments provided by the adoptive parents? The answer is simply that the relative rank ordering of the mothers in IQ was preserved in the rank ordering of the children in IQ (to the extent of $r = .44$) and that the correlation coefficient is unaffected by differences in the means between the predictor and outcome variables.

Environmentalists interpreted the Skodak and Skeels findings in terms of absolute performance levels. Hereditarians emphasized the preservation of the differences in IQ among the children that had been present among the mothers.

There is a formal statistical connection between genetic effects assessed by agreement in rank ordering and environmental effects as reflected in absolute performance levels (Jensen, 1973). For simplicity, let's assume that genetic differences account for 50% of the variation in intelligence test scores and environmental differences account for the other 50%, and there is no correlation between the children's genes and the environments into which they are placed. If the variance in IQ is 15^2 or 225, then the variance of environmental effects equals 112.5 and the variance of genetic effects equals 112.5 also. The square root of each of these (10.61) is the standard deviation of either environmental or genetic effects. Thus, one standard deviation increase in environmental quality is associated with an absolute increase in IQ of 10.61 points. Now, assume that the mean IQs of the biological mothers in the Skodak and Skeels study were properly obtained and the biological fathers, if known, would also average the same IQ as the biological mothers. The mean difference in IQ of 21 points could then be explained if the adoptive home environments averaged about two standard deviations above the mean for the generality.*

While the environmental quality of the adoptive homes was unknown, and quality is extremely difficult to measure in any case, it seems likely that these homes were substantially superior since such families are usually selected for high scores on various environmental indexes. Had the children averaged 40 IQ points more than the biological parents, it would have been very difficult to argue that the heritability** of intelligence was equal to .5, since this would have required that the adoptive homes average about four standard deviations above the generality in environmental quality. This would mean that only one in 10,000 homes would be eligible to adopt a child, if selection of an adoptive family were made only on environmental quality—clearly an implausible figure.

What Is Inherited?

If there is a heritable component to intelligence, what might it be? Unfortunately intelligence test items do not lend themselves to linkage with underlying biological processes. Items like, "How are a pear and an apple alike?," simply do not permit direct translation to brain processes. Because exegeses of individual items on intelligence tests can be interpreted as culturally biased, critics have prematurely concluded that genetic variation in the normal range is not important. This is tantamount to endorsing the view that something currently incomprehensible must be false. Critics often fail to appreciate that it is the aggregate of items, each possessing some fallibility that, when summed, can index reliable genetic variation.

---

* This discussion has been oversimplified. There is some likelihood that the IQs of the biological mothers were systematically underestimated and it is unlikely that the biological fathers had as low a mean IQ as the biological mothers. For a detailed treatment of the Skodak and Skeels study, see Willerman (1979).

** Heritability is defined as the proportion of total variance that can be attributed to genes.

What features of the brain would make good candidates to account for genetic resemblance on intelligence tests? At the outset we must stipulate that there is no unequivocal answer to this question. It seems, however, that a good candidate must be fairly stable in the face of environmental variation. Many of the biochemical and anatomical changes induced by environmental deprivation or enrichment, for example, in the work of Krech, Rosenzweig, Bennett, and Diamond, or in the work of Greenough (1975) might not be the best place to start.

Greenough (1975) has shown that environmentally deprived rats have fewer higher order dendritic arborizations, suggesting a reduced capacity for making interconnections in the brain. These animals were also poorer maze learners, our closest analogue to intelligence in humans.

The data reviewed in Rosenzweig and Bennett (1977) show consistent differences in favor of enriched rats for many aspects of brain size (independent of body weight) and the ratio of RNA to DNA. Diamond (1977) has reviewed the anatomical evidence indicating that enriched rats have greater cortical depth than standard reared or impoverished animals. These enriched animals also have more glial cells and a greater number of synapses than impoverished animals, the largest effect being due to the impoverishment, rather than to the enrichment. The picture that is beginning to emerge is that enrichment increases size, number, and RNA/DNA ratios in many areas of the brain. It is almost as if the brain responds to appropriate stimulation like a muscle to exercise, perhaps both needing further activity to maintain tonus.

It is possible that the differences between genetically more able individuals and others is related to absolute size of brain. There is a consistent repeatable finding that larger brain circumference is associated with higher intelligence (e.g., Broman, Nicholas, & Kennedy, 1975), but such correlations (averaging about .10) do not appear large enough to account for the whole story.

A good candidate for the heritable side of things must be relatively immutable in the light of the vagaries of assignment to different rearing environments. One candidate that has been relatively neglected is neural conduction velocity. It is a seductive one because of the evidence that those who can process relatively simple information more rapidly than others tend to perform better on tests of intelligence (E. Hunt, 1978).

Mice can be bred for neural conduction velocity in the tail (Hegmann, 1975), but it remains to be demonstrated that speed in the central nervous system can be modified by selective breeding. Salamy and McKean (1976) have shown reliable individual differences in the speed of neural conduction in the auditory brainstem of human infants. Speed of conduction at three months and at six months of age correlated .97 for seven healthy infants. The evidence for neural conduction velocity as a critical factor in intelligence is not yet in. One study of children with Down's syndrome showed them to have faster auditory brainstem velocities (Glidden et al., 1976, in Clausen, 1978). Faster speed without intersensory integration, however, might not be beneficial, and the organization of brain processes must be considered as well.

Many investigators have studied EEGs and cortical evoked responses with the idea of obtaining a relatively unbiased measure of brain function and integrity (Callaway, 1975; Clausen, 1978). Findings from these studies are inconclusive when trying to relate brain processes to intelligence. Many cortical processes are especially susceptible to situational and motivational factors, thereby threatening the validity of any one set of findings. It is important that these "extraneous" factors be understood before much progress can be made in this area.

MENTAL RETARDATION AND PSYCHOSOCIAL RISK

The concept of psychosocial risk under relatively "normal" variations in environments is more appropriate to the moderate than to the severe forms of mental retardation or deficiency. My reason for saying this is that a large number of genetic disorders have mental defect prominently associated with them (see Gottesman and Golden, 1978). While it is likely that for many such deficiencies, environmental enrichments can diminish the depth of retardation, it seems unlikely that such retardation can be eliminated through psychosocial remediation. Other environmental manipulations such as diet, prosthetic devices, or biochemical interventions will be necessary here.*

That mild and severe retardation appear to have different causes is well established. Roberts (1952) had shown that the siblings of severely retarded individuals averaged near 100 IQ while the siblings of the moderately retarded averaged only about 80 IQ. The milder form of mental retardation became known as "cultural-familial" retardation, the

---

* Although the study of Skeels and Dye (1939) has been interpreted as indicating that the IQs of some severely retarded can be improved considerably, I think that the proper interpretation of that study is that the retarded infant scores were produced by severe environmental deprivation and were unrelated to impairments in the underlying biological substrate. Evidence in support of this inference comes from the fact that no neurological abnormalities were observed in any of these infants, despite their severe retardation.

hyphen indicating that genetic or environmental factors, or both, could be operating.

Roberts explained his findings by suggesting that severe deficiencies had their origins in rare genetic or environmental events unlikely to be duplicated in the siblings. These rare events included genetic mutations, recessive single gene disorders, perinatal trauma, or infections. The moderately retarded have fewer of these conditions, and depending on one's predilections, it can be argued that the moderately retarded are simply on the lower end of the polygenic continuum for intelligence and hence their siblings are also more likely to be on the lower end. Since the environments of the moderately retarded are usually regarded as undesirable by conventional standards, it is also possible to argue that moderate retardation is due to adverse environmental circumstances. Roberts' design is incapable of distinguishing between genetic and environmental predilections in this regard. Adoption studies of the offspring of moderately retarded individuals would be useful.

The two broad classes of mental retardation should not be construed as hard and fast dichotomies when only IQ scores are used in making analyses. Johnson, Ahern, and Johnson (1976) analyzed IQ data on the siblings of 242 retarded subjects by their degree of IQ retardation. They found that 22% of the 510 siblings of subjects with IQs less than 40 were themselves retarded, whereas 33% of the 335 siblings of the subjects with IQs of 50 or more were themselves retarded. This difference is significant, but not large enough to indicate completely distinct etiological mechanisms. If only siblings of the most severely retarded (IQ < 20) are compared to the siblings of the least retarded (IQs ≥ 60), the distinction does become clearer. Only 16.7% of the siblings of severely retarded subjects are themselves retarded, whereas 39.1% of the siblings of the mildly retarded are themselves retarded.

There is no substitute for finding the etiological mechanism operating in each individual with retardation, and the above analysis is meant only to be a heuristic to suggest that different factors are likely to be more common in some forms of retardation than others and that these factors will vary with the degree of retardation.

Another reason for distinguishing these two broad classes of retardation is the finding that severe retardation is uncorrelated with social class. Thus, children with IQs below 50 are just as likely to come from high as opposed to low social class homes. It is also interesting to note that the incidence of severe retardation has not changed over the past 45 years (Abramowicz & Richardson, 1975).

Established Causes

Chromosomal anomalies are about 50 times more frequent in spontaneous abortions than in newborns, and congenital malformations may be present in 4% to 5% of newborns with careful examination (Langman, 1975). That abortuses have many more malformations and chromosomal anomalies indicates that a good deal of genetic selection is occurring prenatally.

Infections, radiation, and chemical agents can affect the genome itself or can alter the timing of various events during morphogenesis. Table 1 provides a very schematic picture of a few systems during morphogenesis and some major developmental events occurring at particular times. By examination of these and other systems in the newborn, it is possible to identify when a particular developmental aberration occurred and some of its consequences. An abnormal event during morphogenesis can give rise to single or multiple defects, some occurring simultaneously with the initial aberration and others occurring as secondary consequences (Smith, 1976). Many of these defects are those about which little can be done and those affecting the central nervous system are often associated with severe mental deficiency. Examination of family pedigrees can often give clues as to whether transmitted genetic factors are responsible for the abnormalities.

Since abnormalities during morphogenesis can affect multiple and superficially diverse systems, it would be of interest to consider symptoms in many psychiatric disorders as potential aberrations in morphogenesis. For example, Cohen (1978) has reported that women with dark hair and light eyes are more likely to have been hospitalized in a psychiatric facility. Eye pigment and hair color are inherited independently, but both derive from the neural crest, a critical *Anlage* for the development of the central nervous system. Could it be that some defect in embryogenesis could account for this seeming inexplicable finding?

Unknown Causes

The majority of all retardation is of unknown cause, and this applies *a fortiori* to the milder forms of mental retardation. For that reason it has always seemed that the milder forms should be more remediable, and, in fact, it has been those who are at risk for moderate retardation who have been most frequently targeted for enrichment programs.

Table 1

A Sampler for the Timing of Various Events in Morphogenesis

Age (mos)	Central Nervous System	Eye and Ear	Face	Extremities	Other
1	Closure of neural tube; Ganglia V, VII, VIII, and X	Beginning of optic cup and ear invagination	Mandible	Arm buds	Evagination for thyroid, liver and pancreas
2	Optic nerve connection to brain	Eyelids, cochlear duct	Primitive Palate	Tubular bone	Few glomeruli, testes, vascular plexus at vertex
3	Cervical and lumbar spinal regions enlarge	Retina becomes layered	Cheeks	———	Genital ducts; tail degenerated
4	Myelination begins	Scali vestibuli around cochlear ducts	Palate complete enamel and dentine	Bones	Uterus, kidney, dermal ridges
5	———	Ossification of inner ear	Nose ossifies	Nail plates	Lung decrease in mesenchyme
6	Cerebral cortex layered	———	Nares reopen; tooth primordia	———	Lung alveoli
7	Cerebral fissures and convolutions	———	———	———	Vascular components for respiration
8	Myelination within brain	Lacrimal duct canalized	Rudimentary maxillary sinuses	———	———

Modified from Smith (1976)

PREVENTION OF RETARDATION

Obviously, the prevention of retardation is an extremely complicated matter. If genetic or environmentally caused biological defects are already present, the task is one of remediation in an impaired organism. If no defects are present, then remediation might operate in different ways. Most studies of environmental enrichment have involved children who have no known defects save high risk for low intelligence or developmental retardation. When environmental enrichment is applied, however, it is important that any observed improvements be due to "fertilizer" as opposed to "hot house" effects (Vandenberg, 1968). In the hot house growth can be more rapid, but final attainment may not differ from expectation. With fertilizer, ultimate attainment can also be increased.

A few enrichment programs with high risk children, without known biological defects, have been remarkably successful. Skeels and Dye (1939) removed developmentally retarded children under two years of age from an orphanage and had them reared individually by mildly retarded girls in cottages. The "enriched" children 25 years later (Skeels, 1966) had completed a median of 12 years education and all were self-supporting. A contrast group remaining in the orphanage had completed only three years of education and one-third were still wards of institutions as adults.

The children transferred to the cottages were later adopted and the high median education attained by this group was in part attributable to the presumably higher social class rearing. The feebleminded women had higher absolute mental ages than their charges, despite their low IQs. This might not have been detrimental when the children were young, although one would expect that continued rearing by these girls would not have been so beneficial when the children became older. At any rate, these findings appear to demonstrate a fertilizer effect.

What is so perplexing about these findings is that it is hard to believe that these feebleminded mothers provided an enriched environment, except when compared to the deplorable environment in the orphanage (see Skeels, 1966). Rearing by feebleminded parents would seem more akin to the environments of many children at risk for cultural-familial forms of mental retardation. Perhaps the affective component of rearing was especially important since each cottage was proud of its charge and competed to see which could have their child reaching some developmental milestone first.

One of the most interesting modern enrichment studies is that of Heber (1978). In this study 20 children whose mothers were in the mildly retarded range were provided with enrichment from weaning until the children entered public school. At nine years of age the children averaged an IQ of 108 on the WISC, while a control group, not provided enrichment, only averaged an IQ of about 80. Since the formal enrichment program had terminated with school entrance, it seems that a fertilizer effect had also been demonstrated.

Not all such studies have demonstrated fertilizer effects. For example, in a carefully conducted study by Karnes (1973), preschool enrichment produced substantial increases in IQ at the termination of the program. One year after the program there had been a precipitous drop in IQ. Thus, these results look much more like a hot house effect.

Multiple enrichment groups were formed by Karnes in an effort to compare different treatment programs. The most successful program appeared to be the one employing a verbal bombardment approach. At the end of the enrichment program these culturally deprived children had an average IQ of about 113. One year later the mean had dropped about 10 points. It is not readily appreciated that a mean drop of 10 points is psychometrically enormous. For six year olds to drop 10 IQ points at age seven means that they gained only four or five months of mental age during the entire year. This is because (in simplified form) an IQ of 113 at age six is associated with a mental age of 82 months. One year later at age seven, an IQ of 103 is associated with a mental age of about 87 months. The growth rate of these children in mental age was therefore only five months during a twelve month period—equivalent to a 42 IQ.

This value is dramatically lower than the other treatment groups, which also tended to show declines over time, but of a more gradual nature. Can the typical public school environment be so pernicious as to produce the startling depression in growth rate? I think it unlikely. It is possible that intrinsic motivation (Hunt, 1966) for the kinds of tasks called for on intelligence tests had not been established in these children. Hence, the IQ scores are more a parody of high intelligence than the genuine article. In much the same way as it is possible to teach a child of three years the meaning of life so that he can repeat it before friends, it is possible to obtain high IQ scores on intelligence tests without truly understanding the deeper meanings implied by the questions.

The scores in the Karnes study could have been elevated artificially, not necessarily by formal coaching, but by teaching with the test in mind. Items on the Stanford-Binet have become goals for what children are to know at different ages. If teaching were directed by these goals, then the IQ test, instead of sampling only a portion of what the child knows, comes closer to all the child knows or can do.

Between six and eight years of age, the Stanford-Binet introduces new item content. It is possible for a child of six to obtain an IQ of 113 by passing all the items at age six and five of the six items at age seven. But when the child is retested at age seven, he must answer all the items at age seven and all the new items at age eight (or their equivalent at higher ages) to obtain the same IQ. Thus, large changes in item content can account for the precipitous drops over time. For middle-class children, the test items usually represent a smaller sample of what the child knows or can do. Consequently, items passed are not as closely tied to the specific age at testing and reexamination a year later will not be associated with precipitous IQ drops.

The results of the Hunt et al. (1976) study are not yet in with regard to fertilizer or hot house effects because the children are very young. Some performances of enriched children from extremely deprived backgrounds in this study are truly remarkable, but it remains to be seen whether the improvements are maintained over the long run. Acceleration of developmental quotients in infancy are only weakly associated with later performances (for an exception see McCall et al., 1977). For example, Willerman and Fiedler (1977) had eight month Bayley developmental quotients for children who, at age four, averaged over 140 IQ. Correlations between Bayley scores and IQ averaged zero. The scores at eight months of age were only slightly better than those of a control group of children averaging about 108 IQ at age four. Furthermore, culturally deprived groups in the United States do not show developmental lags on standardized tests of infant development (Broman, et al., 1975).

Koluchová's (1976) study showed conclusively that environmental enrichment can have substantial impact on later intelligence. A pair of identical twin boys were reared in an attic under extreme conditions of deprivation by a cruel and disturbed stepmother. The biological father was judged to be of near normal intelligence as was the biological mother. When discovered at age six these twins were extremely retarded. After being placed in a good environment, however, their IQs began to improve and after a few years were near 100. This study was important for three reasons. First, deprivation had enormous consequences for the children's development. Second, improved environmental conditions were associated with substantial increases in intellectual performance. Third, the notion of a critical period for the development of certain intellective functions was challenged.

The first two reasons for the study's importance do not seem susceptible to challenge. The third is more problematic, however. There was no evidence that these children were neurologically damaged and their parents were regarded as being of average intelligence. Hence, it is possible that the rapid improvements in performance of these twins was largely because the underlying brain processes were intact, despite phenotypic performance levels compatible with severe retardation. It is conceivable that preoperational skills had developed in the children at near age-appropriate times, but were not easily detectable in their overt performance.

It seems likely that there are many paths to retardation; some environmental paths can produce phenocopies* of others that might be genetic in origin. One interesting example from the study of schizophrenia illustrates this nicely. Kinney and Jacobsen (1978) reanalyzed data from a group of adult schizophrenics (Kety et al., 1976), dividing them into two groups. One group had a schizophrenic biological relative, the other did not. These authors assumed that those with a schizophrenic relative had their schizophrenia for genetic reasons, while those without a family history of schizophrenia were environmentally produced schizophrenics. Examination of obstetric records indicated an excess of perinatal complications and potential postnatal brain injury among those without a family history of schizophrenia. Also, those without a family history of schizophrenia tended to be born during the first five months of the calendar year. The latter suggests the possibility of some embryological or viral aberration, although season of birth hopelessly confounds prenatal and postnatal events. The point of this example is that it indicates that a seemingly homogeneous diagnosis (schizophrenia) can be associated with underlying heterogeneity. Classification into more homogeneous subtypes may be very important for making progress in this area.

Neurological Damage

Developmental retardation as a consequence of neurological impairment can also be ameliorated by rearing in a high social class environment. Holden and Willerman (1972) followed infants with definite

---

* Phenocopies are environmentally produced events that appear to duplicate genuine genetic phenomena.

neurological abnormality at age one. In infancy these children performed at a very retarded level. At four years of age, only 5% of neurologically damaged infants from a high social class were retarded on an IQ test, but 35% of those from a low social class were retarded. Thus, high social class was capable of substantially affecting the intellectual fates of these children.

It is interesting to speculate on the reasons why so few of the neurologically abnormal children from the higher social class became retarded later. One possibility is that the damage was impressed on a child with greater genetic and biological resources with which to cope. Another possibility is that the higher social class families were more persevering in the intellective and affective education of their children. In effect, some parents can supply necessary ingredients for cognitive growth, if the child cannot obtain that information on his own. From this perspective it is the damaged infant who is more susceptible than the non-damaged infant to environmental stimulation and raises the hope that a substantial fraction of such damaged children can benefit from intense ameliorative efforts.

A GENETIC PERSPECTIVE

In my view there are really important consequences of taking a genetic perspective on psychosocial risk. First, it forces workers to evaluate competing hypotheses about the origins of various categories of impairment. Thus, the idea of following children at risk when they are reared in their own homes is recognized as not generally powerful, because genes and environment are confounded. This is why the idea of using orphanage children, as did Hunt et al. (1976), Skeels and Dye (1939), and Tizard and Rees (1974), is so attractive.

Enrichment programs for the disadvantaged also have considerable merit in this regard. By removing children from the home for large portions of the day, they may effectively disconnect the pervasive influence of home environment from the influence of new environments.

Another important feature of a genetic perspective is that it naturally leads to the dissection of heterogeneity in order to produce more homogeneous subclusters. For example, Herndon, Goodman, and David (cited in Neel, 1955) examined the genetic disorder of gargoylism, a form of dwarfism depicted on Gothic cathedrals. They showed that the phenotype of gargoylism could be dissected into two separate disorders, now called Hunter's and Hurler's syndromes. The important distinction between the two disorders was that Hunter's syndrome followed sex-linked genetic lines in which clouding of the cornea never occurred, while Hurler's syndrome was autosomal recessive and corneal clouding was present in the vast majority of cases. Before this genetic analysis was undertaken, the presence of corneal clouding appeared more variable and was thus less informative about the disease. With the genetic analysis, the picture became much clearer. Psychologists need to do much more of this, because there are many paths to a particular phenotypic outcome and failure to recognize multiple pathways will stymie real progress.

Genetic methods for uncovering heterogeneity are important even in the normal range of intelligence. One such example comes from the work of Bessman, Williamson, and Koch (1978), who studied the siblings of individuals with phenylketonuria (PKU). The genetic defect in this recessive disorder is in the inability to convert the amino acid phenylalanine to tyrosine because of a missing enzyme.

The siblings of PKU cases are especially interesting because two-thirds of them are heterozygote carriers of the defective gene, as are all the mothers of PKU children. These mothers are only half as efficient as normal individuals in converting phenylalanine to tyrosine (although some tyrosine is obtained directly through foodstuffs). The genetically normal children of such mothers can convert the phenylalanine properly, but the heterozygote children are only half as efficient as normal. As a consequence, heterozygote fetuses of heterozygote mothers are doubly at risk for nutritional deprivation—they obtain less tyrosine directly from their mothers and are less able to convert the other nutriments to tyrosine.

It is possible to detect the heterozygote carriers of the PKU gene by means of a biochemical test. When Bessman et al. divided the siblings into the carrier and noncarrier groups and administered IQ tests, they found that carrier siblings obtained IQs at least 10 points lower than their genetically normal siblings. These mean differences were all in the normal IQ range and reveal the importance of genetic variation (and its interaction with nutrition) even among those who do not have very low IQs.

Since tyrosine is especially critical for proper brain development, Bessman et al. suggest that PKU carrier mothers (about one in 50 in the general population) receive dietary supplements of tyrosine, especially during the last trimester of pregnancy when the fetal brain is developing most rapidly. PKU is only one of a number of amino acid disorders affecting intelligence, and it seems likely that similar approaches may be useful in other disorders of this kind.

This analysis highlights the need for understanding intellectual variation within families and not only between one family and another. In the justifiable concern with the large fraction of the population exposed to a variety of environmental abominations, the fact that a substantial fraction of the IQ variation lies within families may have been neglected. Ameliorating inhumane environments associated with poverty and deficient social care will not have the consequence of eliminating all the advantages and disadvantages that come from genetic variation.

3

A Diathesis-Stress Model for the Study of Psychosocial Risks: The Prediction of Infantile Obesity

RAYMOND C. HAWKINS, II

University of Texas

INTERRELATIONSHIP OF PSYCHOSOCIAL AND BIOPHYSICAL RISK FACTORS IN INFANT-ENVIRONMENT TRANSACTIONS

The introduction to this section provided a conceptual framework for the interrelationship of two broad categories of risk factors that contribute to developmental disorders in infancy and early childhood: biophysical and psychosocial risks. The "flowchart" (Figure 1 in the preface) distinguished and summarized both kinds of risks as they characterize the parent, the infant, and most importantly, the caregiver-infant transaction process. The hypothesized developmental outcomes of these risks from this diathesis-stress model were given in Figure 2 in the preface.

This flowchart contains a wealth of complex, speculative interrelationships. To simplify matters, a few summary points are offered. First of all, the influences of biophysical risks (largely genetic, constitutional factors) upon the developing infant are hypothesized to be unidirectional. These direct influences upon the infant, although quite important, will not be emphasized in this paper. More important for our consideration is a second, *bidirectional* influence: the contribution of

This research was funded by grants from the University of Texas Research Institute and from the Institute of Human Development and Family Relations at the University of Texas at Austin.

biophysical factors to early caregiver-infant transaction (cf. Buss & Plomin, 1975).

Certain biophysical characteristics (e.g., biologic/genetic defects or variations, parental temperament, infant temperament) may predispose psychosocial problems in parent-infant transactions. Difficulties in parent-infant transactions occur when particular atypical infants or atypical parents disrupt the reciprocity of the relationship, producing asynchrony in the transactions between the caregiver and infant (Brazelton et al., 1974). For example, small-for-date infants may not be able to emit responses which will elicit appropriate caregiving responses. They may be deficient in providing eye contact, social smiling, and cuddliness, and these deficiencies may then contribute to a less than optimal early learning experience with the caregiver, who may in turn increase vulnerability to subsequent developmental disabilities (Figure 2 in the preface).

In the above case, biophysical risks function as independent variables for longitudinal risks studies (e.g., Mednick & Schulsinger, 1973). Thus, in predictive studies of obesity we may investigate inherited tendencies toward excessive adipose tissue and subsequent psychosocial risks, such as lowered self-esteem, impaired peer relationships, and possible emotional disturbances. The model being described bears resemblance, then, to a diathesis-stress interaction. A genetic predisposition toward excess adipose tissue deposition and subsequent psychosocial stresses combine to increase vulnerability to obesity.

Another way of looking at the biophysical factors, however, would be to consider them as dependent variables. That is, one might examine the effects of psychosocial influences upon the physical growth or constitution of the infant. It is uncommon to find in the literature discussions of biophysical factors as dependent measures. Here the direction of inference is reversed, in the sense that the focus of investigation is directed toward the possible influence of psychosocial risks, specifically the quality of the parent-infant transactions during feeding, upon the infant's rate of physical growth and formation of excess adipose tissue.

PREDICTION OF INFANTILE OBESITY: ASYNCHRONY OF CAREGIVER-INFANT FEEDING AND SLEEPING PATTERNS

In an ongoing pilot study, I have focused upon the infant's rate of physical growth (especially body weight and adipose tissue stores) as determined by biophysical and psychosocial factors in interaction. There are two perspectives I wish to point out. First, it is clear that atypical birth size can be due to genetic or congenital influences. Second, the physical growth of the infant over the first three months of life may be a function of the psychosocial context, as defined above.

One reason for examining physical growth and the rate of relative weight gain and adipose tissue formation in early infancy derives from a developmental continuity assumption and primary prevention orientation. Juvenile onset obesity has been thought to persist into adulthood and pose a significant risk to physical health with related social disabilities (see Bruch, 1973, 1978; Collipp, 1975; Winick, 1975 for reviews). Early intervention efforts, commencing in infancy, have been proposed (Garn, 1976).

Research interest in predicting infantile and childhood obesity would lessen if obesity could be treated easily as the child matures. Obesity has been extremely difficult to treat successfully in adulthood, however. As Stunkard and McLaren-Hume (1959) have stated in a well-known quote:

> Attrition rates in clinics range from 20-80% and only 25% who enter therapy lose 20 lbs.; only 5% lose as much as 40 lbs. Most of these weight losers regain all the lost weight (p. 79).

This quote describes the often recognized "yo-yo" syndrome of body weight. My personal interest in obesity and weight-control derives from my behavior modification treatment program for overweight college students at the University of Texas Student Health Center (Hawkins, Setty & Baldwin, 1977, unpublished treatment manual). For a time there was great enthusiasm for the success potential of behavior intervention approaches for weight-loss. This enthusiasm was based largely on the presumption that these procedures would correct maladaptive eating habits, thus producing not only substantial weight-loss, but long-term maintenance of this weight-loss. More recently, however, at least one review of follow-ups from such behavioral treatment programs (Stunkard, 1977) has found that this claim for permanent weight-loss may be premature. Stunkard cautions that there may be biological limits that may preclude some individuals from maintaining an "ideal" normal body weight. These persons may be quite resistant to weight-loss efforts in adulthood.

Other investigators, however, still reasoning from a behavioral orientation, have implicated early maladaptive feeding experiences as at least a partial explanation for the recalcitrance of the treatment of obesity in adulthood. There is indeed an important distinction between juvenile-onset and adult-onset obesity: The juvenile-onset obese person has been found clinically to be much more difficult to treat successfully (Stunkard & Mendelson, 1967; Grinker & Hirsch, 1972; Rimm & Rimm, 1976). Rimm and Rimm (1976) found, for example, that their most severely overweight women had a two to three times greater likelihood of having been overweight since childhood, and experienced more difficulty losing weight in adulthood, relative to those overweight women who had not become obese as children.

One popular explanation for this tendency for juvenile-onset obesity to be more resistant to treatment is the "fat cell" hypothesis (Hager, 1977). Knittle and Hirsch (1968) theorized that under- or overfeeding in young rats (and by inference, in human infants) causes a permanent alteration in the number of fat cells, as early as the first year of life. There is an increased number of fat cells in the case of this early over-feeding, as well as an increase in fat cell size. Brook, Lloyd and Wolff (1972) conducted a series of cross-sectional studies of humans, including human infants under one year of age, and found that already at the age of one to three years there was a three-fold increase in the number of fat cells in obese children. He did not prove that this adipocyte hyperplasia was due to overnutrition, however. A number of clinical studies have tentatively concluded that the number of fat cells is not reduced by dieting, either in adulthood or as early as age five (Hager, 1977). Once the number of fat cells has been "fixed," dieting merely shrinks cell size. I like to offer the metaphor of "millions of starving little fat cells, crying out for food!" This, then, might be the sort of "biological limit" to which Stunkard (1977) was alluding.

This excess number of fat cells could be predisposed by genetic or congenital factors; however, Knittle and Hirsch (1968) offered the provocative explanation that hyperphasia is due to early overfeeding. This "over-nutrition" hypothesis provided the conceptual base for investigating the relationship between overnutrition in infancy and infantile obesity. Because of the great resistance to treatment of juvenile-onset obesity, many investigators are looking to early infancy to try to identify, intervene, and prevent subsequent weight problems through early dietary management.

The Prediction of Infantile Obesity

The fat cell theory implies a developmental continuity assumption: Fat babies become fat children who, in turn, become fat adults. It is important to determine the relative contribution of genetic/metabolic/ temperament factors and psychosocially based causes (such as learning experiences leading to overnutrition) to developmental obesity.

Genetic Studies

Jean Mayer (1968) summarized the genetic data in terms of the elevated risk for the offspring of overweight parents to become obese by the end of high school: Seven percent of children of normal weight parents are obese upon graduation from high school; if one parent is overweight that risk rises to 40% and if both parents are obese then 80% of these children will become overweight by the end of high school.

These data do not separate genetic from environmental influences, but they do show the extent of the risk factor to be considered. A definitive separation of genetic and environmental factors requires powerful designs such as twin studies and the adoptee methods (see Chapter 2). Hartz, Giefer, and Rimm (1977) have recently reviewed the rationale and mechanics for calculating heritability statistics for obesity, as well as some of the substantive findings.

Borjeson (1976) studied 40 monozygotic (MZ) and 61 dizygotic (DZ) twins between seven and 11 years of age, obtaining measurements of subcutaneous fat. He found a heritability of .5 to .75 for skinfold thickness, i.e., the intrapair differences in skinfolds were much smaller in the MZ relative to the DZ twins.

Withers (1964) utilized the adoptee method to assess genetic contributions to obesity. He found that there was a high degree of correlation between the weight of parents and the weight of their natural offspring, but no correlation between adopting parents' weight and the weight of their adopted children, even if they were adopted at birth. Biron et al. (1977) have since replicated this finding.

Garn's (1976) adoptee study, however, revealed some evidence for familial psychosocial causes for obesity. There were no differences in the magnitude of fatfold correlations in biological parent-child and adopting parent-child pairs, suggesting some role for unspecified environmental factors. Garn's finding should caution us to conduct further twin studies and adoptee studies and then consider the findings together. Twin studies yielding higher heritability estimates than adoptee designs suggest the operation of complex genetic/environment covariations in the etiology of developmental obesity. Garn's data, however, show a substantial correlation between parental and child fatfold measures, strongly supporting the familial transmission of tendencies for individual differences in adipose tissue stores. Hartz et al.'s (1977) study of the heritability of percentage overweight utilizing a sample of prepubescent biologically related and nonbiologically related siblings also found that family environment was an important contributing factor to obesity (accounting for 32% of the variation in the children's obesity). The estimated heritability was low (.12). There are indications, then, that some important life history influences are operative for obesity. The question is whether these influences reflect early overnutrition, underactivity, or some combination.

Review of Longitudinal Studies

Assuming that there is a developmental continuity in obesity from infancy through adulthood, we should find empirical evidence for this continuity from longitudinal studies. The longitudinal evidence is suggestive, but not conclusive:

(1) Parental overweight or excess adiposity predicts relative overweight or excess fatness in infancy and/or childhood (Fisch et al., 1975; Garn, 1976; Charney et al., 1976; Poskitt, 1977; Mack & Johnston, 1976; Poskitt & Cole, 1978). Generally from 9 to 10% of the variance of the infant's fatfold thickness can be predicted from the mother's fatfold thickness (Whitelaw, 1976).

(2) There is a significant relationship between maternal weight gain during pregnancy and the infant's rate of relative weight gain in infancy and childhood (Fisch et al., 1975; Whitelaw, 1976). These data implicate some influence of the intrauterine environment upon tendencies for fatness after birth.

(3) Rate of relative weight gain in the first six months to first year of life predicts excess weight and/or excess skinfold thickness in childhood (Eid, 1970; Taitz, 1971), adolescence (Mack & Johnston, 1976) and even in adulthood (Charney et al., 1976). About 10 to 20% of the variance in relative body weight and skinfold thickness at age seven to 10 can be accounted for by the rate of relative weight gain in the first year of life. More recent and better designed studies (e.g., Mack & Johnston, 1976) have found that the proportion of the variance that could be accounted for approached 35%, i.e., a two to three times greater risk for skinfold thickness at or above the 90th percentile in adolescence (Mack & Johnston, 1976) or for becoming an overweight 20- to 30-year-old adult (Charney et al., 1976), given excess weight gain in the first year of life.

There are three findings, however, that shed some doubt on the continuity assumption for the predictability of childhood or adult obesity from rapid relative weight gain in infancy, and also discredit the early overnutrition hypotheses:

(1) Mellbin and Vuille (1976) have pointed out the controversies and inconsistencies in criterial measures of obesity that have been employed in longitudinal studies. These investigators found little association between rapid weight gain in infancy and later "pure" fatness (i.e., fatness without concomitant increase in lean body mass at age nine to 11 years). They did find a significant relationship between rapid weight gain in infancy and an increased total body mass in relation to height in 10½-year-old boys whether or not this overweight was accompanied by increased fatfold thickness.

(2) Either very slight (Sveger et al., 1975) or no differences (Rose & Mayer, 1968) were found in mean calorie intake between groups of normal and rapidly gaining ("obese") infants.

(3) Poskitt (1977) found no significant correlation between calorie intake in infancy and body weight at age five.

If overnutrition is not the whole story that accounts for early rapid relative weight gain/excess fatness and for persistence of overweight into later life, then what about other explanations?

In a fascinating pilot study, Mack and Kleinhenz (1974) examined the caloric intake, growth, and activity levels of five black infants born to disadvantaged obese mothers living in Philadelphia. These investigators found wide, stable individual differences in these infants' activity levels (as measured by actometers on the infant's wrists and ankles) between 8 and 56 days of age. A strong negative correlation was obtained between growth in relative body weight (i.e., weight/height ratio) and activity level. Those bottle-fed infants who had higher caloric intake and who were less active showed an increased weight for their length. These results suggest that underactivity may be at least as related, if not more related, to infant obesity than is infant overfeeding.

To summarize these findings, then, there is evidence for the developmental continuity of overweight and excess adiposity. This may be due to early overnutrition, but the current evidence for a specific genetic/metabolic influence or for underactive temperament is at least as plausible. A diathesis-stress model would be appropriate for testing in future longitudinal studies.

The Potential Importance of Parent-Infant Feeding Transactions
in the Development of Obesity: Test for the Overnutrition
Hypothesis in Asynchronous Transactions

It is plausible that careful scrutiny of parent-infant feeding transactions in the first three months of life may yield a key to understanding the development of maladaptive eating habits contributing to juvenile onset obesity. Given the possibility of a diathesis-stress interaction, such a longitudinal study of early feeding/sleeping patterns should include equal numbers of infants born to obese mothers and normal weight mothers.

The first three months of an infant's life may be a particularly important period for studying feeding transactions. By the 42nd day postnatally the infant is capable of behaviorally regulating its caloric intake (Fomon, 1974). If one experimentally varies the concentration of the infant's formula by increasing the concentration or diluting it, the infant by this age can compensate for this challenge by adjusting the amount consumed. During the first month of life the infant's biological rhythms (e.g., sleeping/waking, hunger/satiety) also become synchronized with the schedules of the caregiver (Sander et al., 1970). "Irregular" infants exhibit greater asynchrony in early transactions with the caregiver and become at greater risk for later developmental disorders (Thomas & Chess, 1977). One possible outcome of such asynchrony in the feeding context may be infantile obesity.

Hilde Bruch (1973) has proposed a theory for developmental obesity that may help us to identify the form such asynchronies may take in early feeding transactions. Bruch's provocative theory contends that childhood onset obesity stems from faulty learning in infancy. That is, because the mother fails to discriminate her infant's signals of hunger from his cues of other aversive internal states, feeding does not occur specifically in response to the infant's biological need for food, but instead to the infant's cues of negative affective states in general. Thus, overfeeding develops as a learned response to general distress. Bruch contends that as a result of this learning process, the infant confuses hunger with other internal unpleasant sensations. This "confusion" persists into adulthood, accounting for maladaptive eating habits, life-long maintenance of obesity, and secondary personality disturbances (e.g., negative body image and feelings of personal ineffectiveness).

This theory derives from Hilde Bruch's extensive clinical observations, but has not been empirically verified via longitudinal studies with appropriate controls. Clinical evidence for asynchrony in the feeding context, possibly contributing to infantile obesity, is found in a study by Ainsworth and Bell (1969).

Ainsworth and Bell (1969) followed a sample of 26 babies of white, middle-class Baltimore mothers as these babies interacted with their mothers during feeding from birth to age three months. Twenty-two of these infants were bottle-fed. For each mother-infant dyad observed during home feedings, interactions were classified on the following dimensions: type of feeding (breast vs. bottle), timing of the feedings (by mother), determination of the amount of food and the end of feeding, the mother's handling of the baby's preferences for kinds of food, pacing of the baby's intake, and problems related to feeding. This qualitative scoring procedure allowed determination of how the reciprocal responses between mother and infant determined meal frequency and meal size.

Examination of the individual data of the 26 babies reveals some patterns of ingestion that seem consistent with Bruch's theory. For example, two mother-infant dyads were characterized as showing "demand feeding with overfeeding to gratify the baby," i.e., these mothers appeared to treat too broad a spectrum of their infants' signals as "hunger." Thus these mothers coaxed their infants to overeat in a given feeding and to have too frequent meals. These two babies became overweight and began to oversleep. One year later these infants were still relatively overweight. Interestingly, their mothers were not themselves obese. In two other mother-infant dyads, characterized by "scheduled feeding with overfeeding to gratify the baby," the infants seemed to sleep excessively, thus requiring their mothers to awaken them to be fed, at which point they coaxed their infants to overeat. In this latter case, not only did these mothers appear to respond inappropriately to their infants' satiety cues, but also the infants' cues were inappropriate (i.e., sleeping until feeding time rather than signaling mother when hungry). In similar fashion, one can reinterpret the categorization of all the mother-infant pairs of the Ainsworth and Bell study according to the extent to which the infant's and/or the mother's cues were appropriate or inappropriate with regard to feeding initiation or termination (Hawkins, 1977). This post-hoc case analysis yields evidence for asynchronous feeding transactions consistent with Bruch's theory of infant overfeeding and weight gain, and also supports Mack and Kleinhenz's (1974) findings concerning the importance of individual differences in sleeping and activity level.

Design Considerations

Ainsworth and Bell's (1969) findings suggest the importance of a more thorough longitudinal investigation of the relationships of mother-infant feeding transactions during the first months of life to a number of infant characteristics, e.g., infants' caloric intake, relative weight/length gains, fatfold increases, and the temporal patterning of sleeping and feeding. For such a study to provide an empirical test of the diathesis-stress model for infantile obesity presented earlier, particular care must be exercised in selecting the appropriate sample of infants and caregivers and the choice of dependent measures.

Sampling

If certain biophysical conditions, such as an increased number of fat cells, predispose some infants toward developmental obesity, then a sampling strategy should select half the infants to be at "high risk" for excess adipose tissue deposition with the remainder serving as controls. An optimal method would be to select infants separated at birth for purposes of adoption. The biological mothers (and preferably the fathers as well) of the index adoptees would be known to be obese with a juvenile age of onset or manifesting a metabolic disorder such as diabetes, while the biological parents of the control adoptees would have no history of obesity or related disorders. An alternative plan would be to obtain nonadopted infants whose parents are clinically obese and compare this group with control infants whose parents have a normal weight history. This latter strategy would permit analysis of caregiver-infant feeding transactions leading to infant overnutrition, but would be less desirable in that it would not permit separation of genetic and environmental contributing factors.

Other sampling considerations include the parity of the infant and the type of infant feeding. Although Charney et al. (1976) have discounted the importance of birth order as a predictor of developmental obesity, several studies have shown that bottle-fed babies show a more rapid weight gain in the first year of life (Wiel, 1975; Neuman and Alpaugh, 1976) and are less active and more placid than breast-fed babies (Bernal & Richards, as cited by Wiel, 1975). One practical advantage of studying bottle-fed infants, moreover, is that measures of the volume of formula ingested at each feeding may be obtained for correlation with the behavioral measures of caregiver-infant transactions.

One final issue in sampling concerns demographic categories of psychosocial risk where the incidence of obesity may be higher. Stunkard et al. (1965, 1972) and Mack and Kleinhenz (1974) have targeted low social class and black racial background as demographic characteristics elevating the incidence of obesity.

Dependent Measures

Given the complexity of the multiple and interacting factors implicit in the diathesis-stress formulation for infantile obesity, it seems advisable to use several dependent measures in a convergent design. *Anthropometric measurements* (length, body weight, triceps and subscapular skinfold thickness) should be obtained at regular intervals. The dependent measures more crucial for assessing the diathesis-stress model, however, are the measures of infant behavior, caregiver behavior and attitudes, and data from caregiver-infant transactions. At the molar level, in naturalistic contexts, *daily infant feeding-sleeping records* may be kept by the caregiver (Hawkins, unpublished data).* These records of several categories of information pertaining to the infant's feeding and sleeping behavior as well as the caregiver's mood prior to, and immediately after each feeding may be compared with the more objective measures of *mother-infant feeding transactions* videotaped during regularly scheduled home visits and coded according to behavioral categories such as those developed by Brown et al. (1975) and by Dunn and Richards (1977). The advantage of these videotaped data would be to provide the microanalytic detail needed to test Hilde Bruch's (1973) theory about maternal insensitivity to the infant's hunger and satiety signals.

Some additional *subjective rating scales* administered would also be useful. First, to gather information about each parent's prior experience caring for infants as well as their reactions to this pregnancy and childbirth and their expectations about their baby's development, attitudinal measures such as those described in the chapters by Walker and by Pharis and Manosevitz (this volume) could be given. Second, measures of parental and infant temperament (Buss & Plomin, 1975; Carey, 1970; Chess & Thomas, 1977) might provide some preliminary information pertinent

---

* Copies of the Daily Infant Feeding/Sleeping Record (which comprises the behavioral categories of the temporal patterning of feeding and sleeping, duration of feedings, place of feeding, identity of the caregiver and the caregiver's mood prior to and after each feeding, type of food and amount of food ingested per feeding, and numerically coded descriptions of the infant's behavior prior to, during, and after the feeding), with instructions, may be requested from the author.

to the contribution of these biophysical characteristics (i.e., the "matches" vs. "mismatches" between parent and infant temperaments) with regard to the quality of the parent-infant feeding transactions.

Specific Hypotheses

Using this "high risk" design for intensive study of infant characteristics and social, environmental factors in the first three months after birth with follow-up at the end of the first year might permit testing of the following hypotheses:

(1) Each infant's relative weight gain (i.e. increase in weight/length ratio and increase in fatfold thickness) will be directly proportional to each infant's caloric intake and, perhaps, duration of sleeping. That is, "fat" babies will either eat and/or sleep more than will "slim" babies during the first three months of life. At 12 months of age the relative body weight gains and skinfold measures will be proportional to the weight/length ratio and skinfold values taken at age three months (i.e., babies who are fat at three months of age will be more likely to be fat when they are a year old).

(2) More importantly, just as in adults (Hawkins, 1977), infant overfeeding and overweight will be associated with (a) excessive meal frequency, (b) excessive meal size, (c) underactivity (oversleeping), (d) high caloric value of the infant's food (e.g., perhaps more ingestion of solids beginning earlier in life), and (e) any combination of these four behavioral parameters.

(3) The videotapes of the mother-infant transactions should permit identification of those behavioral cues by which the infant signals his mother that he is "hungry" and his mother's response to these signals (i.e., the reciprocal interaction determining meal frequency). Similarly, the tapes may reveal how the mother responds to her infant's satiety cues (i.e., whether there is synchrony or asynchrony in the reciprocal interaction determining meal size). Thus overfeeding and weight gain in early infancy should be specifiable as a function of the infant's inappropriate hunger or satiety cues and/or maternal inappropriate responses to these signals from the infant.

(4) "High risk" infants born to obese mothers should be more likely to show a more rapid relative weight gain and increase in fatfold thickness than infants born to normal weight mothers. Similarly, their daily feeding/sleeping records should show more evidence of overfeeding and/

or oversleeping during the first three months of life, and the videotapes may show more indications of asynchrony in the mother-infant feeding transactions.

Case Study of an Obese Mother-Obese Infant Dyad

In a preliminary pilot study of four infants with overweight mothers, one black infant became marginally obese (i.e., his relative weight and skinfold thickness exceeded the ninetieth percentile at age three months, by Fomon's (1974) norms). Preliminary analysis of this infant's feeding/ sleeping records revealed an interesting difference pertinent to the diathesis-stress theoretical model of infantile obesity. This obese infant's mother reported a distinctive pattern for her infant's behavior during feeding: For 35% of the feedings her baby seemed sleepy or uneager to eat. The other mothers rarely used this behavioral category. The mother was perceiving a difference in her infant's state, but there was no detectable difference in the volume of formula ingested when the baby was rated sleepy compared to when he was rated awake or eager to feed. Is this the case of a temperamentally inactive infant who failed to give his mother clear signals for meal termination? Was this mother trying to overfeed her baby to make him sleep more? Perhaps the micro-analytic detail of the mother-infant feeding transactions on videotape will help provide a tentative answer. This case does bring to mind the clinical descriptions of Ainsworth and Bell's (1969) babies who became obese.

Implications

The studies reviewed in this paper suggest an interrelationship of biophysical and psychosocial risks contributing to developmental obesity in infancy and early childhood. In addition, there is some weaker evidence that the expression of biophysical characteristics (e.g., genetic/ metabolic predisposition for obesity, inactive temperament) is mediated within the psychosocial context of synchrony or asynchrony in early parent-infant transactions. In contrast, little evidence was found for the infant "overnutrition" hypothesis. That only one of the obese mothers' infants became measurably obese in this pilot investigation is consistent with the findings of a recent study by Whitelaw (1977). Whitelaw measured skinfold thicknesses at birth and at one year of age of infants who were obese, thin, or normal at birth, as well as infants of obese mothers and infants of diabetic mothers. At one year of age skinfold thickness did not differ significantly among the groups of infants, and there was no significant relationship between skinfold thicknesses measured at birth and one year of age.

Few investigators have provided a direct test for the assertion that infant overfeeding potentiates long-lasting problems of obesity. The longitudinal "high risk" design for the study of caregiver-infant feeding transactions during the first three months of life, proposed in this paper, would provide such a test.

It seems justifiable to recommend, however, that a longer follow-up period be included in longitudinal studies such as the one just described. So long as the infant's physical growth is being closely monitored by the pediatrician (generally at least over the first 18 months of life), one may not be able to see the contributions of biophysical factors or of asynchronous feeding transactions to manifestations of excessive adiposity (Whitelaw, 1977). Understanding what happens to these children later on during the preschool and school years up to and including puberty is an important endeavor given that one recent British population study by Wilkinson et al. (1977) found that over 50% of children who were obese at age 10 years did not become overweight before age five.

Borjeson (1976), in the twin study of childhood obesity mentioned previously, found that many of the twins increased their body weight and fatfold thickness markedly during the seven- to 11-year-old range. Because the intrapair differences in fatfold were smaller for MZ than for DZ twins, Borjeson attributed this rapid prepubescent increase in adipose tissue to genetically timed physiological "fat spurts." In a design such as Borjeson's where MZ and DZ twins are not reared apart one cannot determine the extent of genetic-environmental covariations. The fascinating implication, however, is that there may be "sensitive periods" for adipose tissue deposition which may be genetically and/or environmentally determined.*

What is the evidence for sensitive periods for adipose tissue deposition? Brook (1972) studied fat cell numbers in children during the first year of life and later. He concluded that the period extending from approximately 30 weeks gestation to the age of one year is the finite sensitive period during which the basic complement of fat cells is determined.

---

* While Brook (i.e. Brook et al., 1975; Brook, 1977) found that heritability for adipose tissue stores was considerably higher for twins over ten years old as compared with estimates for younger twins, it is premature to attribute the prepubescent "fat spurts" to genetic factors exclusively, although it would be reasonable to infer that environmental manipulation to decrease excessive fatness might be more effective when initiated prior to puberty.

This early finding provided the rationale for studying the contribution of early mother-infant feeding transactions to developmental obesity. Salans, Cushman and Weissman (1973), however, found that adipose cells may also proliferate in number later in life during the prepubertal period. Even more provocative are data gathered by Dugdale (1975) regarding patterns of fat and lean tissue deposition in a sample of normal males ranging in age from 26 weeks after gestation to 16 years of age. He found large and cyclical "critical periods" for adipose tissue deposition. Fat deposition was found to predominate during the first year of life, then again during the period between six and 10 years of age, and once again at age 16 to 17. Lean tissue deposition occurred during the intervening periods. Dugdale's data are thus consistent with Borjeson's observation of a marked increase in fatness during the seven- to 11-year-old period in his twin study.

J. McVicker Hunt in his paper on the implications of plasticity for assessment and risk in early development (this volume) referred to a study by Herman Epstein (1974a, b) in which increments in head size (presumably correlated with cognitive-developmental "critical periods") coincided with significant IQ increases during these same time periods. Hunt recommended that learning enrichment experiences should be consistently provided throughout childhood to capitalize on the occurrence of such critical periods for cognitive development, since "plasticity" (or the organism's capacity to make adaptive modifications to novel experiences) may be reversible. In the case of developmental obesity, we may be dealing with plasticity in a "physical" sense: There may be a number of sensitive periods for adipose tissue deposition during childhood and adolescence when the nature of feeding experiences may potentiate excess adiposity (Brook, 1977).

These statements are quite speculative; however, it seems prudent to recommend consistent application of close monitoring of eating habits and the provision of an active lifestyle throughout the developmental period, particularly for children with familial tendencies toward developmental obesity. This viewpoint is well articulated in a quote by Garn (1976):

> There are, of course, innumerable stated explanations for obesity, from infancy to the end of life. If the genes do it (by directing fat storage), if the hypothalamus does it (by regulating eating behavior), or if there is some set point to reset, then the practical solution may arrive neither soon nor simply. . . . If obesity is induced early, in the very first year of life, by overfeeding impressionable fat cells,

then prevention consists of dietary management. . . . In this event, preventative therapy may be limited to the first year of life and to the pediatric patient alone. If obesity is learned by continuing exposure to the environment of eating and inappropriate hunger-free eating behavior, then management goes beyond the infant or child to include the entire family, and not for just a year but for years to come (p. 466).

As of now, the answers to these suppositions are still very uncertain. Considering developmental obesity in its psychosocial context, however, is clearly indicated for future longitudinal studies and prevention efforts.

Part II

DEVELOPMENT OF EARLY PATTERNS OF PARENT-INFANT INTERACTION: THE ROLE OF THE PARENT AND OF THE INFANT

The preceding section presented alternative orientations for psychosocial risk research in pregnancy and early infancy: the individual differences approach, the social environmental approach, and a diasthesis-stress model. The present section focuses explicitly on psychosocial risk within the context of parent-infant interactions. The bidirectionality of influence is assumed in the three chapters contained in this section. Factors that account for differing characteristics of parents and infants in their interactive behaviors are explicitly related to differing patterns of interaction within dyads. These interactive behaviors may be determined by environmental and genetic or other biophysical factors. While these later factors are often only implicitly recognized in this section, they are involved in the transactional processes addressed here since they contribute to the qualitative features of parent-infant interactions.

The three chapters presented in this section focus on current understanding of the processes by which mother and infant achieve a "fitting together" or joint regulation of behavior. Each chapter shares a common concern with the psychosocial risk inherent in relationships in which mother and infant behaviors lack interactive synchrony. In describing the development of synchronous and asynchronous interactions, all three investigators utilize modifications of communication theory in their conceptualization of the prelinguistic interactive behavior of mothers and infants. Tronick and Field view prelinguistic communication as a special case of more general models of communication, but Thoman argues for a more limited view of the parallels between prelinguistic interaction and later linguistic forms of communication. While each of these researchers provides a different theoretical framework to explain behavioral data, the overall goal of each is to explain how infants and mothers develop interactive patterns.

Starting from a general systems perspective, Thoman employs a naturalistic approach to the study of mother-infant interaction. She reports data on mother-infant mutual adaptation under a variety of circumstances which are typical in routine caretaking. She observes the "fit" of mother and infant characteristics, examining the patterning, changes and continuities in the behavioral organization over time of individual dyads. Thoman focuses on the processes by which interactional behaviors are integrated and points out the recurring individual differences in specific mother-infant pairs under study. In presenting her data Thoman points out that her naturalistic observations of mothers and infants do not conform well to adult communication theory.

Field extrapolates from adult-to-adult conversational roles to the interaction between mothers and infants. She delineates constraints imposed on mother-infant interaction by the infant's immaturity. These constraints include, but are not limited to, noncontingent responding, extended latencies of response, and a need to shut out excessive stimuli. In the observation of various high risk dyads, Field's research identifies the role that biophysical risk factors (e.g., premature birth) may play in influencing quantitative and qualitative aspects of interaction. In the examination of interaction in these high risk dyads, Field implicitly adopts a diasthesis-stress model to explain the development of asynchronous patterns of interaction between mothers and infants. Field further presents promising evidence of intervention methods which alter asynchronous interactions under laboratory conditions. She concludes with a cautionary note against premature intervention despite the apparently determinate role of early patterns of interaction in shaping later infant development.

Using a model of joint regulation of communicative acts to study the sharing of functions in time, Tronick examines mother-infant interaction in terms of the structuring of communicative goals and rules. He defines joint regulation of behavior as "mutual recognition of the other's ongoing intentionality or direction of behavior as it relates to one's own." Tronick conceptualizes the mother-infant dyad as interacting cybernetic systems and sees interactive competence as the most significant adaptive experience for the infant. The processes involved in mutual regulation of behavior are viewed as providing the bases for the infant's self-awareness and empathy, and are thus fundamental to the ability to develop reciprocal obligations. In his paper Tronick thus provides an explanation of the role that parent-infant interactions play in the development of later infant competence. Like Thoman, Tronick argues that early patterns of parent-infant interaction affect later development of the infant. Unlike Thoman, Tronick fits communication theory to his data without difficulty.

One of the most significant problems faced by these and other investigators of patterns of parent-infant interactions is the lack of refined measurement and analysis techniques with which to study infant-adult interaction. In the three studies presented the conceptualization of communicative processes whereby joint regulation is achieved does not provide clear and logical operational definitions of the relevant units of analysis. Thoman argues for the importance of attending to the simultaneity of interactive behaviors. Tronick and Field focus more on the sequences and contingent relations among interactive behaviors of dyadic partners. These and related issues pertinent to methods of measuring and quantifying interactional patterns are further addressed in Section V, "Methodological Issues in Assessing Infant Characteristics and the Quality of Parent-Infant Interactions," of this volume.

Judging the most appropriate theoretical orientation or the most productive observational strategies for characterizing mother-infant interaction is premature at this point. Further, prescribing the form of clinical intervention is equally premature. What can be gleaned at this point is evidence for continuity between early interactive patterns and later infant development and, further, the modifiability, under laboratory conditions, of interactive behaviors of high-risk dyads. Further research is needed, however, to clarify the nature of the connection between early interactive patterns and later infant development, as well as the form and content of intervention appropriate for asynchronous dyads.

4

Disruption and Asynchrony in Early Parent-Infant Interactions

EVELYN B. THOMAN
University of Connecticut

Along with a growing demand for intervention at earlier and earlier ages, there is a growing need for identifying those infants who are in need of, and can be helped by, intervention measures. At the same time, there is also an increasing recognition of the difficulties of assessment at very early ages for the purpose of predicting developmental outcome. McCall, Hogarty, and Hurlburt (1972), in a review of studies involving early assessment for prediction of later development, conclude that until three years of age prediction is unreliable. A review by Lewis (1973) draws a similar conclusion. More recently, a report by McCall (1976) indicates some correspondence in relative test performance over the first two years, but he summarizes the problem: "The changes in relative position from one age to the next are more impressive than the similarities" (p. 100). It has generally been found that prediction is most reliable at the extreme low end of the continuum (Honzik, 1976), and that the extreme values are most responsible for the relatively high relationships reported in some studies. In extreme cases, of course, the biological damage to an infant from prenatal, perinatal, or early postnatal events is sufficiently severe that assessment for screening purposes is readily achieved with or without systematic procedures.

A major problem for assessment is posed by the infant without apparent anomaly who has been exposed to stressful circumstances in the prenatal or perinatal period, such as anoxia or prolonged labor as iso-

---

The research described in this paper was supported by the William T. Grant Foundation, and NICHD Grant HD-08195-01A2.

lated events or in combination with prematurity. As Parmelee, Kopp and Sigman (1976) point out, some infants with known risk status develop normally, whereas others have developmental difficulties at a later age. The challenge is to identify those infants who need continued surveillance and may at some future time be in need of clinical intervention.

A second major challenge for assessment is that of identifying infants who are born without any known previous stressors and appear to be fully normal very early in life, but go on at a later age to have developmental dysfunction. The need is to identify these infants at as early an age as possible for purposes of intervention aimed at prevention or reduction of disability.

And the final challenge for developmental assessment is to be able to depict the developmental status of individual infants or children within the normal range. Reliable discriminations among normal infants is a prerequisite for a reliable indication of the nature and extent of deviance of any infant with abnormal characteristics.

The major obstacle to prediction of developmental outcome is posed by the developmental process itself, which is not unitary in nature nor linear over time. Furthermore, each individual infant has a unique developmental course (Wohlwill, 1973). An infant neither functions nor develops within a vacuum, and strategies for assessment which do not take this into account have proved to be futile. The most widely used assessment for newborns, the Brazelton Scale (Brazelton, 1973c) very clearly reflects a recognition of this important point. Rather than subject the infant to a standardized sequence of prescribed stimuli, the scales are based on test items which are presented in accordance with the infant's state or arousal level at any particular moment during the course of the test. The nature of the items include responsiveness to social as well as inanimate stimuli, all of which are conditions to which the typical infant must adapt during the course of naturally occurring events.

The recent emphasis by many researchers on mother-infant interaction reflects a recognition that an understanding of the developmental process and assessment of the infant must take into account an assessment of the environment in which the infant lives. The developmental process represents an ongoing integration between the characteristics of the infant and environmental experiences as they interact with the infant's characteristics. Expressed more explicitly, each individual infant has a unique organization of sensitivities and responsiveness to environmental events, and each family provides a unique set of environmental experiences for their infant. Any serious attempt at assessment for descriptive or predictive purposes must take into account the dynamic events that are involved in the developmental process for any individual infant.

Our approach to the assessment problem does not, at this time, include an effort to devise a practical, general-use and quickly applied testing instrument. Rather, we are taking a very different route to assessment by providing very intensive and empirical descriptions of infants in their natural environments. Our objectives are to identify the adaptive behaviors of each infant studied, the ways in which these adaptive behaviors fit with those of the mother, and to depict the short-term stability or changes in the patterning of their relationship variables. Where judgments of an infant's coping capabilities can be made, these judgments constitute an assessment. Where the interactive behaviors of mothers and infants are found to be demonstrably facilitative or interfering for the infant's developmental status, it is possible to assess, or evaluate, the relationship. The long-term predictive potential for such assessments is still another issue. Our immediate concern is to provide information on the nature of the earliest development of the infant and the mother-infant relationship. Reliable information on early functioning in the setting in which an infant is adapting should have significant implications for an understanding if not prediction of later development.

Parenthetically, it should be stated that an emphasis on the mother as the major figure for social interaction during the early weeks is not an expression of a lack of regard for the father's role. Parke (this volume) and others have provided impressive evidence for the significance of the father's interaction with the infant. Our studies begin at the time of the infant's birth, and, for the population we have sampled, the primary caretaker at that time is typically the mother. During the course of our observations, when the father is present and interacting with the infant, he is the one who is observed. This is not a frequent occurrence, however, and not sufficiently frequent to provide useful data. However, since we have dedicated ourselves to taking the baby out of the vacuum for study, fathers are included whenever they "take over."

DEVELOPMENT OF THE EARLIEST PATTERNS OF INTERACTION

It seems reasonable to assume that the neonate's behavior and activity during its initial social encounters reveal adaptive behaviors derived from genetic and prenatal influences. These adaptive behaviors are modified during early development during the maturation processes and interaction with the mother or caregiver. The evolving interaction reflects a basic process which involves the infant's input into the mother-infant system and thus the infant's role in its own growth process. If this is so, then our ability to measure these patterns during the early days may allow us to begin to identify antecedents to subsequent development. Thus, to begin to understand the factors that influence the development of an infant, it is necessary to describe the ongoing process of mutual modification of mother and infant from the inception of that relationship.

Very few studies of mother-infant interaction have given attention to the development of the relationship from the earliest days after the infant's birth. Consequently, little is known about the early stages of interaction or about how these early patterns may lead to more stable ones that become established over time. Our previous studies of mother-infant interaction have suggested that some very early interactive patterns may be responsible for later interactional patterns as well as for the behavior characteristics that develop in the child (Thoman, Turner, Leiderman, & Barnett, 1970; Thoman, Barnett, and Leiderman, 1971; Thoman, Leiderman and Olson, 1972). These studies indicate that infants give cues during feeding from the first day of life and that mothers may vary markedly in their sensitivity to their infant's cues during feeding interaction. Specifically, during feeding interactions during the first three days of life, primiparous mothers were found to show greater persistence in trying to get the infants to feed, greater inconsistency in terms of changing activities from feeding to nonfeeding ones, and much greater stimulation of their infant during the course of the feeding. Other evidence (Brody, 1966) indicates that these early patterns of feeding interaction persist through the latter half of the first year. Likewise, characteristics found in mothers and their first and later born infants are similar to those that have been reported in studies of mothers interacting with first and later born children at older ages. Mothers are generally more attentive to firstborns (Koch, 1954); mothers are more directive of the firstborn (Lasko, 1954; Stout, 1960); and they exert more pressure on the first child for achievement and responsibility (Davis, 1959; McArthur, 1956; Rosen, 1961; Sampson, 1962; Sutton-Smith et al., 1964). Mothers are also more inconsistent in their training of the firstborn (Hilton, 1968; Sears et al., 1957); and they interfere more with the first child (Hilton, 1968). The prelude to these behaviors is indeed found in our observations of primiparous and multiparous mothers with their newborn infants.

In any mother-infant relationship, characteristics of both the mother and infant contribute to their ongoing process of mutual adaptation. This mutuality has long been a consideration for infants with developmental problems.

DEVELOPMENTAL DYSFUNCTION AND MOTHER-INFANT INTERACTION

Greenberg (1971) describes the interactional behavior of mothers and infants with atypical behaviors, and he reports ". . . a linking of atypical behavior, atypical development, disturbed and often withdrawn mothers, negligence and abuse in the care and treatment of babies . . ." (p. 416). This study began when the children were two and a half years of age. However, if we are to understand etiology of developmental difficulties in infants, it is critical that we explore the relationships that may accentuate or diminish difficulties in the developmental process of infants much earlier than this age. For example, in research concerned with relating emotional deprivation in very young children and their failure to thrive, Leonard, Rhymes and Solnit (1966) found marked inadequacy in the mother-infant relationships. The mothers expressed feelings of inadequacy and they appeared incompetent in terms of dealing with the feelings and other activities of their infants. These women were, in fact, failing to thrive in their development as mothers. The authors observed that developmental characteristics of the infants may have also contributed to the maternal-child difficulties. "Thus, each infant and mother contributed reciprocally to the other's failure to thrive as well as the faulty relationships between them" (p. 610).

The nature of interaction failure is further illustrated in a study of colicky infants. Carey (1968) found that mothers of infants who cried excessively provided a great deal of stimulation for their infants, but these efforts failed to comfort the infants. The primary characteristic of the maternal caretaking activities was its inconsistency, which apparently derived from uncertainty about the role of the mother. This uncertainty was clearly expressed prior to the onset of excessive crying in their infants. Even though these mothers stimulated their infants, their stimulation was in no way designed to match the needs of the infant or infants. Either (a) the infants did not indicate their needs by the behavior exhibited, or (b) the mothers failed to perceive the infants' behaviors as cues for their own caretaking behaviors. Disruption of this process by any of several means—such as premature birth, unresponsive or disorganized responses of the infant, or inadequate mothering—should serve to exaggerate the infant's difficulties in the course of development. Our research and that of others has indicated that the mutual adaptation —or maladaptation—of mother and infant begins from the time of birth.

These considerations suggest the general rule that the earliest organization of the mother-infant system occurs as a function of the capacities of both the mother and her infant; the infant's capabilities for indicating its status, signaling its needs and responding to maternal interventions; and the mother's ability to perceive cues provided by her infant and to respond appropriately to these cues.

A COMMUNICATION MODEL FOR EARLY INTERACTION

The major assumption for our model of mother and infant interaction is that it constitutes a communication system from the time of birth. It is the nature of this communication network that must be explored. Our position is that, during very early mother-infant interactions, linguistic models are not yet applicable in an attempt to understand the nature of mother and infant communication. The earliest communication has characteristics which are unique to this stage of development, requiring special explanatory principles rather than ones derived from functioning at a later age. The newborn infant is biologically designed for survival in a social environment and is thus a "born communicator." The cue-giving capabilities of infants have long been of interest (e.g., Ainsworth, 1967; Call, 1964; Robson, 1967). But the nature of the earliest communication has not been considered in terms of how it may differ from the organization of cue-exchanges which occur sequentially as in verbal exchanges at a later age.

Primarily, the earliest communication is essentially affective in nature. That is, "information" in the traditional sense is not intentionally being transmitted, whether communication takes the form of vocalization, of gesture, or of contact body movements. The sensory systems of the human infant are remarkably well developed, and the communication process consists of multimodal sensory stimuli provided by the holding, moving, talking, looking, and other forms of interventions given simultaneously by the mother and baby during any interaction. The simultaneity of cue-giving behaviors is an important quality of these exchanges, with variations in temporal overlap—a "feathering" of behavioral events (to use a descriptive term from Golani, 1978).

The mutual cue-exchange of mother and infant has been described as a dance by Gunther (1961), and others. That is, it is possible for a mother and infant to achieve a rhythm of interaction in which each can lead or follow or anticipate the actions of the other and thereby exhibit simultaneous communicative behaviors as is the case with two partners dancing. Stern (1977) very eloquently describes the simultaneity of mutual behaviors of mother and infant, and he has examined these patterns in great detail both in vocal (Stern & Gibbon, 1978) and visual (Stern 1974) modalities.

A variety of research techniques may be needed to thread out the related patterns and their changes over age. A number of investigators have been engaged in fruitful research beginnings in this area (Brown et al., 1975; Dunn & Richards, 1977; Beckwith et al., 1976).

A very molecular approach has been taken by Tronick, Adamson, Wise, Als and Brazelton (1975), Condon and Sander (1974b), and Stern (1971, 1974a, 1974b). Using time-lapse photography and frame-by-frame analyses of films, they have demonstrated temporal relations between the behaviors of mothers and infants. In these analyses, behaviors are found to occur either simultaneously (i.e., in the same time-frame) or so close together sequentially that it is impossible to view the behaviors in an initiator-responder framework. Their research emphasizes again the importance of observing the behaviors of both members of the system simultaneously if the behavior of either member of the pair is to make any sense. This evidence for a much more complicated communication network between mother and infant than has previously been assumed, opens new vistas in the area of empirical study of the infant as a social and feeling being.

Almost certainly the principles involved in the early affective communication between mother and infant differ from those involved in later linguistic communication. We are not the first to maintain that the principles applied to the study of language are not applicable to early communication. Chomsky (1967) has taken a very strong stand on this issue, contending that the nonlinguistic communication of animals and infants has no continuity with the nature of language. Without limiting ourselves to Chomsky's formal linguistic framework, we should heed his warning that very different principles may apply to linguistic and prelinguistic communication. This may continue to be the case at a later age when nonlinguistic communication continues to develop concurrently with the acquisition of specialized, conventional verbal forms of communication but according to different principles.

The importance of rhythms is another facet of nonverbal communication that may relate both to the simultaneous exchange and the affective quality of early interaction. Rhythms may be very molecular moment to moment ones or they may be of longer-durations—minutes or hours (Ashton, 1976; Sander et al., 1978; Tronick & Brazelton, 1978; Brazelton, 1974b, 1977; Stern, 1977; Tronick et al., 1975). These are potentially derived in part from the infant's own endogenous rhythms. As these and other researchers have pointed out, a major task of the mother and the infant is to synchronize their separate rhythms. When this occurs, one can say very subjectively that the nature of the interaction on a moment-to-moment basis or over longer time spans is truly like a dance. Progress has been made by each of these researchers toward depicting the qualities of the "dance."

The importance of nonverbal communication and the rhythmic patterning of cues has been emphasized as a means by which each partner comes to have expectations for the behaviors of the other member of the dyad.

MAJOR STRATEGIES FOR THE LONGITUDINAL STUDY OF MOTHER-INFANT INTERACTION

The very general objectives of our research with infants and their mothers are: (1) to identify individual characteristics of infants from the time of birth; (2) to describe the nature of the mother-infant interaction in terms that depict their capacity for synchrony; and (3) to identify the effects of the mother-infant interaction on the developing behaviors of the infant. These objectives are congruent with our purposes already indicated, namely, to provide some understanding of the developmental processes during the infant's earliest weeks of life, both with respect to the infant's own behavioral organization and with respect to the social network the infant interacts with, and to identify individual patterns of developing mother-infant relationships.

With these objectives in mind, the research is guided by simple but relevant strategies:

First, as indicated in the objectives listed above, developmental study of the infant and of the mother-infant relationship is begun at its inception, that is, within 24 hours after the infant's birth. Only by observing the infant separately and with the mother from the time of birth will it be possible to identify the initial characteristics of the infant and his contribution to the mother-infant relationship. Also, only with such early observations, followed by successive observations repeated over relatively short time intervals, will it be possible to infer the relationship of the infant's adaptive capabilities and characteristics of the mother-infant interaction.

Second, the mother and infant are observed under circumstances which are as natural as possible. That is, they are observed in the hospital immediately after the infant's birth, and they are observed in the home during their usual routine, without any interventions or contrived situations. In this way, and to the extent that the effect of the presence of an observer is minimized, it should be possible to describe real mothers and infants interacting in their real world. Infants are observed alone when they are left alone by the mother, and the mother and infant are both observed when they are together.

Finally, our studies of mothers and infants involve intensive observations, in terms of total duration of observation, frequency of behavior recording, and number of behaviors recorded. This aspect of our research is the result of more than a decade spent in developing observational procedures and recording techniques. We have found that a whole day's observation (seven hours) enables us to record the mother-infant interaction in the variety of circumstances under which it typically occurs— e.g., feedings, caretaking activities, baby naps, periods of intermittent social interaction, and even periods when the mother may be focused on housework despite auditory cues from the infant. Successive weekly observations of seven hours' duration provides measures that reliably describe individual infants and mother-infant behaviors (Thoman, Becker & Freese, 1978; Thoman et al., 1978).

CODE-RECORDING BEHAVIORS IN NATURAL-LIVING CIRCUMSTANCES

An important aspect of the intensity of the observation is the large number of behaviors that are recorded. The code-recording procedure is based on a number of principles which enable us to record a great deal of information with minimal time and motion. The nature of the code is very much like a language, with nouns, action words, and modifiers. Intensive training for weeks or months is required to use this code-recording system reliably. In fact, we believe that we have fulfilled the request made by a noted pediatrician, Dr. Carlton Gajdusek (1968). He calls for a notational system for behaviors such as Laban dance notation served for body movements, a "cipher language," as a taxonomic sorting of ". . . observations on what stimulation a child receives from the environment and what response to it he makes—e.g., his environmental experiences and his behavioral response . . ." (p. 13), and he concludes most enthusiastically: "if pediatric research gives us a new notation and representation for 'those first affections' of perception, it will have contributed to more than the remedy of the ailments of man, but, as the arts, to the joys and means of his existence!" (p. 14). This dramatic statement is a rare bit of reassurance of the importance we have placed on the ability to record as many of the behaviors of the mother and infant in their natural circumstances as possible.

While there are some behaviors which infants emit that may be considered universal as cues within the mother-infant communication network—crying or smiling, for instance—it is not reasonable to expect to understand the complexities of multi-modal communication by focusing on these cues alone. The same holds for maternal behaviors. The vocabulary of behaviors that are important in each relationship may differ. It is necessary, therefore, to record as many cue-behaviors as possible in order to identify in each individual relationship those that may serve most potently. An example of this principle is given in our report (Thoman, Becker & Freese, 1978) of one mother-infant relationship in which the baby's open-eyed REM was responded to as wakefulness. On numerous occasions, the baby was fed immediately following an episode of open-eyed REM, and accordingly, the feedings were very brief as the baby was unresponsive (obviously asleep) on these occasions. In fact, most mothers seem to be unaware of the occurrence of open-eyed REMs. In the case of this one mother-infant pair, the dynamics of their interaction surrounding the feeding would remain a mystery without a record of this specific behavior.

Given the subtleties of the early nonlinguistic communication, it is necessary to record a large number of behavioral actions any—or many—of which may serve as cues by each member of the dyad for the other. Only extensive data from each dyad can reveal which behavioral cues are relevant and which are not relevant for that particular pair. At the same time, extensive data can reveal which behavioral cues may be common to all pairs of mothers and infants, to subgroups of mothers and infants, or occur uniquely within a single mother-infant pair.

Several factors make it possible to reliably record a very large number of mother-and-infant behaviors. First, many of the coded behaviors occur only in limited contexts. For example, behaviors such as Suck Stimulation, Not-Sucking, and Not-Attached (see Table 1) occur only when the infant is feeding or has been given a pacifier. Secondly, the detail with which certain variables are recorded varies within the observation. For instance, distinctions among the sleep states are made only when the infant is alone in the crib. Also, the variables include a number of totally inclusive and mutually exclusive categories of behavior which require code-recording only when a change occurs within the category. For example, an infant's position is coded as Prone, Up, at Shoulder, or Supine. Once a position has been recorded, it is not re-coded until the position changes. Finally, economy in recording is aided by the use of standard inferences which eliminate the actual marking of some variables. For instance, if the mother carries the infant, this implies that the infant is being moved, and consequently the move category is not marked.

BEHAVIORS RECORDED

Very generally the kinds of behaviors we record in the home during the early weeks are designed to give information about the infant's behavioral states throughout any observation, including: sleep states, state-related behaviors, and respiration during periods of time in the crib; maternal behaviors that describe her location with respect to the infant, the position in which she holds or places the infant, stimulation given to the infant including tactile, movement, vocal, gestural, and visual attention; and the nature of her activities during periods of caretaking interaction including feeding, changing, or bathing the baby.

The infant's state provides an ongoing developmental characteristic for assessing the relationship between mother-infant interaction and the infant's development. State is an ubiquitous expression by the infant at all times, at all ages, although the quality of expression and organization of state parameters change with age. Individual differences in state organization (Thoman, Korner & Kraemer, 1976; Thoman, 1975a) reflect both environmental and maturational influences (Thoman and Becker, 1978). ". . . the differentiation of behavioral state becomes the central developmental characteristic of the newborn" (Sameroff, 1972, p. 210).

It should be noted that *all* behaviors are regarded as characteristics of the mother-infant relationship, even though it is necessary to record some as mother behaviors and some as infant behaviors. The activities of each member of the dyad are considered to be a function of the total inter-active system. Even when the infant is asleep, as indicated in the description given earlier, there may be an exchange between the partners. And characteristics of the sleep states may reflect the immediately previous interaction during the infant's wake period, as well as the ongoing rhythmicity attained in the relationship.

Behavior and Context

This view of relationship variables has major implication for using the behavioral data. A variable may consist of a single behavior or any combination of behaviors. For example, mother behaviors such as pat, or pat *and* caress, or pat *or* caress may each be considered as variables. Either baby sucking, or sucking while alert may be considered as a variable. Combinations of mother and baby behaviors may also be considered as variables for analysis. For example, vis-à-vis involves both members of the dyad; the mother may be holding the baby and providing any of a variety of forms of stimulation, while the baby is in any of the behavioral states that are recorded. Thus, any cluster of these co-occurring mother and baby behaviors may be considered in combination as a variable to be assessed for its frequency, duration (number of episodes) or variability in duration. Defining and analyzing data from a wide variety of combination variables is the unique potential that is derived from having recorded a large number of behaviors throughout an extended period of time.

Another way of viewing the behaviors as variables is to consider the context in which they occur. For example, mother talking while the baby is crying is very different from mother talking while the baby is quietly alert. Thus, mother talking can be considered with either crying or alert as the context, or background variable. By the same token, the same variable can serve as the context for different behaviors on the part of either member of the dyad. For example, while the mother is holding the baby, the baby can either be crying or can be in a quiet alert state. It can be seen that any combination of behaviors of one or both members of the dyad can be measured within the context of a wide variety of other behavioral combination variables. Again, this potential is available because of the large number of behaviors of both mother and infant that are recorded.

It may be well to make a more explicit distinction between assessing combinations of variables and assessing one variable within the context of another one, i.e., using the second variable as the background variable. Figure 1 shows a bar graph representing a seven-hour observation. During 27% of this particular observation the mother was holding the baby.

During 15% of the observation the baby was alert, and the baby was alert 42% of the time the mother was holding the baby. There were also alert periods when the mother was not holding the baby. If epochs of *Baby Alert and Mother Holding* are counted, they constitute 11% of the observation; however, if *Mother Holding* is the background variable, then baby alert is 42% of Mother Holding time. Thus, whether the total observation or a portion of the observation is identified as the background variable, the percentage measure will differ. This distinction is a very important one for analyzing the mother-infant process, and it will become more clear as the data are described in the sections that follow.

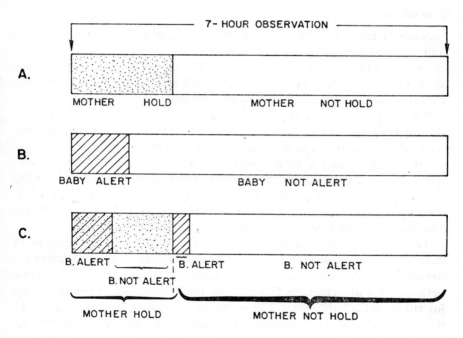

FIGURE 1. Relational measures of mother and baby behaviors: Percent of the total observation that the mother is holding the baby: Hold (Total) = 27%. Percent of the total observation that the baby is alert: Alert (Total) = 15%. Percent of the total observation that the baby is alert while the mother is holding him/her: Alert & Hold (Total) = 11%. Percent of the total observation that the baby is alert while the mother is not holding him/her: Alert & Not Hold (Total) = 3%. Percent of the time when the mother is holding the baby that he/she is alert: Alert (Hold) = 42%. Percent of the time when the mother is not holding the baby that he/she is alert: Alert (Not Hold) = 13%.

In the remaining section of this paper, additional details of our procedures will be described, data from the total group of 20 subjects will be summarized, and comparison data for one individual mother-infant pair will be presented. One purpose is to demonstrate that the patterning of relationship behaviors for individual mother and infant pairs can be reliably described during the early weeks of life. A second purpose is to demonstrate that the quality of an interaction can be described quantitatively by comparing the single subject with the overall patterning shown by a comparable group of subjects.

A STUDY OF TWENTY INDIVIDUAL MOTHER-INFANT RELATIONSHIPS

Procedures

Some of the procedures for this study have already been referred to, and a more complete description of the methodology has been given elsewhere (Thoman, Becker & Freese, 1978; Thoman, Acebo, Dreyer, Becker & Freese, 1978). However, a few additional details may give a more coherent picture of how the data were obtained.

The subjects were twenty primiparous mothers enrolled in the project during their last trimester of pregnancy, and their infants born at full-term without perinatal or early postnatal problems.

Prenatal assessments of mothers were obtained from interview and questionnaires. Mothers and infants were observed in the hospital during the early postpartum period (Freese, 1975), during two feedings while they were together, and during one interfeeding period while the infant was in a crib in an observation room.

The first home observation was made when the infant was eight to 14 days of age, with subsequent home observations made at approximately weekly intervals. Each observation consisted of a continuous seven-hour period. Two observers participated in the observation, each recording for three and a half hours. The changing of observers in the middle of the observation was accomplished without interruption of either the observational procedures or ongoing household activities.

During the observation period the observer avoided interaction with anyone in the household. She selected locations which permitted a clear view of the infant's face but where she was as unobtrusive as possible in the household setting. Wherever the infant was moved the observer followed. During long sleep periods when the infant was in the crib, the observer remained with the infant and recorded sleep patterns. It was made clear beforehand, however, that though the observer remained with the baby she in no way acted as a "baby-sitter" in the mother's absence.

Throughout each seven-hour observation the occurrence of any of the 75 mother or infant behaviors (presented in Table 1) were code-recorded every 10 seconds. A small electronic timing device provided the observer with a signal through an ear microphone every 10 seconds. At each signal the necessary codes were recorded, with no formal pause in the observational process. In this way, nearly continuous recording of the occurrence of each behavior was possible.

TABLE 1

Mother and Infant Behaviors, Birth to Five Weeks

Mother's Location
  Out
  Far
  Near
  In contact
  Holding infant
  Carrying infant
  Holding infant at shoulder

Infant's Location
  Crib
  Cradle Board
  Other

Infant's position
  Prone
  Supine
  Upright

Mother-Infant activity
  Changing infant
  Feeding infant
  Bathing infant
  None of these

Feeding inputs
  Breast or bottle
  Water
  Solids

Maternal Stimulation
  Pacifier
  Suck-stimulation (during feeding)
  Positioning infant for en face (eyes
    are open)
  Looking at infant

Infant Behaviors
  Not attached to nipple (during feeding)
  Not sucking (during feeding)
  Vocalize (nonfussy)
  Smile
  Frown
  Grimace
  Burp
  Bowel movement
  Spit up
  Hiccup
  Gag
  Jitter
  Hand-mouth
  Suck hand or fingers
  Grunt
  Yawn
  Sneeze
  Cough
  No body movements
  Small body movements
  Large body movements

Infant States
  Sleep
    Active
    Quiet

  Wake
    Drowse
    Daze
    Alert
    Waking active
    Brief fuss
    Sustained fussing
    Crying

TABLE 1 *(continued)*

Talking to infant
Smiling or laughing at infant
Patting
Caressing
Moving
Rocking
Immersing baby (during bath)
Mother detaches baby from nipple
(during feeding)

Indefinite

Eyes Closed (when mother holding infant and sleep state cannot be judged).

Sleep Behaviors
Rapid eye movements (REMs: brief, sustained, REM-storm)
Eyes open (briefly, as during REM)
Mouthing
Rhythmic mouthing
Sucking
Jerk
Startle
Sigh
Sigh-sob
Occurrence of any infant behavior listed above

Reliabilities among the three observers who carried out these observations were calculated for each variable using the following formula:

$$\frac{2 \text{ (number of agreements)}}{\text{number of occurrences recorded by both observers}}$$

The interrater reliabilities among the three observers for variables to be analyzed for this report ranged from .75 to .99.

The data to be described came from the four observations on weeks two to five. For the 20 mother-infant pairs, more than 200,000 10-second epochs were recorded over the four home observations, with presence-absence information on 75 behaviors during each epoch.

Variables Analyzed for Mother-Infant Pairs
On Weeks Two, Three, Four, and Five

From the list of recorded behaviors presented in Table 1, combinations of mother and/or baby behaviors were selected as relationship variables most relevant for describing the pair. Variables were defined from behaviors occurring concurrently within each epoch. Some variable combinations are obvious from their labels; the components of others need to be specified, including the following:

Total Observation. The number of epochs in any home observation.

Caretaking. The mother-infant pair is engaged in one of the following activities: feed, change, or bathe.

Social Interaction. *All* of the following are occurring: (1) the infant is in the awake state; (2) the mother is holding or carrying the baby; and (3) the mother is not engaged in a caretaking activity.

Mother Looking and Baby Awake. While the baby is awake, the mother is looking at the baby's face and holding him/her in the en face position, but the infant is *not* looking at the mother's face.

Stimulating. The mother is engaged in *any* of the following maternal stimulation variables: pat, caress, move, or rock.

The remainder of the variables analyzed were either single variables or combination of variables taken directly from Table 1, such as *Hold or Carry,* or *Fuss or Cry,* or *Drowse or Daze,* or *Change or Bathe.*

Stability of Mother-Infant Behaviors During the Early Weeks

Absolute frequency of occurrence is usually not the appropriate measure for assessing these relationship variables. First, the total number of epochs in an observation was never exactly equivalent to the 2520 that make up a seven-hour period ($\bar{x} = 2495$; s.d. $= 110$); and second, as already indicated, many of the variables constitute a portion of some context behavior which was itself a component of the total observation. Figure 1 illustrates the definitional description of some of the variables: the baby's alertness can be measured as a percent of the total observation, written as Baby Alert (Total); it can be measured in terms of the percent of time the baby was being held by the mother, written as Baby Alert (Mother Holding); or it can be measured when the mother is not holding the baby, Baby Alert (Mother Not Holding). Although each variable assesses the baby's alertness, they may or may not be highly correlated, and each may be very important for depicting the characteristics of individual mother and infant relationships.

Table 2 presents summary values for the measures of concern for this report. The group means are based on means for each of the 20 individuals over the four weekly observations. The four weekly observations permitted assessment of individual differences among mother-infant pairs for each of these measures of the interaction. An analysis of variance for repeated measures was used to assess individual differences as well as changes over weeks, and sex effects. There were no significant sex effects

TABLE 2

Mean Percent (of Base Variable) Over Weeks 2, 3, 4, and 5, for Pair *M* and the Group of 20 Mother-Infant Pairs; Standard Error of Measurement; and Lower Bounds Reliability Coefficient

	Pr. M	$\bar{X}_{20}$	SEM_{eas}	r_{tt}
Baby: Behavioral States				
Wake (Total)	38.6	34.5	4.8	.50
Alert (Total)	19.2	14.5	2.6	.72
Fuss or Cry (Total)	3.0	4.1	1.2	.73
Drowse or Daze (Total)	15.3	13.3	2.4	.21[a]
Episodes of Sleep 5 min	3.0	2.7	0.5	.39[a]
Quiet Sleep (Sleep)	42.0	33.0	3.4	.70
Quiet Sleep$_A$ (Quiet Sleep)	89.9	87.0	5.5	.49
Mother and Baby: Interacting Situations				
Caretaking (Total)	11.9	14.3	2.3	.80
Caretaking (Hold or Carry)	25.0	43.2	5.7	.82
Hold or Carry (Total)	28.5	26.9	4.0	.84
Social Interaction (Total)	13.7	10.4	2.4	.73
Social Interaction (Baby Awake)	35.0	29.5	4.9	.80
Baby States During Interaction				
Alert (Social Interaction)	31.8	44.0	7.3	.71
Fuss or Cry (Social Interaction)	12.8	9.9	3.9	.76
Drowse or Daze (Social Interaction)	53.8	40.4	6.4	.73
Alert (Feed)	21.3	25.7	8.0	.75
Drowse or Daze (Feed)	71.5	45.6	8.0	.65
Alert (Change or Bathe)	76.1	52.1	11.7	.60
Drowse or Daze (Change or Bathe)	3.3	6.0	3.7	.46
Fuss or Cry (Change or Bathe)	6.1	27.5	10.3	.62
Mother: Stimulation During Interaction				
Talking (Social Interaction)	43.0	46.1	6.2	.86
Stimulating (Social Interaction)	86.0	81.2	4.6	.74
Looking (Fuss or Cry)	70.6	60.9	9.2	.78
Talking (Fuss or Cry)	46.5	41.2	7.5	.84
Stimulating (Fuss or Cry)	58.8	35.4	7.8	.82
Mother: Affectionate Stimulation				
Caress (Total)	13.3	8.4	1.5	.83
Pat (Total)	8.0	3.5	1.0	.79
Mutual Visual Attention				
Vis-à-vis (Total)[b]	2.3	2.6	0.8	.59
Vis-à-vis (Mother Looking and Baby Awake)[b]	8.5	12.4	3.6	.71

[a] $p > .05$
[b] Significant increase over weeks, $p > .05$

for any of these variables. For two variables, there were significant monotonic trends over weeks: Vis-à-vis (Total) and Vis-à-vis (Mother Looking and Baby Awake). The latter variable refers to those epochs in which the mother was looking at the baby while maintaining the en-face position—while the baby was awake but not returning the mother's visual gaze. The mean rate of each of these variables increased over the four weeks of observation. There were significant individual differences for all but two of the interactive variables: Drowse or Daze (Total) and the Number of Episodes of Sleep lasting five minutes or longer. The results of these analyses provide evidence for significant stability across weeks for most of the variables listed in Table 2.

Table 2 also presents the total-test reliability (reliability over observations) for each variable based on the formula $r_{tt} = (1 - 1/F)$ and the standard error of measurement based on the formula $SEM_{eas} = s.d. \sqrt{1 - r_{tt}}$. The very high, lower-bounds reliability values shown in Table 2 indicate that the mean scores across the four weekly observations reliably measure behaviors of each individual mother-infant pair over this period of time. Each of these reliable measures are, therefore, potential predictors of later behavior.

Patterning of Behaviors in the Mother-Infant System for the Group of 20 Infants

It can be seen from Table 2 that babies during the first five weeks of life spend about a third of the day awake: a little less than half of the wakeful time is spent in alertness, and slightly less of the wakeful time is spent in a drowse or daze. These normal babies fussed or cried only about 4% of the seven-hour period, that is, averaging 102 epochs or approximately 17 minutes per day. During the epochs when the babies were fussing or crying the mothers were looking at them much of the time (60.9% of Fuss or Cry epochs); they were talking to the infants 41.2% and stimulating them 35.4% of the fuss-and-cry time. The distribution of talking and nontalking is very similar when social interaction is a context variable: Talking (Social Interaction) = 46.1%. However stimulation is distributed very differently during social interaction and when the baby is crying. Stimulation (Social Interaction) = 81.2%; Stimulation (Fuss or Cry) = 58.8%. Stimulation includes patting, caressing, moving or rocking the baby. It is somewhat surprising that mothers generally do more of these kinds of stimulation during social interaction periods—which may also include epochs of fussing and crying —than they do during fussing or crying as the context variable. This may in part be due to the fact that fussing or crying occurs more during caretaking activities (27.5% of Change or Bathe) and relatively little during social interaction (9.9%).

Characteristics of the infants' sleep are also depicted in Table 2. They typically had less than three naps during the day (sleeping periods longer than five minutes). The sleep was distributed 33% in Quiet Sleep and 57% in Active Sleep. Quiet Sleep$_A$ composed most of the infants' Quiet Sleep (87.0%) time. This variable refers to Quiet Sleep periods when the respiratory pattern is judged to be highly regular from breath-to-breath (Thoman, 1975a). During Quiet Sleep$_B$, respiration shows some irregularity and may include episodes of brief apnea.

It can also be seen from Table 2 that mothers spend approximately 14% of the seven-hour day in caretaking activities and a little less than that proportion in social interaction. Mothers spend 26.9% of the day holding their babies; and 43.2% of this time is used for caretaking purposes. The remainder of holding time is used for social interaction or for holding the baby while the baby is asleep. It should be noted that the definition for Social Interaction requires that the baby be awake. Overall, the mothers and babies were engaged in social interaction only 29.5% of the baby's waking time.

Table 2 indicates those activities of mothers that are associated with the baby's state organization. It can be seen that the babies were more likely to be alert when the mother was caretaking—changing or bathing—than during social interaction or feeding. During feeding the babies were more likely to be in a drowsy state.

And finally, Table 2 presents the total amount of affectionate stimulation given by mothers throughout the day. These values are relatively low: caressing 8.4% and patting the baby 3.5% of the seven-hour day. During many of these epochs the two are occurring simultaneously, so that the two percentages are not additive. Vis-à-vis (Total) is also relatively low, 2.6%, but during a much greater period of time, 12.4%, the mothers make themselves available for vis-à-vis. Both of these latter variables are ones that show a significant increase over weeks, as already indicated.

These data give a picture of the distribution of mother and infant behaviors over their seven-hour day. Such a detailed description of mother-and-infant behaviors has not been presented before.

The Relating Process in One Mother-Infant Pair

Mother-infant pair *M* was selected for detailed description because of some specific characteristics of the infant that appeared to the observers to be a real impediment for the mother-infant relating process. The baby was an extreme example of the noncuddly type described by Schaffer and Emerson (1964). When the baby was held, he showed obvious signs of distress; his state was more generally that of a drowse or daze rather than alertness, or even fussing or crying. One would not expect these behaviors to be part of an interactive system that could develop optimally. A baby's visual responsiveness to the mother is a most rewarding behavior for her ministrations and attention and these rewards were clearly lacking from this baby. We have described these aspects of the baby's behaviors in previous reports (Thoman, Acebo, Dreyer, Becker & Freese, 1978; Thoman, 1975b). However, the present report focuses on the details of the mother-infant interaction from data analyses that illustrate our pattern approach to assessing an individual baby and an individual mother-infant relationship.

Interaction Profiles for Mother-Infant Pair M

The mean values over weeks for mother-infant pair M on each of the variables assessed are presented in Table 2 so that the percentage levels can be compared with those for the total group of 20 babies. Since this pair was separated from the group for special consideration *post hoc,* they were included in the total group analyses.

In order to provide an overview of the comparisons of mother-infant pair M with the total group, a profile method of presentation is used. The strategy of comparing an individual with a normative group is commonly used in clinical assessment. With the group mean as a baseline, each of the measures for mother-infant M in Table 2 were transformed to z-scores and plotted to indicate deviations from the mean of the group. The resulting series of profiles is presented in Figures 2, 3, 4, 5, and 6. Because each measure had a very high reliability score, it is appropriate to use the data in this fashion to depict the variations of an individual subject. The standard error of measurement is also included, however, to emphasize the extreme deviation of some of the measures for pair M. This procedure was designed to highlight the characteristics of relationship M.

Figure 2 presents a profile of Baby M's behavioral state organization. From this figure, it can be seen that overall Baby M was awake and alert more than most babies and not very fussy. This much of the description is not consistent with that given earlier in our explanation for choosing this baby as a subject—in which the amount of drowse and fussing by the baby was emphasized. However, it can be seen that baby *M* did exhibit, throughout the observation, a greater amount of drowse and daze. Subsequent analyses will further clarify this apparent paradox.

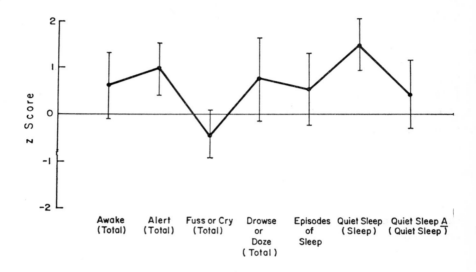

FIGURE 2. Profile of behavioral states for Baby *M*, compared to the group on each measure.

Figure 2 also gives a clue to the baby's sleep organization. Despite the fact that Baby *M* had less sleep time (as indicated by the greater wakefulness), the number of episodes of sleep were greater than the average for the group. A most dramatic aspect of this baby's sleep was the very high percent of quiet sleep. The implications of this characteristic will be discussed later. The final characteristic, Quiet Sleep$_A$ (Quiet Sleep), is a measure of regularity of respiration during quiet sleep. Baby *M* was relatively high on this measure, indicating fewer periods of erratic respiration during quiet sleep. The characteristics presented in Figure 2 are mixed ones with respect to any assessment of the baby's behavioral state organization: although erratic in his sleep-wakefulness, his sleep states showed a high degree of inhibitory control, generally considered to indicate a higher maturational level.

If we now focus on the mother's side of the interaction, Figure 3 presents characteristics of the relationship in terms of how the mother distributed her caretaking and noncaretaking time. It can be seen from Figure 3 that Mother *M* spent relatively little time in caretaking activities, that is changing or bathing or feeding, in comparison to other mothers. A most notable characteristic is that despite the fact that she held or carried the baby somewhat more than other mothers, a much *lower* proportion of the time she held the baby was for caretaking purposes. Mother *M* held her baby primarily for noncaretaking activities. This characteristic is also reflected in the portion of the profile indicating that she and the baby spent a very high percentage of their time in social interaction—whether this was measured as a percent of the total observation or as a percent of the infant's waking time. This profile clearly indicates a mother who is giving a great deal of attention to her baby not required for changing, feeding or bathing him.

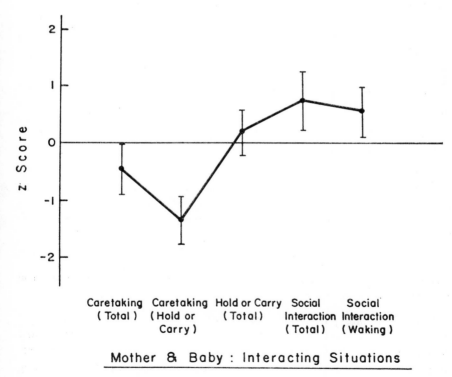

FIGURE 3. Profile indicating maternal activities, compared to the group on each measure.

The next figure, Figure 4, relates Baby *M*'s states to the mother's activities. The first notable characteristic of the baby in this regard is that
he was alert less than the other babies when he was with the mother,
during social interaction and during feeding. This is quite inconsistent
with the high degree of alertness depicted in Figure 2. However, it must
be noted that the apparent discrepancy is accounted for by the very great
amount of alertness shown by Baby *M* when he was being changed or
bathed and when he was alone in the crib. His differential alertness
under these different circumstances has been described in detail in
previous reports (Thoman, 1975c; Thoman, Acebo, Dreyer, Becker &
Freese, 1978). Rather than being alert, Baby *M* was either fussing or
crying or he was drowsy during social interaction; during feeding he was
in a drowsy state a great deal.

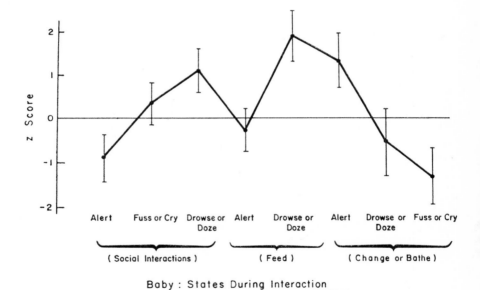

Figure 4. Profile of Baby *M*'s behavioral states during social interaction, feeding, and
caretaking.

Baby *M*'s state patterns become comprehensible when they are separated into circumstances when the mother is holding the baby and those
when she is not. For instance, during social interaction and during feeding the mother is holding the baby, whereas during changing or bathing
the mother typically is not holding the baby. Note that when being

changed or in the bath Baby *M* was highly alert and fussed and cried very little. The pattern of measures suggests a synchrony between the mother and baby when the baby was *not* being held.

Figure 5 returns to the mother's side of the interaction, with a description of her stimulation of the baby. In general, Mother *M* was high on all forms of stimulation and especially high when the baby was fussing and crying. In view of the baby's fussiness especially during social interaction, it appears possible that her stimulation was excessive or inappropriate. However, the patterning of the baby's states just described suggests that her stimulation when the baby was irritable was not inappropriate, though it was apparently ineffective in soothing him. The baby's general aversion to being held is most apparent in the data.

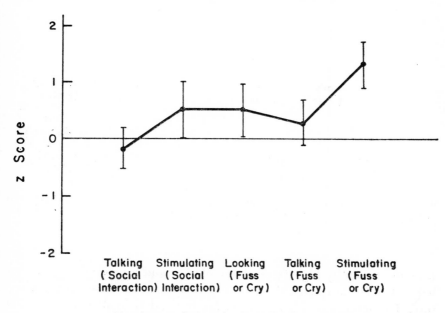

Mother: Stimulation During Interaction

FIGURE 5. Profile of Mother *M*'s maternal attention variables during social (non-caretaking) interaction, and when Baby *M* was fussing or crying.

The stimulation variables in Figure 6 are presented separately because they are worthy of special emphasis. It can be seen that Mother *M* patted and caressed her baby a great deal throughout the day, when compared with the group of mothers. Her affectionate stimulation was consistent

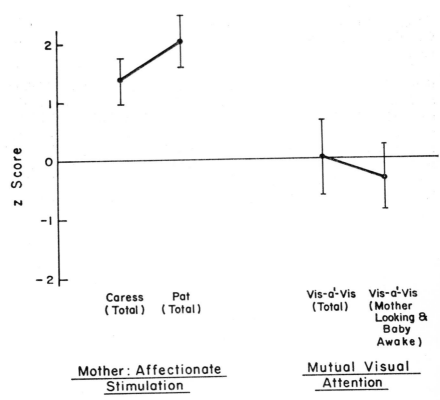

FIGURE 6. Levels of caressing and patting by Mother *M;* and level of mutual visual looking and of unilateral visual attention by Mother *M.*

with the generally high level of stimulation and attention she gave her baby. Their mutual visual attention provides a somewhat different picture. The level of vis-à-vis between Mother and Baby *M* is close to that of the total group. However, the mother was very persistent in her efforts to achieve vis-à-vis with the baby, as indicated by vis-à-vis (Mother Looking and Baby Awake). Although, by definition, the baby was awake during these periods of being placed in the en-face position, he did not return her gaze. This characteristic of the interaction is again consistent with the baby's aversion to being held, since at this age vis-à-vis almost invariably occurs when the mother is holding the baby.

DISCUSSION

The analyses of 30 complex interactional variables for the 20 subjects gives a rather detailed description of how mothers and babies spend their day together during the first five weeks of life. The variables analyzed include combinations of behaviors of mothers and babies occurring concurrently; they also include behaviors of both members of the pair under a variety of circumstances. Naturalistic studies of mothers and infants have typically not involved such detailed information in such a short age span. In fact, because of the brief age span covered by these observations there was not a developmental change over weeks on most of the measures. Thus, stability over weeks was a major finding with respect to mother-infant relationship measures over this time period.

The data from the total group of normal subjects provided a background distribution as a frame of reference for portraying the relating process of one mother-infant pair. Observations over four successive weeks permitted assessment of reliability of the measures, and the very high reliability, along with the general finding of stability over weeks, permits the conclusion that these measures could be averaged over weeks to provide a reliable description of individual infants or mother-infant pairs. It was with the use of such data that we described the mother and infant of special interest for this report.

The use of profiles constitutes a non-linear approach to assessing a developing infant. A look at the profiles taken as a whole makes it clear that no single variable nor even the long list of variables considered separately could provide a meaningful portrait of this mother and infant pair.

As the picture of the subject described in this report indicates, deviance on any single measure is not necessarily "all bad." In fact, the unusual behaviors of the baby in this study were possibly counteracted by unusual behaviors on the part of the mother, namely the very great amount of attention and gentle affectionate stimulation she gave the baby. This interpretation is supported by follow-up assessment and observations. At one year the baby's mental developmental quotient, assessed by the Bayley Scales, was 112. Even more relevant is evidence for his social-emotional development. During three weekly home observations at one year, this baby cried less than any other in the group of 10 observed at that age. Although the mother and baby interacted at about the same overall level as the other mother-baby pairs, their interaction clearly reflected an adaptation to the baby's early avoidance response to body contact. Their actual body-to-body contact was extremely low; physical contact consisted primarily of the baby's body being in contact with the mother's legs on occasions that the baby approached her. Other forms of interaction replaced intimate physical contact of this pair, including looking, talking, and touching. While the mother did not differ from the total group in the percent of time she was available for interaction with the baby, the baby was very low with respect to crying as an attention-seeking behavior when no interaction was ongoing. In numerous ways, the mother seemed to be allowing the baby to pace the interaction. Thus, all indications from our observations suggest the development of a highly adequate and synchronous relationship, one that should continue to be facilitative of the baby's development.

The data bank accumulated from the observations of the twenty subjects through the first year offers the possibility for profiles of each individual pair, using the same variables, or additional ones. In each case, the objective would be to identify the most salient characteristics of the particular relating pair. Commonalities among subgroups of infants with similar profiles should give far greater information on developing infants and mother-infant relationships than analyses derived from summary statistics for the group as a whole.

A current extension of this project is relevant to the present volume, namely, the addition of infants born with risk status. Infants born prematurely or small-for-dates are now being included. These subjects will offer the opportunity to assess differences in the early relating process among mother and infant pairs with a wider range of expected outcomes. Individual analyses of data from each of these infants are of special importance, as their patterns of deviations from the normal group should give clues as to whether there are disruptions in their early developmental course. Neither the mothers nor the babies to be included in our project will have apparent deviances or medically diagnosed handicaps at full-term gestational age. Thus, clues to disruption must come from the intensive observations that are made in the study.

Because of the very intensive nature of the observations for assessment in our project, the procedures are not considered in the category of an assessment "tool," although assessment is a primary objective. We have already identified some patterns that place infants at risk (Thoman, Miano & Freese, 1977; Thoman, 1978) from studies of normal infants, and our expectation is that the inclusion of risk infants in our studies will provide the opportunity to explore a larger number of patterns that may potentially place an infant or a relationship at risk.

In conclusion, we believe that the intensive study of individuality among infants will increase our understanding of development—a process which can only occur in individuals rather than groups, and which reflects the interactive effects of experience and endogenous changes. A focus on developing individuals can potentially provide a common ground for those concerned with "basic research" and those concerned with clinical assessment and intervention. A coalition of these interests, expressed in an emphasis on assessment and prediction for the individual infant, should lead to research providing a greater understanding of normal developmental processes and of developmental dysfunction, as well as information on the complexity of measurement that may be necessary for identifying difficulties along the developmental course.

5

Interactions of High-Risk Infants: Quantitative and Qualitative Differences

TIFFANY MARTINI FIELD
Mailman Center for Child Development

The importance of early social interactions has been highlighted recently by longitudinal studies of high-risk infants suggesting continuities between early interaction patterns and later development (Beckwith et al., 1977; Brown & Bakeman, 1979; Clarke-Stewart, 1973; Field, 1979b; Jones, 1979; Pawlby & Hall, 1979). In addition to suggesting continuity, these studies provide a developing picture of normative and disturbed interaction patterns. This chapter will review some of these patterns.

Generally, the high-risk infants of interaction studies have been designated as lying on one of two, not necessarily separate, continua: reproductive casualty (Pasamanick & Knobloch, 1966) and caretaking casualty (Sameroff & Chandler, 1975). An arbitrary classification, for example, places premature and Down's syndrome infants along the former continuum and infants of lower-class or teenage mothers along the latter.

Although increasing numbers of investigators are studying the peer interactions of these infants (Field, Goldberg, Stern & Sostek, 1980), this chapter will focus on infant-adult (usually infant-mother) interactions. The specific interactions reviewed are those of mother-infant feeding and face-to-face play during the first several months of life. The rationale for this seemingly narrow focus is that the earliest social interactions have typically been observed in the context of feeding and face-to-face play, most usually with the mother as social partner. The time span selected relates to the observation that face-to-face interactions peak around three months and at around five to six months infants become more "turned-on" to interactions with objects (Cohen & Beckwith, 1976; Piaget, 1953; Trevarthen, 1975) and thus are more difficult to engage in face-to-face play.

In all of the studies to be reviewed, behavioral measures were recorded on film or videotape for both infant and parent, and occasionally psychophysiological measures such as heart rate were simultaneously recorded. In some of the studies only contemporaneous developmental measures were reported, while in others follow-up data enabled an assessment of continuities between early interaction patterns and later development.

Since the data converge to suggest some consistent patterns, we are taking the liberty to generalize about normal and disturbed or optimal and nonoptimal interactions. One generalization that can be made from the data is that the interactions of high-risk infant-mother dyads are quantitatively and qualitatively different.

QUANTITATIVE DIFFERENCES IN INTERACTIONS OF HIGH-RISK INFANTS

Quantitatively speaking, high-risk infants from either the reproductive or caretaking casualty continuum tend to be unresponsive or hypoactive. At the same time, their mothers tend to be hypoactive or hyperactive. In the case of interactions with reproductive casualty continuum infants, the mothers tend to be hyperactive, while in the case of interactions with caretaking casualty continuum infants, they tend to be hypoactive. Thus, in the context of our previous examples, the mothers of premature and Down's syndrome infants are typically hyperactive during interactions (Brown & Bakeman, 1979; Field, 1977a, 1977b, 1978c; Goldberg, Brachfeld & DiVitto, 1979; Jones, 1980), while mothers from lower socioeconomic status groups tend to be hypoactive (Field, 1980; Kilbride, Johnson & Streissguth, 1977; Sandler & Vietze, 1979).

A model which can be borrowed from the arousal level, information processing or performance literatures to characterize this quantitative difference is that of an inverted U function. Maternal hypoactivity and hyperactivity are at the extreme ends of the inverted U function with infant behaviors or the optimality of interaction varying on the Y axis as a function of the amount of maternal activity.

The Inverted U of Early Interactions

There is a long history of mapping performance on an inverted U-shaped function. The independent variables, depending on the theory, include drive, anxiety, or arousal level (Fiske & Maddi, 1961; Spielberger, 1966). The theory predicts that, at high levels of drive, anxiety or arousal, a subject's performance becomes disrupted due to over-responding, often to irrelevant cues. At low levels, a low rate of behavior occurs and hence a low level of appropriate responding.

More recently, a number of authors have described a discrepancy hypothesis in terms of an inverted U function (Kagan, 1971; Schaffer, 1974). The discrepancy hypothesis states that an event which activates existing schema but which cannot be assimilated produces a state of arousal. A moderate level of arousal will produce attention, and probably accommodation. The level of arousal predicted under the discrepancy hypothesis is believed to follow an inverted U-shaped function, with low discrepancy producing rapid assimilation, moderate discrepancy resulting in probable accommodation, and very discrepant events producing either little attention and/or negative affect.

In adopting this model for early interactions, we are proposing that minimal or excessive maternal activity (hypoactivity or hyperactivity) contributes to nonoptimal interaction, probably as a function of its effects on infant arousal levels. Maternal behaviors commonly reported as frequencies, durations or proportions of interaction time, including talking, smiling, exaggerated facial expressions, head nodding, tapping, poking, caretaking and game-playing, can be plotted on the X axis. The frequently reported infant behaviors, including looking, vocalizing, smiling, cycling, squirming and fussing, can be plotted on the Y axis. Typically, the quantity of positive infant behavior varies from high to low as the quantity of maternal behavior varies from moderate to the extremes of high or low. This relationship can be described as an inverted U function, plotting optimality of interaction or, more specifically, plotting commonly recorded infant behaviors such as gaze activity or type of vocalization on the Y axis. An illustration of this relationship appears in Figure 1.

Behavioral Data to Support an Inverted U of Early Interactions

Reproductive casualty continuum infants and hyperactive mothers. In terms of activity levels, the interactions of reproductive casualty continuum infants and their mothers are frequently characterized by hypoactivity or hyporesponsivity of the infant and hyperactivity of the mother. These dyads are often described as the infant being less active and responsive, and the mother exerting more effort or appearing to try harder to engage her infant.

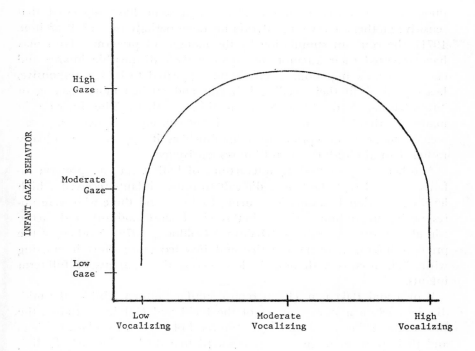

FIGURE 1. The relationship between amount of maternal vocalization and amount of infant gaze.

The reproductive risk group whose interactions have been most commonly studied is the preterm infant with or without perinatal complications (Brown & Bakeman, 1979; Beckwith et al., 1976; DiVitto & Goldberg, 1979; Field, 1977a, 1977b, 1979b; Goldberg, Brachfeld & DiVitto, 1979). Comparisons between term and preterm infants suggest that the preterm infant-mother dyad experiences more difficulty interacting.

For example, a recent study on early feedings of preterm and term infants revealed that the preterm infants were more distractible during feeding and their mothers less sensitive to infant feeding behaviors and rhythms (Field, 1977b). The mothers of preterm infants, unlike those of term infants, stimulated their infants continuously, failing to reserve their stimulation for the nonsucking periods when the infant was otherwise unoccupied and free to interact. Although some have suggested that sensitive mothers reserve stimulation for these periods (Kaye & Brazelton, 1971), the constant stimulation by the mothers of preterm infants may have reflected their attempts to organize their distractible infants and encourage milk ingestion. Their infants appeared to be less responsive, less organized in their feeding behavior and elicited more coaxing or "stimulation-to-feed" behavior from their mothers. The increase in maternal stimulation in response to infant unresponsiveness, however, seemed to be counterproductive, inasmuch as it appeared to enhance rather than diminish the infants' unresponsiveness.

Another study of feeding interactions of both term and preterm infants reported that the "more difficult to rouse" infants received a high level of functional stimulation during feedings, and those who were unresponsive to auditory stimulation received more auditory and tactile stimulation during feedings (DiVitto & Goldberg, 1979). Mothers of the preterm infants were more active and invested more effort interacting with their infants with notably less success than parents of full-term infants.

Brown and Bakeman (1979) report similar findings. Unlike the middle-class, white mother samples of the Field and Goldberg studies, the Brown and Bakeman sample was comprised of lower-class, black mothers and their preterm infants. They reported that during the early feeding interactions preterm infants (versus term infants) were less active and were viewed as less responsive. Mothers of the preterm infants were more active generally and, in particular, were more persistent and were more likely to initiate and continue behavioral episodes than mothers of full-term babies. They exerted more effort, and their interactions were more stereotyped or less varied. Thus, the burden of maintaining the interactions fell disproportionately on the mothers of the preterm infants (Brown & Bakeman, 1979).

Not unlike the feeding interactions, the face-to-face interactions of preterm infants during the first few months of life have also been characterized by hypoactive, hyporesponsive infants and hyperactive mothers (Field, 1977a, 1979b). In our studies of face-to-face interactions, the preterm infants were less responsive and showed more aversive behaviors (gaze aversion, squirming and fussing) and their mothers were more stimulating in all modes (visual, tactile, auditory and vestibular) during both the infant's eye contact and gaze aversion periods. Similarly, the mothers of postterm infants, who also gaze averted, squirmed and fussed, were typically hyperactive or overstimulating. A follow-up of these infants at two years (Field, 1979b) suggested that the mothers who were overactive during early face-to-face interactions were overprotective and overcontrolling during later interactions with their infants. The infants who were visually inattentive during the early interactions were verbally unresponsive and showed language delays during the two-year interactions.

Floor play interactions of eight-month-old and one-year-old preterm infants and their parents studied by Goldberg et al. (1979) featured less playing and smiling and more fretting by the infants. The parents of the preterm infants spent more time being close to, touching and demonstrating toys than parents of term infants.

The picture that emerges from these analyses of different types of interactions (feeding, face-to-face and floor play) at different stages during the first two years of life among preterm infants and their parents is a vicious cycle of the infant being relatively inactive and unresponsive, the parent trying to engage the infant by being more and more active or stimulating, which in turn leads to more inactivity and unresponsivity on the part of the infant. Although the parent's activity appears to be directed at encouraging more activity or responsivity of the infant, that strategy is counterproductive inasmuch as it leads to less instead of more infant responsivity.

Other groups for which similar phenomena have been observed include the Down's syndrome infant and the child with cerebral palsy. Analyses of interactions between Down's syndrome infants and their mothers suggest that the infants engaged in less eye contact and initiated fewer interactions (Jones, 1980). Their mothers were simultaneously noted to be more active and directive during these play interactions. Similarly, cerebral palsied children have been noted to exhibit fewer interactive behaviors, and their mothers are more active and controlling during interactions (Kogan, 1979).

The above authors have speculated about the frequently observed hyperactivity of the mothers of unresponsive infants labeled "at risk" due to perinatal complications and/or handicapping conditions. The most vague interpretation suggests that the frustration of receiving minimal responses from the infant leads to a kind of aggressivity on the part of the mother. Another notion is that the mothers are more active to compensate for the relative inactivity of their infants, perhaps "to keep some semblance of an interaction going." A third relates to the mother's wanting her child to perform like his agemates, and attempting to encourage performance by more frequent modeling of behaviors. Still another interpretation is that the mothers view their infants as fragile and delayed and as a result tend to be overprotective. Overprotectiveness in the extreme is construed as overcontrolling behavior. Although direction of effects or causality cannot be derived from these studies of interactions, the data have evoked considerable concern since the behaviors of these dyads appear to persist over the early years of the child's life.

Caretaking casualty infants and hypoactive mothers. Infants who have been designated as being at risk for "caretaking casualty" include those born to adolescent mothers, lesser educated and lower-class mothers. In addition, some have viewed multiple birth infants (e.g., twins) and later born infants as having potential interaction problems related to their caretaking situations. Frequently, these infants, not unlike the "reproductive casualty" infants, are unresponsive, although their mothers, unlike the mothers of the "reproductive casualty" infants, are typically hypoactive or hyporesponsive.

A study comparing the interactions of white, middle-class and black, lower-class adult and teenage mothers and their infants revealed a very low level of activity on the part of the teenage mothers (Fields, 1980). They were less active, less verbal, less contingently responsive and played "infant" games less frequently. This was observed for both white, middle-class teenage mothers whose infants at birth received optimal Brazelton interactive process scores and for black, lower-class teenage mothers whose infants were more developed motorically (based on the Brazelton at birth and the Denver at three months). Thus, without respect to their infants' initial social responsivity and initial (as well as contemporaneous) motor development, the teenage mothers were relatively inactive. Although the infants were not "difficult" neonates, as was the case for the preterm infants, they engaged in less eye contact and emitted fewer contented vocalizations when they were three months old. Since our analyses yielded rates at the opposite extreme of those of the preterm infant-mother samples, we revised our interaction rating scales to incorporate the hypoactivity, hyporesponsibility features of these mothers. (See Field, 1980 for interaction rating scale.)

Another study of lower-class, black teenage mothers and their neonates suggested that during neonatal-mother feeding interactions maternal age was not a contributing factor except for a tendency of the teenage mothers to be less verbal during their interactions (Sandler & Vietze, 1979).

Class comparisons of early interactions have frequently revealed that both lower-class infants and their mothers are less active, particularly verbally, than their middle-class counterparts. As early as the first month of life, lower SES infants received significantly less verbal stimulation from their mothers in both a lulling and chatting fashion, and their mothers cared for them without talking to them (Kilbride, Johnson & Streissguth, 1977).

Similarly, studies of older infants reveal less activity among lower-class mothers and infants than among middle-class dyads. Lewis and Wilson (1972) reported less smiling and vocalizing among the lower-class infants. No differences were reported for the frequency of mother vocalizations, although those of the middle-class mothers were more contingent. In addition, Field (1980) reported less activity, verbal interaction, contingent responsivity and less frequent playing of infant games among lower-class, black mothers than among white, middle-class mothers.

A cross-cultural study comparing British working- and middle-class mothers with American lower- and middle-class mothers suggested that both in England and the U.S. the lower-class mothers engaged in less verbal and imitative behavior and less game-playing during early face-to-face interactions (Field & Pawlby, 1980). Their infants were simultaneously less verbal, smiled less frequently, and engaged in less eye contact. Interactions of slightly older infants (10-month-old infants) and their lower-class mothers also featured less verbal activity and fewer reciprocal vocalizations (Bee, VanEgeren, Streissguth, Nyman & Lockie, 1969; Tulkin & Kagan, 1972).

Similarly, less educated mothers are reported to talk less frequently, use less positive language, respond with less contingent vocalizations and give less specific communications when engaging in face-to-face talk with both their one- and eight-month-old infants (Cohen & Beckwith, 1976).

Two other groups reported to receive either less eye contact or less verbal stimulation include multiple birth infants (twins) and higher birth order infants. A few investigators have reported differential behavior on the part of mothers and their twins. Stern (1971), for example, reported less maternal eye contact with one twin who later exhibited behavioral problems. Kubicek (1979) also reported less eye contact between one twin and his mother. In this case, the twin experiencing less eye contact was later diagnosed as autistic. A study of monozygotic twins and their mothers by our group suggests that the mother is typically less active with the second born twin (Field, 1978b). However, in the case of prematurely born twins or twins discordant in birthweight, the mother was typically overactive with the twin who had the lowest birthweight or who experienced the most perinatal complications.

Birth order effects typically favor the first born. Kilbride et al. (1977), for example, reported that later born infants received significantly less frequent and sustained interactions during the neonatal period with respect to looking, verbal, tactile, caretaking and play behaviors. Jacobs and Moss (1976) also found comparable birth order differences in maternal interactions with three-month-old infants.

The dynamics contributing to lesser maternal activity and stimulation in these groups are unclear. In some of the studies neonatal assessments as well as developmental assessment made at the same time as the interaction assessments of these infants (e.g. Field, 1980) revealed no particular lags in development or interactive deficits which might contribute to the lesser responsivity of their mothers. The mother's condition itself, e.g., a depressed socioeconomic status or multiple infants/children to care for, may leave the mother with less time and energy for interaction. A similarly simple explanation for the lesser activity of teenage and less educated mothers may be a limited repertoire due to lesser experience or exposure to the infants, the literature on infancy and appropriate infant stimulation.

Whatever the cause, the low levels of stimulation are disconcerting given the reports that mothers of infants/children who were later diagnosed as schizophrenic or autistic engaged in less eye contact during early interactions (Massie, 1978) and that mothers of abused infants engaged in less verbal and physical interactions with their infants (Dietrich & Starr, 1979).

Manipulated Interactions and an Inverted U

Although mother and infant activity is a simultaneous, reciprocal phenomenon, rendering any statement about direction of effects mere speculation, interventions have focused on the easiest-to-teach partner, the mother. Experimental manipulations illustrate that interactions can be varied by altering the mother's activity level.

One manipulation which alters maternal activity involves changing the mother's visual stimulus (Trevarthen, 1975). Mothers began interacting with their infants, but suddenly were face-to-face with an adult appearing in a one-way mirror. The mothers altered the rate and pacing of their vocalizations from the typically slow pace reserved for infants to more adult-paced verbal activity. This manipulation resulted in infant gaze aversion. Asking the mother to remain stonefaced in another manipulation invariably resulted first in active attempts by the infant to engage the mother, followed by waning interest and ultimate gaze aversion (Tronick et al., 1978).

A manipulation which had an opposite effect, namely that it increased infant gaze, involved asking the mother to "count slowly" while interacting (Tronick et al., 1978). This instruction effectively slowed down and diminished the activity of the mothers and enhanced infant attentiveness.

A series of manipulations has been tried in our lab (Field, 1977a; 1979b). The manipulations were generally effective at modifying both the amount of the mother's activity and the infant's attentiveness and vocalization. An attention-getting manipulation, asking the mother to keep her infant's attention, dramatically increased the amount of her activity and decreased the amout of her infant's gaze and contented vocalizations. Conversely, asking the mother to imitate her infant's behavior effectively diminished maternal activity and elicited more infant gaze. An order effect, when using these two manipulations during the same session, suggested that mothers who were given the imitation instruction first learned that it was an effective attention-getting device and used it during the attention-getting situation. Thus, the manipulations revealed an inverse relationship between maternal activity and infant attentiveness or gaze.

Other manipulations, including the mother's repetition of her phrases and the mother's silencing during her infant's gaze aversion, also resulted in decreased maternal activity and increased infant attentiveness (Field, 1978c). Similarly, during a feeding manipulation in which the mother was asked to remain silent during her infant's sucking periods, the infant also spent more time looking at her. These manipulations, however, were only effective in those dyads whose spontaneous interactions featured considerable maternal activity and infant inattentiveness, e.g., those of preterm infants and their mothers.

In the case of hypoactive mothers, we have manipulated the activity level of the mother by simply giving her a nursery rhyme song to sing or teaching her a wordy version of some popular infant game such as "tell me a story," "I'm gonna get you," "So big," "itsy bitsy spider," "peek-a-boo," or "pat-a-cake." Typically these mothers' verbal, tactile and facial activity increases with these songs or games, and the infants' attentiveness and contented vocalizations correspondingly increase (Field, 1979a).

The most observable, measurable effect of these manipulations is the variation in frequency of maternal and infant behaviors. An attention-getting instruction invariably elicits very high activity levels in the

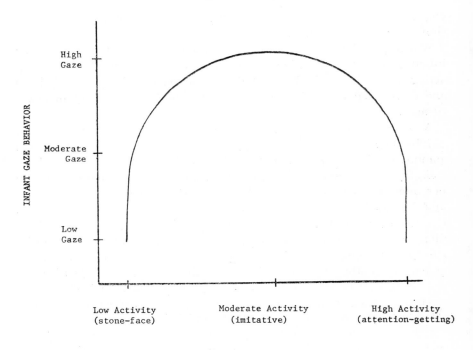

Manipulations of Maternal Activity

FIGURE 2. The relationship between manipulations of maternal activity and infant gaze.

mother and very low activity and attentiveness or nonoptimal activity such as gaze averting or fussing in the infant. The extreme of that, the stone-faced, inactive mother, also elicits inattentiveness in the infant. If the mother's activity level tends to be high, an imitative instruction seems to lower her activity to a moderate level; if her activity level is low, giving her an infant game to play or song to sing facilitates a more moderate level of activity. In both cases, the infant engages in a greater amount of eye contact and contented vocalizations. These manipulations of maternal activity and their effects on infant activity can be superimposed on an inverted U curve, as in Figure 2.

Psychophysiological Data to Support an Inverted U
of Early Interactions

In the context of the arousal or activation model (Fiske & Maddi, 1961; Hebb, 1949), high or low levels of stimulation are considered to be arousing. High arousal levels in either an over or under arousing situation are thought to be experienced as aversive. In an aversive situation we might expect to find elevated heart rate (Graham & Clifton, 1966).

In mother-infant interactions characterized by high activity level of the mother and low activity-low attentiveness of the infant, the arousal model would predict elevated heart rate or at least elevated heart rate as compared to heart rate characterizing more modulated interactions. To assess the physiological effects of the previously described manipulations, we simultaneously monitored heart rate activity. Since there are no discrete stimulus presentations and since stimulus behaviors occur with such rapidity during interactions such that heart rate does not have sufficient time to return to baseline for a stimulus-locked analysis of heart rate, we used tonic heart rate or heart rate averaged across the interaction as compared to baseline heart rate.

The stone-faced manipulation of Tronick et al. (1978) and our attention-getting and imitative manipulations were used. Tonic heart rate of both the mother and infant paralleled their behaviors. In the less active mother/more attentive infant imitation interaction situations, heart rate was slightly below baseline for mothers and infants. And in the high activity/attention-getting and no-activity/stone-faced situations, heart rate was significantly elevated for both mothers and infants (Field, 1978a).

Certainly the mothers' greater attentiveness during imitation (in order to observe the infants' behaviors to be imitated) and the infants' greater attentiveness in this situation may have contributed to more frequent decelerations, a heart rate parallel of attention (Graham & Clifton, 1966). Conversely, the high activity level during attention-getting and the physical or emotional strain of remaining stone-faced in the no-activity situation may have contributed to heart rate accelerations of the mother. Similarly, the infant's head aversion, squirming and fussing during those situations would elevate infant heart rate as a function of physical movement. Alternatively, or at the same time, the mother's overstimulation may have been aversive for the infant, and the infant's gaze aversion, squirming and fussing may have been aversive for the mother. While videotapes of smiling infants have been shown to trigger only negligible

changes in autonomic arousal of mothers, gaze averting, fussy infants are
perceived as aversive and elicit elevated heart rate, diastolic blood pressure and skin conductance increases in mothers (Frodi, Lamb, Leavitt
& Donovan, 1978). These increases were especially apparent when the
infant being viewed was described as "premature." Whether the heart
rate elevations during our manipulations were a function of increased
activity level or increased arousal associated with the mutual aversiveness
of mother overstimulation and infant inattentiveness, they are suggestive
of increased arousal in both mother and infant. In this way, the heart
rate levels appear to conform to the U curve depicted in Figure 3.

A comparison of preterm and term infant-mother dyads experiencing
these manipulations revealed not only greater activity on the part of the
mothers of preterm infants and lesser attentiveness on the part of the

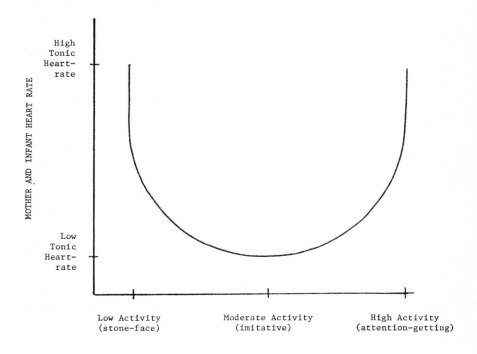

Manipulations of Maternal Activity

FIGURE 3. The relationship between manipulations of maternal activity and infant-
mother tonic heart rate.

preterm infants, but also characteristically higher heart rate levels of both preterm infants and their mothers, despite equivalent baseline levels of the term and preterm dyads (Field, 1979b).

Thus, quantitative differences can be seen in both the behavioral and physiological activity of the high-risk infant-mother dyads during early interactions. A number of arousal theorists such as Hebb (1949) have emphasized the quantitative aspects of stimulation as being more important than the qualitative aspects. An inverted U function model based on quantity of behavior or heart rate levels is perhaps parsimonious for our purposes, but also simplistic in light of the qualitative differences also observed in the early interactions of high-risk infant-mother dyads.

QUALITATIVE DIFFERENCES IN INTERACTIONS OF HIGH-RISK INFANTS

Qualitative differences in early interactions appear in the organization of interaction, interpretation of interaction signals and development of conversation rules. A number of investigators have elaborated on these features of interactions between adults (Chapple, 1970; Duncan, 1972; Jaffe & Feldstein, 1970; Kendon, 1967) and between adults and infants (Brazelton, Koslowski & Main, 1974; Stern, 1974b; Tronick et al., 1978; Tronick, Chapter 6, this volume).

In the adult interaction literature, Jaffe and his colleagues have elaborated on the rhythmicity of dialogues between adults (Jaffe & Feldstein, 1970). Kendon (1967) and Duncan (1972) have analyzed conversations by listener-speaker roles and the signals that announce switching of roles. Chapple (1970) has focused on initiation-dominance patterns in interaction, and via experimental transients or disturbances has illustrated how interaction asynchrony may occur either by latency of responses or by interruptive actions.

In the infant literature, Brazelton et al. (1974) have outlined phases of interaction between infant and mother including: (1) initiation, (2) orientation, (3) state of attention, (4) acceleration, (5) peak of excitement, (6) deceleration, and (7) withdrawal or turning away. The mothers' roles to facilitate these interaction phases include: (1) reduction of interfering activity, (2) setting the stage, (3) creating an expectancy of interaction, (4) intensifying her infant's attention, and (5) allowing for reciprocity.

Tronick et al. (1978) more recently have described similar phases of interaction including: (1) initiation, (2) mutual orientation, (3) greeting, (4) play dialogue, and (5) disengagement, and in this volume he describes three behavioral states (engaged, monitor and disengaged) and three joint interactive states (match, conjoint and disjoint). Brazelton et al. (1974) and Tronick et al. (1978) have then plotted synchronous and asynchronous interactions and their variations during these phases and states of interaction.

From these elaborations and from those of the adult literature we can extrapolate some conversation rules which are basically similar for both adult-adult and adult-infant interactions. The ways in which they differ appear to relate to the limitations imposed by the infant's less mature arousal regulation and information processing abilities and less developed behavior repertoire. These limitations, deriving from the infant's lesser maturity and experience with interaction, place a disproportionate burden of monitoring and sustaining the interaction on the adult interaction partner. These unusual demands placed on the adult have been variously described as the infant's unreadable signals, unpredictable and unresponsive behaviors (Goldberg, 1977). A similar elaboration suggests that the challenges posed by the infant during early interactions relate to his (1) disorganized rhythms, (2) undeveloped response repertoire and (3) non-contingent responses (Field, 1978c). Thus, there are important modifications of an interaction rule system posed by the immaturity of the infant.

Phases and Rules of Interactions: Modifications and Violations

For the purposes of simplicity we have labeled three phases of interaction: (1) initiation; (2) involvement and (3) termination. Within these phases a number of rules appear to be established and followed including: (1) speaking the same language; (2) relating to the same subject or playing the same game; (3) taking turns; (4) monitoring the partner's interaction rhythms and signals; (5) emitting readable signals, and (6) contingently responding.

There seem to be a number of ways in which these interaction rules are modified and sometimes violated during infant-adult interactions:

Initiations. Initiations are less evenly distributed between the partners of an infant-adult interaction than an adult-adult interaction; namely, they are more frequently made by the adult than the infant. Because of the infant's unstable state organization, the adult partner tends to assess the infant's readiness to interact prior to initiations. Then, realizing that the response latency of an infant is longer than that of an adult, the adult will often wait longer for an infant to respond to his initiations. When initiations are made by the infant, they are often made in the visual system (as opposed to the more common verbal or gestural initiations made by adults in interactions together). A simple turning toward or looking at the mother is often interpreted as an initiation or at least a readiness to interact.

In addition to less frequent initiations by the infant, failures to respond to initiations commonly occur. These are signaled by the infant's failure to look at the mother when she speaks. Not having the adult's motoric ability to turn or walk away from an initiation, the infant has only his gaze, head turning or fussiness to signal his rejection of an initiation.

The stress of receiving too few or too many initiations has been documented during manipulated adult-adult interactions by Chapple (1970). In one experimental manipulation, the experimenter remained silent, which was increasingly stressful for the subject, who continued to make initiations without a response from the experimenter. In another manipulation, the experimenter continued to make initiations to the subject without letting the subject get a word in edgewise, an equally stressful situation for the adult subject.

This phenomenon is frequently observed in interactions between hypoactive, hyporesponsive, high-risk infants (such as the preterm) and hyperactive mothers. The mother persists in initiating when her infant is not responding to her initiations. The stress apparently felt by the infant receiving continuous initiations is manifested by excessive gaze aversion and fussiness. Tronick's stone-faced manipulation is an example of the situation in reverse, the mother being unresponsive and the infant making continuous initiations.

The infant first makes a series of overtures to the stone-faced mother and then finally averts gaze and turns to other activity. An experiment in nature is the hypoactive, depressed-looking mother who rarely initiates. The infant, himself, then rarely initiates, and the net effect is a failure to go beyond the initiation stage of an interaction (Field, 1978c).

Speaking the same language. Speaking the same language in infant-adult interactions has been affectionately referred to as talking "baby talk" (Ferguson, 1964). Several have noted the speech modifications of mothers as they shift from talking to an adult versus an infant. Trevarthen's (1975) manipulation nicely demonstrated that a mother while talking to her infant, if suddenly faced with an adult, will alter the pacing of her verbalizations from an "infantized" to an adult pace. Stern (1974b) has elaborated on a number of language features which characterize adult speech to infants or "infantized" behavior. These include exaggerated facial expressions, prolonged vowel sounds and higher pitched vocalizations. Other behaviors unique to the adult-infant interaction are adult limitations of infant behaviors (Field, 1977a; Pawlby, 1977). These have been interpreted as attempts by the adult to approximate behaviors which can be readily assimilated by the infant inasmuch as they are already in the repertoire of the infant (Field, 1978c; Pawlby, 1977; Piaget, 1953).

When adults are engaged in an attention-getting interaction with their infants, their typical "infantized" behaviors often disappear. Thus, for example, the mother of the unresponsive preterm infant is frequently so preoccuppied with getting her infant to attend or respond that her "infantized" behaviors drop out of her repertoire. Similarly, her imitative behaviors are less often observed, perhaps because her infant emits fewer behaviors for her to imitate. Infantized and imitative behaviors are also less frequently observed in the depressed-appearing, lower-class mother (Field & Pawlby, 1980). Infantized, imitative behaviors may derive from a spirit of fun and from being sufficiently involved with the infant to lose awareness of an interaction observer who might be seen as intimidating by the lower-class mother. When the observer expressly invites the mother to imitate her infant, however, the imitation appears to expand the mother's seemingly limited repertoire and to elicit more attention from the infant.

Relating to the same subject or playing the same game. Relating to the same subject or, in infant parlance, playing the same game, is considered an important rule for infant interactions. Since the infant's behavioral and game repertoire is limited and varies with developmental age, age-appropriate adjustments are accordingly made by the mother (Field, 1979a; Gustafson & Green, 1978; Sroufe & Wunsch, 1972). For example, as infants become more mature, games shift from those employing primarily tactile stimulation to those employing verbal behavior (Sroufe & Wunsch, 1972) and also shift from those in which the infant assumes a passive role to those in which the infant assumes an active role (Crawley, Rogers, Friedman, Jacobson, Criticos, Richardson & Thompson, 1978; Gustafson & Green, 1978).

In our culture, there are several infant games which appear to be universally popular. Variations of these are observed in England (Field & Pawlby, 1980). However, in that country the singing of nursery rhymes seems more popular than the infant games observed in the U.S.

One very popular game is "tell me a story." The mother invites her infant to tell a story. The infant coos and the mother treats that as a piece of information and responds by saying, "Oh, is that right and then what happened?" as if they were relating to the same subject. Similarly, the infant's smiles and laughter are treated by the mother as engagement in the same game when she plays "itsy-bitsy spider," "crawling fingers," "so big," "I'm gonna get you," "peek-a-boo" and "pat-a-cake." All of these games are highly repetitive with simple and stereotyped roles for both parent (fathers and mothers) and infant. They typically are interspersed throughout the parent-infant interaction and in duration appear to approximate the infant's attention span. As the infant appears to habituate to one game, the parent sensitively introduces a variation on that game or shifts to another (Field, 1979a).

Another form of relating to the same subject is the mother's verbal "highlighting" and expanding on the infant's behaviors (Jones & Pawlby, 1975). For example, mothers frequently comment and elaborate on whatever the baby is doing such as "Yuk, you spit up. You're so funny. Whenever you get happy, you spit up, all the time."

Relating to the same subject or playing the same game appears to be problematic for some groups of high-risk infant-mother dyads. The mother of the preterm infant, for example, frequently introduces developmental age-inappropriate games such as "peek-a-boo" to an infant who is eight-weeks post expected date of delivery (Field, 1979c). Given mothers' reports that they tend to think in terms of their infants' chronological age rather than developmental age, this finding is not surprising. The problem for the lower-class, lesser educated or teenage mother is that her game repertoire is more limited (Field, 1979a; Field & Pawlby, 1980). In addition, the games they play lack the rich verbal content which typically accompanies infant games. When given directions and some lyrics for a game, however, these mothers manage to become more active with infants and in turn elicit more eye contact.

Some consider that infant game-playing during face-to-face interactions facilitates the infant's understanding of the structure of interactions and development of turntaking (Field, 1979a; Gustafson & Green, 1978).

Turntaking. A number of infant interaction researchers consider that turntaking is one of the most important conversation rules to be learned by the mother (Brazelton et al., 1974; Field; 1978c). Turntaking poses subtle difficulties for the mother due to the relatively infrequent initiations of the infant to "take a turn" and the relatively latent responses of the infant to the mother's offering of turns. Both failures to initiate and latency of responses have been observed as interaction stresses in the adult literature (Chapple, 1970). Since the infant frequently does not clearly signal an intent to take a turn, the mother is often observed taking her baby's turn as well as her own. To avoid stealing all turns the mother frequently has to actively elicit the infant's initiation of turns and modify her expectancy about response latencies. The structure of infant games facilitates this process.

Using again the examples in the extreme, the hyperactive mother of the preterm infant and the hypoactive lower-class mother, the former mother often doesn't let her infant get a word in edgewise. The preterm infant's rare and latent responses perhaps contribute to a mental set that the infant is not going to respond, so the mother responds for him, taking turns for both herself and her infant. Long silences, failures to elicit responses and abortive conversations have frequently been reported to us as frustrations felt by these mothers. In contrast, the lower-class mother in the face-to-face situation rarely initiates turntaking sequences except when invited by the observer to play infant games. The infant in this example also does not have the opportunity to learn the turntaking rules of conversation. Failure to initiate turns or stealing the infant's turns in either case is a kind of control or domination of the conversation and robs the infant of the opportunity to learn the turntaking rules of conversation.

Monitoring signals. Monitoring the infant's interaction rhythms and signals so as to modulate the pacing, form, and intensity of stimulation is perhaps the sine qua non of the mother's role in interactions. This is a characteristically different role for infant-adult than adult-adult dyads. While the adult listener almost invariably monitors the behavior of the adult speaker (Kendon, 1967), the roles are reversed in infant-adult interactions. In infant-adult interactions the adult who is usually the speaker is constantly monitoring the infant (Field, 1978c; Stern, 1974) while the infant who is typically the listener is alternately looking toward and away from the speaker. Thus the onus of monitoring signals is on the mother.

Since the signal repertoire of the infant is most developed visually, gaze and gaze aversion of the infant provide the principal cues rather than verbal and gestural cues which prevail in the adult signalling system. Most typically a turn toward the mother or eye contact made by the infant is interpreted and responded to as a readiness to interact signal. The significance of the infant's gaze aversion is subject to interpretation. Although some have attributed the infant's turning away to an habituation phenomenon and describe it as a signal to the mother to introduce a new game or conversation, others have suggested that turning away serves as a time-out or pause from the conversation so that the infant may process the information or modulate arousal experienced in the previous looking period (Brazelton et al., 1974; Field, 1979c). We have made the latter interpretation since heart rate acceleration accompanies the looking away behavior. If the infants were seeking out additional or different stimulation, we might expect to find heart rate deceleration (a component of orienting) instead of acceleration, typically associated with an aversive arousing situation. Certainly the infant's excessive gaze aversion is aversive for the mother, as evidenced by her report, her behaviors and her elevated tonic heart rate (Field, 1979b).

Just as the very active mother of the preterm infant rarely lets her infant get a word in edgewise, she also rarely lets her infant get a break in edgewise to process information, modulate arousal, attend to something else or just take a break from the conversation. During feeding interactions, mothers of these infants do not tend to reserve their stimulation for the breaks in sucking activity when the infant is otherwise unoccupied (Field, 1977b). During face-to-face interactions they are rarely silent during the infant's looking away periods. Often interpreting the infant's gaze aversion as rejection, they accelerate their activity or move their faces to the infants' new angle of gaze to retrieve their attention. Continual "face thrusting" in response to gaze aversion frequently leads to squirming and fussing in the infant, signals which typically emit soothing and low keyed behaviors in the mother, but in more disturbed interactions lead to accelerated activity on the part of the mother.

In contrast, the hypoactive mother frequently does not pick up on the infant's gaze signal or does not interpret it as a readiness to interact; thus the interaction, rather than being interrupted or terminated, as in the previous case, never gets started.

The more positive signals of the infant (cooing, smiling and laughing) are also subtle nuances which must be closely monitored. Accelerated activity on the part of the mother during laughter of the infant is sometimes observed to heighten the infant's arousal level such that laughing quickly turns to crying. Close monitoring of these signals is considered critical to contingent responsivity.

Contingent responsivity. Contingent responses are those which occur within a given time of the stimulus behavior and/or are similar in kind (modality or form) to the stimulus behavior, suggesting that they are direct responses to the partner's behavior. A number of interaction researchers have suggested that responsivity must be contingent so that the partner to the interaction can feel that he has some influence on the interaction (Lewis & Goldberg, 1969; Watson, 1967). If the mother's response is appropriate and occurs within a few seconds of her infant's behavior, it is more likely to be perceived by the infant as a direct response to his own behavior. Many of the previously mentioned responses which are sensitively timed by the mother such as a smile to a coo or ceasing activity when the infant resumes sucking or looks away can be seen as contingent responses to the infant's signals. Most frequently, infant behaviors such as smiling and vocalizing are followed by similar behaviors on the part of the adult (Gewirtz & Gewirtz, 1969; Lewis & Wilson, 1972). Other ways in which mothers contingently respond are by highlighting and imitating their infants' behaviors, imitations being very effective contingent responses inasmuch as they are both similar to the stimulus behavior and typically occur with extremely short latency. Infant behaviors such as smiling, cooing and sustained eye contact are viewed by the mother as contingent responses to her behaviors and encourage more of the same game when the infant responds in such a way.

Contingent responsivity has been viewed as one of the three Rs of infant-adult social interactions since it appears to be a critical component for sustaining interactions (Field, 1978c). The importance of this interaction rule is dramatized by disturbed interactions. The hyperactive mother often fails to contingently respond in her pacing of behaviors, for example, by failing to slow down and modulate her activity as her infant becomes fussy or failing to cease her activity when her infant turns away or resumes sucking. Perhaps the frequency with which she fails to elicit a response leads her to expect fewer responses and to thus override them with her own activity when they do occur. Being somewhat preoccupied with getting her infant to attend or to feed, many of the other responses of her infant appear to go unnoticed.

In many ways contingent responsivity can only occur when there is close monitoring of interaction signals. Since the infant does not typically monitor his mother's signals closely in the visual mode, he seems to depend on his mother's verbal signals. Although the infant, by virtue of his limited verbal repertoire, may not respond in the same modality (verbally) to his mother's verbal signals, his visual responses (looking toward mother) often follow immediately upon her verbal signals (Field, 1978c). However, the mother may view the infant's visual response to her verbal behavior as a less contingent response and thus derive less satisfaction from the response. Although most mothers of high-risk infants show the necessary prerequisite for contingent responsivity, that of close visual monitoring of the infant's behaviors, many fail to contingently respond.

Termination of interactions. The termination phase, not unlike the initiation phase of interactions, seems to be subtly controlled by the infant. Just as the infant signals a state of readiness for the start of an interaction and a state of involvement during the interaction, he also signals the end of an interaction. The infant's cues for the termination phase are usually less subtle than those of the initiation phase. Although he cannot walk away from an interaction, the infant can just as dramatically announce the end of an interaction by a repertoire of termination signals including yawning, gaze and head aversion, squirming out of the infant seat, fussing or crying.

Less extreme forms of these behaviors often signal pauses or breaks from the interaction, although they are sometimes interpreted by the mother as termination signals. As the infant's schedules (feeding and sleep-wakefulness) become more regular, the very time of day lends saliency to his termination signals. Only the very insensitive mother fails to read these quite obvious signals.

To summarize, then, the qualitative differences between typical and disturbed interactions vis-à-vis phases and rules of conversation appear to be more subtle than the quantitative differences. They are more difficult to measure and analyze than the quantitative behavioral frequencies, proportions and conditional probabilities. But when forced to characterize differences between harmonious and disturbed interactions, it is often subtle qualitative differences that the interaction observer describes. Since the qualitative differences interact with quantitative differences, newer models and measures may be required to advance our understanding of early interaction disturbances.

EVIDENCE FOR CONTINUITIES BETWEEN EARLY INTERACTIONS AND LATER DEVELOPMENT

The importance of understanding early interaction disturbances is highlighted by recent data suggesting continuities between early interactions and later development. In most of the prospective studies of high-risk infants it is too soon to determine whether some of these quantitative interaction differences predict later interaction or developmental differences. However, there are a number of recent studies which suggest that the differences seen in high-risk infant interactions are not confined to the neonatal or early infancy periods.

Follow-up studies of preterm infants, for example, suggest that those who show interaction disturbances early in infancy experience difficulties later in infancy. In one longitudinal study, infants performing at lower levels on sensorimotor assessments at nine months had experienced less mutual gazing at one month, fewer interchanges of smiling during gazing and less contingent responses to distress at three months, and less general attentiveness and contingent responses to nondistress vocalizations at eight months (Beckwith, Cohen, Kopp, Parmelee & Marcy, 1976). For the two year longitudinal follow-up of this group of preterm infants, the best predictor of developmental status at two years was the pattern of interaction observed during the first few months (Sigman, 1978). Similarly, Bakeman (1978) reports that interactions as early as three months during feedings are significantly correlated with teacher ratings of peer interactions as late as three years.

Our data, as already mentioned, suggest that the mothers who were more active and less sensitive to their infants' gaze signals at four months were issuing more imperatives and were overprotective or controlling during interactions at two years. The preterm infants of these mothers were less attentive at four months and were manifesting behavioral problems such as hyperactivity and language delays including a shorter mean length of utterance at two years (Field, 1979b). For other infants on the reproductive casualty continuum, Jones (1979), reporting on Down's syndrome infants, and Kogan (1979), reporting on cerebral palsied children, suggest similar continuities.

For children on the caretaking casualty continuum, such as infants with attachment disturbances (Blehar, Lieberman & Ainsworth, 1977) and lower-class children (Clarke-Stewart, 1973), similar continuities between early interactions and later development have been observed. Dunn (1977c) has suggested that mothers' speech at 13 months is positively associated with IQ scores on the Stanford-Binet at four and half years. Further, Pawlby and Hall (1979) have reported significant correlations between the frequency of early interactions between infants and mothers from disrupted families and the three year language and speech development of the infants.

In many ways these continuities seem ominous, but lest we hastily conclude that continuities suggest intervention, a number of caveats might be made regarding these data, impressions and interpretations. First, all of the above studies are based on group data. As in any group there is considerable variability or individual differences, as many exceptions as there are rules. Second, the data are limited in time and scope, and the observation, measurement and analysis techniques limit any connotations of causality. The state of the art is relatively undeveloped.

Third, the kinds of quantitative and qualitative differences discussed may be culture or group-specific. For example, infant interaction data from non-Western cultures such as French Polynesia (Martini, 1980; Sostek, Zaslow, Vietze, Kreiss & Rubinstein, 1980), Africa (Keefer, 1977) and even Western cultures such as England (Field & Pawlby, 1980) suggest that eye contact and social games are not a goal for all mothers. Similarly, the preterm infant-mother interactions, given the difficulties presented by the infant, and the lower-class mother-infant interactions, given the difficulties presented by the socioeconomic condition, may comprise a culture-specific set of interaction patterns. Consistent with these caveats, the continuities found between early interactions and later development do not necessarily mean we should intervene, particularly since interventions at this stage may be premature.

6

The Primacy of Social Skills in Infancy

EDWARD TRONICK
University of Massachusetts

An understanding of the organization of behavior in any species must focus on its members' most central adaptations. Adaptations can be viewed as the solutions a species develops for the problems posed by the external environment. These problems are posed in two domains—the domain of exchanges with the inanimate environment and the domain of exchanges with the animate environment that is composed of members of the same and other species. For any given species, the relative importance of each domain varies in a species-specific fashion. Each species survives and develops by evolving a unique set of adaptations to a unique mixture of problems in each domain. For example, if one wanted to understand the organization of vegetative reproducing species such as protozoa, the focus would be on their evolved tropisms to temperature, light, acidity and other physical features of the environment. This is because their unique pattern of adaptations is aimed primarily at regulating exchanges in the domain of the inanimate environment. In the human species, the solution to problems of survival and development have been shaped around regulating exchanges in the animate domain. This is evidenced by the species-specific configuration of human adaptive features—food sharing, tool manufacture, division of labor and coordinated tasks, male-female reciprocity, the mother-infant dyad and culture with its elements of symbolic communication, rule giving and following. All of these involve regulating exchanges with conspecifics. An understanding, then, of the organization of human behavior must thus first and foremost focus on the adaptations that our species has evolved for regulating joint activities.

This perspective has several implications. It suggests that each member of our species functions primarily as a communicator and that our most central adaptation is our communicative competence. This competence makes for the skillful regulation of all our cooperative endeavors. Moreover, this communicative competence not only allows us to function in our cooperative contexts but is fundamental and underlies our competence in manipulating the inanimate environment as well. This allows for the viewing of communication with conspecifics and manipulation of objects as a process of skill development, with the communicative skill preceding and generating the object-related skills.

Furthermore, from a developmental perspective, it appears to me that, following the establishment of physiological regulation, the infant's next task is to develop a set of skills for regulating joint exchanges. This is a necessary developmental step, because without the ability to regulate interaction the infant would be unable to regulate object-oriented interactions. Such skills are developed during interactions with adults that have no functional goal. Their goal is the successful establishment of regulation per se. The developmental task is to fulfill a set of constraints that insure incorporation into the species.

This paper will explore three aspects of joint activity. First, the *process* by which mother and infant are able to coordinate their behaviors during face-to-face interaction is described. Second, *forms of disturbance* in the interaction that disrupt appropriate coordinations are discussed. And third, the *consequences of disruptions* on infant development are presented.

JOINT REGULATION OF MOTHER-INFANT INTERACTION

I wish to present a model of the process underlying the joint regulation of activity in which the mother and infant, or any two human communicants, are viewed as two interacting cybernetic systems. The two systems utilize a shared set of generative communicative rules. These communicative rules generate the communicative behavior of each participant *and* predictions about the other's communicative behavior.

When two people come together in an interaction, they must share a goal as to what they want to do together. Let us say it is to have a dialogue. Given this goal, they must have a lexicon of communicative acts whose meanings they share. For example, frowns mean stop and smiles mean continue. They must also share a generative interactive syntax that has a format which specifies one's own communicative performance and a prediction of the partner's communicative performance, e.g., when I am talking, you will be listening.

When an interaction is appropriately coordinated, the sequence of communicative acts emitted by each partner conforms to the prediction each of them has made about the other's behavior. One communicant talks while the other communicant listens, just as each of them had predicted. It is this mutual matching of communicative acts and predictions that is the basis of joint regulation. When prediction and behavior do not match, the interaction is disordered.

However, there is one other condition required for well coordinated joint activities: temporal coordination. Two communicators may share the same goal, lexicon of communicative acts and interactive syntax, but if they cannot act in a temporally coordinated fashion, the interaction will fail to be coordinated. Just recall the last time you and a partner started talking at the same time (and realize how seldom it actually happens). Or, if you want to try an experiment, try mouthing words each time someone starts to talk to you and note the disruption.

In summary, this description indicates what goes into the coordinated regulation of joint activity. The critical feature is a sharing of functions in time. The regulation of joint activity depends on shared interactive goals, a shared lexicon of communicative acts, shared interactive rules, and shared time. Partners generate their own behavior and predictions of their partner's behavior. This conformation or disconformation is the basis of regulation.

The investigation of mother-infant synchrony is a somewhat special case of joint regulation of communicative acts. First, language is not yet part of the interaction. Second, the participants probably do not share the same temporal domain. They are at very different developmental levels.

Condon and Sander (1974b) have approached the problem of temporal coordination by extending work on adults back to infancy. Condon (Condon & Ogston, 1967) has described two types of synchrony: self-synchrony and interactive synchrony. In self-synchrony, changes in direction of an adult's movement are coordinated with the phoneme boundaries of his speech. In interactive synchrony, two adults interact and the changes in direction of their body movements are synchronous with the phoneme boundaries of their partner's speech. Thus, their movement changes are coordinated.

Further, this synchrony extends to the system of mutuality between the organism and the environment. Condon (1974) has recently shown that some autistic children are out of sync with environmental events. Their reaction to an environment event is delayed. They react to what has happened several hundredths of a second in the past, rather than to what happens in the immediate present.

Condon and Sander (1974) have demonstrated that infants are capable of interactive synchrony in that they can coordinate their movements with adult speech. Such synchrony is remarkable since phoneme boundaries are psychological rather than physical entities and may be as short as one-tenth second in duration. Several studies (see Eimas, 1975) suggest that infants may structure speech into phonemes, but it seems well beyond simple explanation that infants are able to process events and respond to them as quickly as interactive synchrony requires.

It may be that infants integrate the rhythm of speech much in the way that adults synchronize themselves with the melody of music, but at the moment there is no clear explanation of the phenomenon of infant interactive synchrony. Certainly, more developmental work is required to follow up on a hypothesis that the ability of the newborn to self-synchronize and to interactively synchronize—its coherence, so to speak—may be a crucial measure of the intactness of its central nervous system.

Our research, on the other hand, has focused on communicative synchrony between infants and adults (Tronick, Als, & Brazelton, 1977a). We sought to answer the question of whether infants and adults are able to synchronize the changes in their communicative acts. To do this we videotaped face-to-face interactions between mothers and their 80- to 90-day-old infants and then described their communicative acts. Thus, eye direction, facial expression, head direction, etc. were described on a second-by-second basis. Every act for every second was then given a ranked score reflecting the positive or negative affective tone of that act. For example, smiles had a higher positive rank than frowns, looking toward was more positive than looking away. The ranked scores were then summed separately for mother and infant and the *relationships* between these summed scores were established. It must be emphasized that the scaling was not done to scale the interaction or to scale each participant. Such scaling is fraught with problems. Rather, the scaling was performed to allow for examination of the relational aspects of the interaction.

This relational aspect was analyzed by correlating the summed scaled scores for each mother and infant pair. High positive correlations would indicate mother and infant changing in the same direction *at the same time* in terms of their affective tone. High negative correlations would indicate that they were changing in opposite directions *at the same time,* and low correlations would indicate that there was little or no relationship between their changes in affective tone.

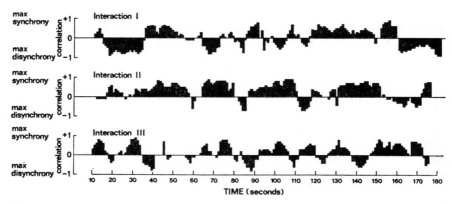

FIGURE 1. Ten second "running" correlations of infant and mother scaled sum scores (from Tronick, Als & Brazelton, 1977a).

As shown in Figure 1, there was a striking result. Correlations were often high and positive, but they were also often high and negative. Mother and infant were able to synchronize their displays but, paradoxically, they could be changing in exactly opposite affective directions. It may be as complicated a task to be out of phase with your partner as to be in phase, but it certainly does not possess the quality of being appropriately coordinated.

To analyze the question of appropriateness, the data were reanalyzed in the following manner. Three behavioral states were defined for mother and infant: (1) Engaged—the communicator is looking toward his or her partner with a bright or smiling face and may be vocalizing or gesturing; (2) Monitor—the communicator is looking toward his or her partner with a neutral or sober facial expression with no vocalization or gesturing; and (3) Disengaged—the communicator is looking away from his or her partner with a cry, frown, or sober facial expression and may be crying, or gesturing. Then three joint interactive states were defined: (1) Match—the communicators are both in the same communicative behavioral state, engage-engage, disengage-disengage, monitor-monitor; (2) Conjoint—the partners are in engage and monitor, or monitor and disengage; and (3) Disjoint—the partners are in engage and disengage. When the three interactions were analyzed in this fashion, it became

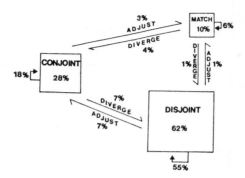

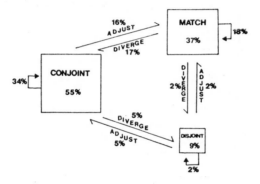

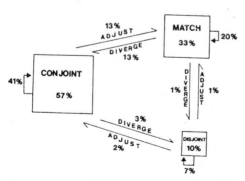

FIGURE 2. Proportion of time in different joint interactive states and the types of state transitions (from Tronick, Als & Brazelton, 1978).

clear that, although the interactions might be synchronous, their coordinations were significantly different (see Figure 2). Interaction I is primarily disjoint and conjoint and interaction II is primarily matched and conjoint. Interaction III is somewhat less matched than interaction II but much less disjoint than interaction I (see Tronick, Als, & Brazelton, 1980).

These analyses demonstrate the extent to which mother and infant were able to appropriately coordinate their communicative behavioral states. Such coordination goes beyond synchrony in that it focuses on the relational appropriateness of the infant and mother behaviors.

What process underlies mother-infant communicative coordination? The answer, I think, lies in the joining of two cybernetic systems and the critical feature has to do with the mutual following of shared interactive rules. Such a model is suggested by studies which demonstrate the consequences of an inability to jointly follow these interactive rules.

FORMS OF DISTURBANCE IN FACE-TO-FACE INTERACTIONS

Some time ago we did an experiment in which the mother was asked to distort the normal interaction with her infant by establishing an *en face* position with the infant but to remain otherwise still in face and body (Tronick, Als, Adamson, Wise, & Brazelton, 1978). It was hypothesized that if the infant only has schemas for interesting displays, this change might be boring or interesting. However, if the infant has a set of interactive goals and a set of interactive rules that are used to make predictions about the mother's behavior, then the infant should attempt to reinstate a rule confirming interaction. That is exactly what happened.

As the mother seated herself in front of her infant, the infant would establish eye-to-face contact and smile at the mother (see Figure 3). When she failed to respond the infant sobered but then might smile again. Following these greetings, the infant would begin a sequence of behaviors that involved looking toward the mother with a bright face, looking away, although probably monitoring her with peripheral vision, and then looking back toward her, again with a bright face, only to look away again. This elicitation sequence was repeated a varying number of times, but eventually the infant would turn and remain away, often engaging in self-comforting behaviors. There were three phases in the infant's reactions. The first was the normal geeting, the second an elicitation phase, and the third a withdrawal and averting phase.

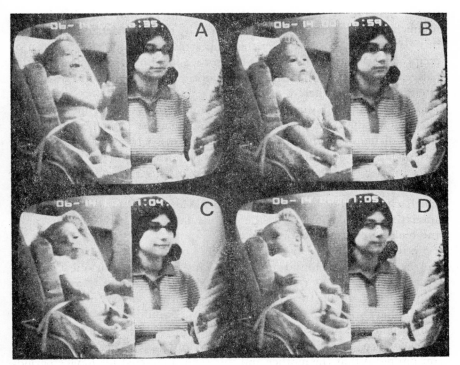

FIGURE 3. Sequential photo of infant's reaction to mother in still face (from Tronick, Als, Adamson, Wise & Brazelton, 1978).

The interpretation follows the model of interactive rules. The infant and mother appear initially to share a goal for mutual playful interaction. The mother apparently is enacting the goal by seating herself in an *en face* position. The infant responds with the normal greeting on his side and with the prediction that she will go on to the next stage of play. When she fails to move on, the infant, still holding to the goal of mutual play, attempts to re-elicit the expected interaction. When that fails, the infant changes goals, withdraws, and turns to self-comforting behaviors. It is a strong emotional reaction.

Brazelton, Koslowski and Main (1974), Stern (1971), and Massie (1975) have observed similar phenomena and have seen more long-lasting consequences. Brazelton et al. (1974) in their studies of face-to-face play of mothers and infants, and of infants with objects, uncovered a crucial pattern of interaction. Using frame-by-frame analysis, they found that a mother, by not pausing during an interaction and allowing the infant to respond, produced turning away by the infant. They interpreted this pattern as a violation by the mother of the basic cyclic pattern of reciprocity. Most significantly, mothers who habitually engaged in this pattern had infants who, as they developed, deployed less and less visual attention to the mother.

Field (1977a and this volume) has found this to be a more general phenomena than we previously thought. She has looked at the interactions of mothers with three-month-old infants who were either premature or post-mature. She found that mothers of these infants did not give their infants enough pause time and the infants responded by turning away. When she had the mothers imitate their infants—a maneuver which changes the mother's rate of behavior and thus gives the infant more time to take his turn, the infants looked at their mothers more and had more positive expressions.

Stern (1977), in his observational study of the interaction of a mother and her twins, also found a rule violating pattern. With one twin, the pattern was one that repeatedly resulted in his turning away and, one might suggest, being turned off. The sequence is shown in Figure 4. As the mother would approach the infant, he would begin to turn away and then, as the infant would start to turn toward the mother, she would begin to turn away. Thus, there was a vicious cycle. The cycle was time-consuming so that the mother and this twin interacted for longer periods of time than the mother and the other twin did, but it was an unsatisfying interaction.

This pattern is important because it constitutes an important adaptive experience for the infant. Further, it seemed to become a pattern with which the infant began to approach other situations. At 15 months this twin was more fearful and dependent than his brother. He refused prolonged eye contact and regularly performed gaze aversion in social situations. This pattern was clearly consistent with the earlier pattern.

Massie (1975), in an ingenious study, did frame-by-frame analysis of home movies parents had taken of their infants prior to the diagnosis of autistic-like psychosis. In some sense, the films serve as prospective account of the early natural history of psychosis. Massie found a pattern of interaction in which positive approach by the infant produced turning away by the mother, followed by turning away of the infant and then turning toward the infant by the mother (see Figure 5). He felt that their interaction violated a basic biological rule of mothers and infants seeking eye-to-eye contact. Moreover, he suggested that the pattern was para-

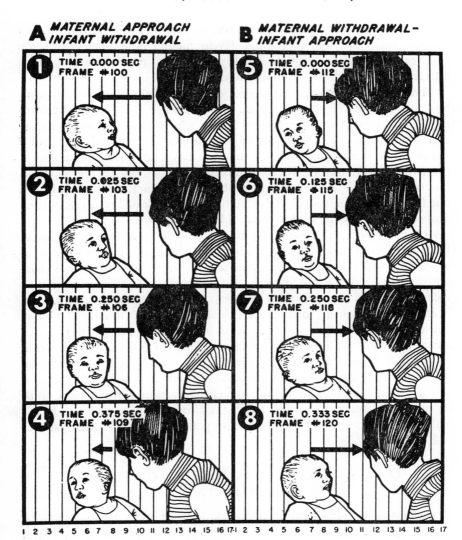

FIGURE 4. Pattern of approach withdrawal between mother and one of her twins (from Stern, 1971).

doxical, with the mother signaling through her holding and touching of the infant the message, "Respond warmly to me but don't look at me." At three years, when this infant was brought into a therapeutic setting, she no longer engaged in eye-to-eye contact with anyone and clearly behaved in an autistic-like fashion. Except for some flaccidity in infancy, this child showed normal developmental milestones during the first year and Massie is understandably tempted to attribute her aberrant outcome to this pattern of interaction.

These observations suggest a more general definition for what is meant by "appropriate" in an interaction. "Appropriate" is the mutual following of interactive rules that have a format which specifies who does what and when to do it. It is a rule of joint activity. "I act this way and I predict that you act that way." In the well-coordinated interaction, a participant's communicative act conforms to his or her partner's prediction about his or her act. In these observations, mother and infant did not follow the same rule at the same time. In each case, as in the Beatles' song, one said "Hello" as the other said "Goodbye."

Although these rules are elaborated, I do not think they are learned. Learning would allow for the mixing and matching of any of a diverse set of combinations to become appropriate. But these observations demonstrate that only certain patterns are permissible. First, to violate such rules is to violate a constraint inherent in the organism. Second, even in the earliest of social interactions this same pattern is found. The burst-pause pattern of sucking is reciprocal to the pause-act pattern of maternal behavior as Kaye and Brazelton (Kaye, 1977) have shown. Third, as has been argued for language learning, it is hard to imagine how an infant would learn the complicated and uniquely ordered sequences seen at three and four months in face-to-face interaction without some built in constraint and capabilities. Rather, I think these latter patterns are elaborations of the basic format of one partner "on," the other partner "off" structure.

CONSEQUENCES OF DISRUPTIONS ON INFANT DEVELOPMENT

To understand the developmental impact of these interactive rule-violating experiences on the infant, they must be placed in an evolutionary perspective. Bowlby (1969a) has suggested that attachment arises out of an adaptation to predation. I think that the significance of the interactive system goes beyond so singular a cause.

All species develop a system of mutuality—a set of mechanisms for sharing a territory, signaling to defend against predators, signaling in dominance relations, signaling in courtship, etc. Thus, adaptation from an evolutionary perspective and learning from an ontogenetic perspective

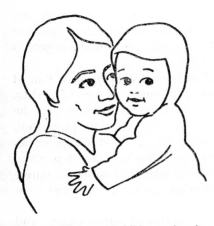

Figure 1. Mother and child are relaxed. Mother touches baby's cheek.

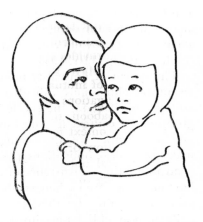

Figure 2. Child turns her head and eyes toward mother's face. Mother's expression tenses and her eyes shift away from child's face. Child tenses.

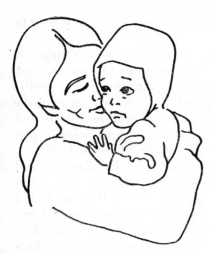

Figure 3. Mother shifts her head backward and to the side of the child's face, blocking child's facial approach and obstructing eye contact. Mother relaxes. Child appears dejected.

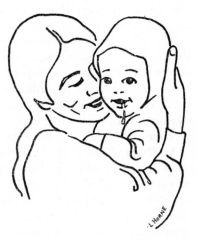

Figure 4. Mother and baby resume original postures, not in eye contact. Child's expression shifts from dejection to pleasure and drooling appears when mother pats child's head.

FIGURE 5. Pattern of interaction between mother and child analyzed from home movies (from Massie, 1975).

can be seen as the development of mutual relations with the animate and inanimate environment. This notion holds true to the extent that the environment provides constraints that have significance for the organism (Ashby, 1958; Mayr, 1963).

The system of mutuality most central to human adaptation is that of reciprocal obligations (Mead, 1934). For the human, as for the gorilla, chimp, and baboon, the species' most characteristic features is that the group is the context for subsistence activities—reproduction, protection, and socialization of the young (Fishbein, 1976). What competencies make reciprocal obligations possible? In answering this question, there is an interesting concurrence of answers that makes it possible to analyze how meanings are exchanged, how interactions are structured, and what skills are required for these tasks.

Reciprocal obligations involve the capabilities of self-awareness and empathy. Self-awareness is the ability to take another's point of view, while empathy is the ability to accurately perceive the emotional experience of another. In Piaget's framework these abilities are slowly constructed during the child's first two years of life. To be reciprocally obligated one must be aware of the effects of one's behavior on others and to act in ways that would be satisfying to yourself, were you to be in other's place.

The philosopher Habermas (1969), in analyzing communication and the exchange of meaning, has said that the communicator's primary task is to understand the message-carrying displays of the other and to modify his own actions in accordance with the other's expressed intent while fulfilling his own intentions. Communication is not monologic but dyadic. Thus, communicative competence allows the interlacing of perspectives between communicators (Tronick, Als, & Adamson, 1979).

As Ryan ((1974) notes, these analyses of reciprocal obligations and meaning emphasize the fundamental nature of the mutual recognition of particular kinds of intention by the speaker and the listener. And if one does not want to talk of intentions, one can substitute a mutual recognition function. However, the fundamental aspect is that something, some function, must be shared between two interactants that results in a mutual recognition of the other's ongoing intentionality or direction in behavior as it relates to one's own. The sharing is the intersubjective structure.

This way of characterizing the process or coordination makes the analysis of interactions a problem of the analysis of the components of skilled performance or what has been called communicative competence.

When interaction is looked on as a problem of the joint organization of serially ordered behavior, connections are again made with the concept of reciprocal obligations and the exchange of meaning.

Lashley (1951) has analyzed skill performances and argued that three conditions must be fulfilled. First, there must be the arousal of an intention or goal in the presence of an appropriate object. Second, there must be a set of organized units of behavior or adaptive acts. Third, a syntax or set of rules for organizing these acts is required. For example, when presented with an object within reach, an infant extends his/her arm, opens his/her hand and then closes it on the object. The skillful infant does not, although the younger infant does, open his/her hand, and then close it and then extend his/her hand only to bat at the object. A syntax aroused by an intention organizes the sequencing of the components for achieving the goal. Cybernetic systems made up of a control element, a comparator for input and goal, and a corrective response have been used to model these performances.

In joint interaction, these same conditions must be fulfilled but, in addition, as we have seen, the two communicators must share goals, interactive rules, and communicative behaviors, and then use these rules to generate their own communicative behavior as well as a prediction of their partner's behavior. Thus, the reasons why I see communicative skills as being the basis for other skilled performances are that first, by three months of age, long before the infant is skillful with objects, he is able to skillfully regulate social interaction with organized social behaviors. Second, the regulation of joint activity is, in fact, more complicated than interaction with objects, since objects after all do not change goals or switch rules. Interaction requires shared functions. Third, from an evolutionary perspective and from work I have done with older infants, it is evident that objects are incorporated into social interaction and not social interaction into object play. In these ways, I think skillful performance with objects borrows its competencies from the competence for the joint regulation of behavior.

Bruner (1971, 1975) has argued that language has many isomorphic relations to joint action and to skilled performances in general—and it is easy to see why. Skilled performances involve syntax, components and goals. Language, as Lashley (1951) noted, is a form of serially ordered behavior. But the skillful regulation of joint activity is more complicated than performances with objects and possibly as complicated as language, since it, too, requires the sharing of the rules that govern it. Objects do not require such rule sharing and, although language does, the organism, prior to language, already has one shared system of rules. How much easier now to learn a second set. In this sense, I think it can be said that skillful performances with objects and language borrow their competencies from the capacity for the joint regulation of behavior.

But our understanding cannot simply be one of the attainment of competencies. In disturbed interactions the infant expresses a strong emotional reaction, a reaction of hopelessness, that eventually becomes a highly disturbed pattern of withdrawal; on the other hand, when the interaction is appropriate, as Stern (1971) points out, joy is the result. The rules of social interchange and the communicative acts that enact those rules can be viewed as the infant's initial and biologically primary adaptive system, in much the same way as later cognitive abilities are an adaptive system. This adaptive system is the basis for ontogenetic adaptation.

When these rules are not followed, a helplessness is learned by the infant which goes beyond the learned helplessness of infants with objects that they have learned they cannot control. The infant is caught in a biological double bind. The infant is adapted to act to achieve reciprocity, for his dependency makes this a biological imperative. When reciprocity is not achieved, the infant can try to continue to elicit the normal reaction and in disturbed situations continue to fail, or just as disastrously, the infant can give up. In either case, the infant learns that his/her actions have no effect and that the situation requires a giving up of the goals of mutuality. The infant develops a pattern of behavior that precludes human interchange and in such withdrawal a denial of the child's self is produced. Where confirmation of intersubjective goals occurs, patterns of greater and greater complexity are elaborated and a confirmation of self takes place. Such self-evaluations are learned in the context of social interactions and then become the patterns that the infant takes into all of his or her environmental transactions.

Part III

ISSUES IN PSYCHOSOCIAL RISK: PARENT-INFANT SEPARATION, EARLY INTERVENTION, AND BIO-ETHICAL CONSIDERATIONS

This section deals with issues related to family adaptation to the newborn. Characteristics of parents which affect the early social environment of the infant, and characteristics of the infant, especially biological ones, are described as these affect the parents and family. The importance of parental expectations about the infant and situations in which these expectations are violated are presented.

Penticuff examines the reactions and stresses of the family whose newborn is critically ill. The role of the father as a significant interactant with the baby is described in the chapter by Parke. In the last portion of this section Friedlander presents a controversial position statement about the need for alternatives for families of infants born with serious congenital anomalies. Fletcher, Diamond, Hawkins, and Bugen present brief reactions to the Friedlander paper.

In the Penticuff chapter, recent research dealing with the effects of separation, extended mother-infant contact, and family stress within the immediate postpartum period are reviewed. Penticuff concludes that current research has not taken into account the totality of factors which impinge upon the developing infant-parent relationship in situations of life-threatening illness of the neonate. Implications of a variety of stressors in the early postpartum phase on incorporation of the infant into the family are presented and their relationship to later parenting adequacy are discussed. Research is presented which indicates the potential importance of intervention to encourage the development of relationships between families and their sick babies.

The second chapter of this section also deals with issues in intervention to facilitate development of relationship between the infant and parent, specifically, the father. Parke describes his research on the sig-

159

nificance of the father's role in early infant cognitive and social development. He points out that fathers receive little support within labor and delivery and postpartum units of modern-day hospitals. Parke argues, however, that the allocation of roles is a right and responsibility of the family itself, and should not be prejudiced by the opinions of workers within the health care system. He describes specific intervention strategies aimed at allowing fathers to appreciate the importance of their role in interacting with the infant and to recognize the infant's capabilities and limitations within the newborn period.

The final portion of this section presents issues which were raised in the course of diverse discussions in the symposium series about the quality of life of families and infants in cases of serious impairment of the infant's developmental potential. The perspective presented is not one of research, but rather comes from the varied experience in working with families by several of the symposium contributors. The circumstances described are those in which the infant's biological condition is such that he/she lacks many capabilities for establishing a reasonable relationship with his/her parents and family. In these cases, even the most positive attempts at effective intervention do not enhance the infant's capacities, nor do they ameliorate the infant's constant requirements for care to sustain life.

The Friedlander paper describes the anguish of parents of the seriously impaired infant and broaches the possibility of decisions to withdraw life-sustaining treatment. Bugen documents the double-edged sword of parent's grief at the ending of the newborn's life versus the stress of his continued existence. Two pediatricians who must deal with this decision on a day-to-day basis present current perspectives on medical treatment or nontreatment of seriously defective newborns. Finally, some cautions and alternative suggestions are presented by Hawkins.

Unlike the papers of the preceding sections, some of the papers in this section present views of ethical issues for which we have no empirical data. We clearly lack consensus about the resolution of the ethical dilemmas which confront parents and helping professionals in the treatment or nontreatment of infants born with serious impairments. Although the presentations in this section describe a variety of views of health professionals on these issues, the reader will find that the major questions go unanswered and, ultimately, remain a matter of personal values, moral intuition and judgment. The contributors to this section unanimously agree that, regardless of the decision made, regardless of whether the infant's life is maintained or ended, the family requires the most skilled and knowledgeable supportive intervention available.

7

Disruption of Attachment Formation Due to Reproductive Casualty and Early Separation

JOY HINSON PENTICUFF

University of Texas at Austin

Because of the extreme dependence of the human neonate on the physical and emotional support of others, the development of an affectional bond between parent and infant is essential if the infant is to grow and develop to his potential. Attachment between parent and infant is a process which has received extensive attention in theory and research, but is not yet very well understood. Bower (1977) reviewed the classic studies of the 1940s and 1950s which have provided the groundwork for current concepts about the attachment process. These early studies did not investigate attachment per se, but instead documented the influence of separation which occurs *after* maternal-infant bonding has taken place. These studies viewed attachment in terms of the impact of long-term separation on the child's physical, cognitive, and affective development. The early researchers generally concluded that insufficient or separation-disrupted ties between mother and child often resulted in the child's juvenile delinquency and decreased ability to sustain satisfying emotional relationships with others.

In contrast, more recent investigations have examined disruptions of the attachment process which occurs *before* affectional bonds have been strongly established. These recent studies have been, for the most part, conducted within special care nurseries, in which separation occurs shortly after birth and may continue for weeks or months. Follow-up of infants discharged from premature and high-risk nurseries has shown that these infants are at much greater risk for abuse, neglect, relinquishment, and nonorganic failure-to-thrive than are infants who have not required neonatal hospitalization.

Hunter et al. (1978) found a 3.9% incidence of child abuse and neglect among infants discharged from a regional neonatal intensive care unit. This incidence among premature and ill newborns is nine times that reported among infants who have not required neonatal hospitalization. Similarly, retrospective studies by Elmer and Gregg (1967), Klein and Stern (1971), and Lynch and Roberts (1977) suggest that rates of maltreatment in premature infants are three to five times the expected rate. Nonorganic failure-to-thrive, considered by Shapiro et al. (1967, p. 1) to be "impairment of the mother's capacity to nourish both in the concrete and in the psychological sense of the word," has been found in a disproportionately large number of infants who had previously experienced neonatal hospitalization (Helfer, 1974; Barnett et al., 1970). This increased incidence of significant disorders in parent-infant attachment seen in situations which have involved separation of parent and infant within the neonatal period raises questions for which there are, at present, few answers.

One of the most important questions has to do with whether the increased incidence of disruption in attachment is due primarily to separation per se, or whether the fact of serious illness in the newborn also produces stress which may disrupt the attachment process. Both of these issues will be discussed and relevant research presented below. Because of the paucity of separation studies which have investigated separation of mothers and their healthy, full-term infants, it will be seen that it is difficult to examine the effects of separation without the confounding effects of other variables which also operate when a neonate is seriously ill.

In an effort to understand how attachment occurs and what factors may disrupt the attachment process, investigations of maternal behavior in nonhuman mammals have often been utilized. Despite the obvious limitations of such studies for drawing firm conclusions about human processes, consideration of the effects of separation on attachment behavior across species offers some insight into the possible biological aspects of this process. In goats, sheep, and cattle, when a mother is separated from the newborn in the first hour or the first few hours after delivery, she will exhibit disturbed mothering behavior upon reunion. These behaviors include such things as butting the offspring away, failure to care for her young, and feeding her own and other babies indiscriminately (Hersher, Richmond, & Moore, 1963; Klopfer, Adams, & Klopfer, 1964; Moore, 1968). In contrast, when there is no separation for the first four days and the mother and infant are separated on the fifth day for an equal period of time, the mother easily regains the maternal behavior characteristic of her species when the pair is reunited (Moore, 1968). From these and other animal studies, and from studies of hormonal levels at antepartum and postpartum in human mothers, it has been hypothesized that there may be a "sensitive period" immediately after delivery during which the mother is optimally able to initiate an enduring and unique relationship with her infant.

Other studies suggest that disruption of tactile contact, more than visual contact, may be central to the breakdown of early mothering behavior. Harlow et al. (1963) studied rhesus monkey mothers who were not allowed to touch their infants but were allowed to see and hear them. After two weeks of deprivation of tactile contact, these mothers spent less and less time viewing their infants. It was concluded that mere viewing was not sufficient to maintain maternal interest. The possibility that this finding might be relevant to mother-infant relationships in humans is clear when one considers that in many special care nurseries it is common for parents to be allowed to view their infants but not to touch or hold them for days or even weeks.

When the infant is hospitalized shortly after birth, separation of parent and infant involves removing the newborn from the normal newborn nursery or from the mother's room, in the case of rooming-in, and admission of the infant to a special care nursery. This intensive care area may be in the same hospital in which the delivery occurred, or it may be a regional center many miles away. If the parents are able to visit the infant frequently, their separation may be categorized in terms of the modalities of interaction available to parent and infant. Barnett et al. (1970) have devised a system for rating levels of interactional deprivation based on whether parents were able to only view their infants, to view and touch their infants, to also hold and rock their infants, etc. The fewer sensory modalities which could be utilized in the interaction, the more complete was the interactional deprivation.

For obvious ethical reasons, there have been very few studies of early separation of healthy human newborn infants and their parents. Indeed, routine complete separation of parent and infant in the first few days after delivery exists only in the high-risk and premature nurseries of the Western world. However, because usual hospital practice allows less than full-time contact between mothers and their healthy newborns, it has been possible to extend the amount of contact between mother and infant within the first several postpartum days and to compare later maternal behavior of extended-contact and control mothers. Klaus et al. (1972) conducted such a study involving two groups of 14 primiparous mothers matched as to age, marital, and socioeconomic status. Their infants did not differ significantly in sex and weight and were normal, full-term babies. The extended-contact group was allowed extra contact with their nude infants in the mother's bed and under a heat panel to ensure maintenance of adequate infant temperature. These mothers were given their infants for one hour in the first two hours after birth and for five extra hours on each of the next three postpartum days. The control group of mothers had only the routine contact with their infants which is customary in most hospitals: an initial glimpse of the baby immediately before the infant is placed in the transitional nursery, a brief contact for identification six to eight hours later, and subsequent contact of 20 to 30 minutes every four hours for feedings. To assess the possible effects of the 16 hours of extra contact provided the experimental group, at one month of age the infants and mothers in both groups returned to the hospital and three measures were obtained. In the first, a measure of caregiving, two questions were asked and then given a score of 0 to 3, with 0 indicating little caregiving and 3 indicating maximal caregiving. The questions were as follows: When the baby cries and has been fed and the diapers are dry, what do you do? Question two: Have you been out since the baby was born? How did you feel? If the mother answered "yes" and indicated that she did not think about the baby while away, a score of 0 was given. Three was scored if the mother did not go out or if she thought about the infant during her absence. Mothers in the extended-contact group more frequently picked up their infants when they cried and tended to stay at home with their babies more than the control group.

A second measure was an observation of the mother's performance during a physical examination of her baby in which the mother was rated as follows: 0—remained seated and detached during the examination, 1—remained seated but watched, 2—sometimes stood and watched, 3—continuously stood and watched. In addition, when the infant cried, the mother was rated as to whether she attempted to soothe the baby. Extended-contact mothers more frequently stood and watched during the physical examination and were more likely to soothe their infants than were the control group mothers.

The third measure was a time-lapse filming of the mother-infant interaction during a feeding. The filming was accomplished using a one-way mirror, although the mothers were informed that they were being photographed. The first 600 frames (at a speed of one frame per second) were analyzed by researchers naive as to the mothers' assignments to experimental or control group and 25 maternal characteristics were scored. These included caretaking skills such as position of the bottle and measures of affection such as extent of ventral body contact, *en face* position, and stroking, kissing, bouncing, and cuddling. Extended-contact mothers engaged in more *en face* and more affectionate behaviors than did mothers in the routine contact group.

A further observation of these groups of mothers and infants when the infants were one year old was conducted to determine whether the differences were maintained. Mothers and infants were observed through a one-way mirror in seven situations: (1) an interview, (2) physical examination of the infant, (3) brief separation of mother and infant, (4) photographs of mother and infant, (5) free play, (6) Bayley developmental testing of the infant, and (7) filmed feeding of the infant. Extended-contact mothers were found in their responses to the interview questions to be more focused on their babies than were the control group mothers. During the physical exam, seven of the 14 extended contact mothers spent 31 to 40 of the total 15-second time periods beside the examination table assisting the pediatrician, while only two of the control group did so. Further, extended-contact mothers soothed their infants in response to crying and kissed their infants more frequently than did control mothers. Other observations of the two groups did not reveal statistically significant differences, with the exception of the infants' Bayley developmental index. The mean scores were 98 for extended-contact infants and 93 for control infants, thus lending support to Rubenstein's (1967) observation that maternal attentiveness is related to the infant's cognitive development. Kennell et al. (1974) point out that these data substantiate the notion that the interaction between mother and infant within the first several postpartum days may have a significant influence on the process of maternal attachment. However, these investigators have recently placed less emphasis on the concept of an optimal or "sensitive" period for maternal-infant bonding early after delivery (Klaus, 1978). One may reason, however, that medical practices which preclude mother-infant interaction for significant amounts of time within the neonatal period risk the possibility of disruption of the initial mother-infant acquaintance process and thus may jeopardize bonding.

Other studies of separation have involved premature and ill infants who were necessarily separated from their mothers for medical reasons. One such study conducted in England (Whiten, 1975) involved 10 mothers and infants who had been separated when the infants were between two and 14 days of age because of the newborns' illness. These illnesses were short-term and the infants were considered to be medically normal at discharge from the special care nursery. The duration of hospitalization did not exceed two weeks in all cases. A control group of 11 mothers and infants, matched as to age, marital status, infant birthweight and sex, who had not been separated were included in the study. When the two groups of infants were three weeks old, the mothers were asked to keep diaries of their baby's behavior for a 24-hour period. The baby's crying, fussing, time spent out of the crib, being fed, time asleep, drowsy, and awake were recorded by dividing the day into five-minute intervals. Analysis of the mothers' records showed that the mothers in the separated group recorded over twice as much crying from their babies as did the mothers in the nonseparated group. The separated babies were not only reported to cry more frequently but also to cry for a longer period on each occasion. Although the nonseparated mothers intervened to soothe their infants with about equal frequency, the mothers of the separated babies intervened to soothe their infants for a smaller proportion of their infants' crying time.

Observations of the mother-infant interaction at one and two months revealed significant differences in the amount of time the mothers and babies spent smiling and looking at each other, with the separated group looking and smiling less. Similar observations at three and four months indicated that most of the differences between the two groups had disappeared. This study raises several interesting questions which relate to the difficulty in attempts to parcel out the effects of separation from the effects of neonatal illness severe enough to require the infant's hospitalization. Even though the infants in this study were considered to be fully recovered from their early illnesses and did not require prolonged hospital stays, it is reasonable to assume that their hospitalization was cause for serious concern on the part of their parents. Indeed, although the infants were judged to be free of disease at discharge, their mother's records may be interpreted to indicate an increase in fussiness, irritability, and decreases in consolability and quieting which may reflect subtle deficits in the infants' state organization due more to preceding illness than to the effects of separation.

Other findings have been reported for mothers and infants who experienced early separation due to prematurity. In a study conducted in the United States, Seashore et al. (1973) investigated behaviors judged to indicate maternal attachment such as close bodily contact between mother and infant, looking and smiling at the infant and interaction excluding feeding and other routine caretaking. In addition, maternal self-confidence was assessed by means of self-report. This measure required that each mother compare herself with several other potential caretakers—father, grandmother, experienced mother, pediatric nurse, and doctor—in calming baby, understanding what the baby wants, showing affection to the baby, diapering, feeding, and bathing the baby. Three groups of mothers and infants, matched as to age, marital and socioeconomic status, were studied. One group delivered premature infants who remained in a special care nursery for three weeks or longer following birth. While these infants were in the hospital, the mothers were allowed only to view them from the nursery window and were not permitted to touch or hold their infants. The second group consisted of mothers who also had delivered premature infants requiring confinement to the special care nursery. However, these mothers were allowed into the nursery to touch and handle their infants. The third group consisted of mothers of full-term infants for whom no separation occurred. The three groups were followed for 21 months after the infants' discharge from the hospital. Results showed significant differences between separated and nonseparated mothers in that separated mothers spent less time caressing, holding, and smiling at their infants than did the nonseparated mothers. However, separation did not affect the amount of time spent in playful noncaretaking interaction with the infant. In the early observations of the separated and nonseparated mothers of premature infants, there were only minor differences in maternal behavior of the two groups. However, at one year, the mothers who were given contact touched their babies more than those who had been denied contact.

Results of the maternal self-confidence measure showed that separation lowered self-confidence only in primiparous mothers, and that self-confidence in these mothers increased over time. At the one- and 12-month assessments there were no significant differences in maternal self-confidence of the three groups. At the follow-up one year after the infants' discharge, it was found that the effects of separation on maternal attitudes and behavior had almost disappeared. However, when observations were made at 21 months, the investigators were surprised to find that of the 18 families in the premature, separated group, there were five divorces; of the 17 premature, contact families, there were two divorces; of the 21 full-term families, there were no divorces. The investigators concluded that "separation in the newborn period does have an effect, albeit nonspecific, by acting through the family as a stress that created disequilibrium in the nuclear family structure" (Seashore et al., 1973, p. 230).

In another study utilizing premature or ill infants and involving an experimental manipulation of maternal contact with the ill infant, Klaus and Kennell (1970) investigated the effects of separation on attachment behavior. Mothers in the Early Contact group were permitted to enter the special care nursery, place their hands inside the infant's isolette and carry out simple caretaking tasks beginning within five days after the infant's birth and continuing throughout hospitalization. In the Late Contact I group, mothers were not permitted to enter the nursery until the infant was 20 days of age and thus were only able to view their infant through the nursery windows without being able to touch, smell, or hear the infant. In the Late Contact II group, mothers were not permitted to enter the special care nursery until the infants reached 30 to 40 days of age. A control group of mothers of full-term, healthy infants was also studied. Analysis of the behavioral data was accomplished in two phases. In the first analysis, a comparison was made between the two experimental groups considered to be most divergent: Early Contact and Late Contact II. All of the mothers in the study were matched as to age, marital status, and socioeconomic level and infants in the experimental groups were also matched as to birthweight, sex, and medical condition. In the comparison of the Early and Late Contact II groups, three observations were made: (1) during the mother's fifth visit to her infant in the discharge nursery, (2) in the home one week after discharge, and (3) in the pediatric follow-up clinic one month after discharge. Results showed that mothers in the Early Contact group were more skillful in caretaking than the Late Contact II mothers only in the first observation. While attachment behavior (smiling at the infant, caressing the infant, looking at the infant) of the Early Contact group occurred more frequently than in the Late Contact II mothers, this difference reached statistical significance only at the third observation.

In a second analysis of the data, the Late Contact I and Early Contact mothers were compared using filmed feeding observations. Mothers in the two groups were asked to allow filming as they fed their infants immediately before their infant's discharge from the hospital. Time-lapse photography was utilized and frame-by-frame analysis of the first ten minutes of each feeding was accomplished. Twenty-five activities were recorded which were similar to those described in the Klaus et al. (1972) study cited previously. The Late Contact I mothers held their infants with less ventral contact, changed position less, burped their infants less, and were not as skillful in feeding as were mothers in the Early Contact group. These differences were maintained when the mothers and infants were again filmed during a feeding at one month after discharge.

CONCLUSIONS

Studies of the effects of separation within the neonatal period have generally provided evidence that early, prolonged deprivation of contact between mother and infant results in disruptions of behaviors which are thought to be characteristic of human maternal-infant bonding, such as ventral contact with the infant, the *en face* position, caressing, kissing, cuddling, and smiling at the infant. In addition, animal studies indicate that separation within the first several hours or days postpartum may seriously disrupt attachment in certain mammalian species. Follow-up of infants discharged from special care nurseries provides grim statistics which show that infants who have required hospitalization within the neonatal period are three to nine times more likely to suffer maltreatment and failure-to-thrive than are healthy, full-term infants.

Thoughtful analysis of these fragmented pieces of data, however, requires that a more comprehensive conceptual framework be applied than those given in the studies presented above. It must be pointed out that prolonged separation of parent and infant occurs only within the high-risk and premature nurseries of industrialized nations. Further, because of the strong trend in this country toward the regionalization of neonatal care for critically ill newborns, there will be increasing numbers of parents who experience interactional deprivation because the majority of regional units do not provide facilities, space, or special training of nursery staff to enable parents to do much more than view their infants through the nursery for days, weeks, or even months. However, the conceptual framework to be applied cannot be limited merely to a notion that deprivation of interaction *per se* will inevitably result in disruption of the development of enduring affectional bonds from parent to infant. It is necessary to consider what the parent brings into the parenting situation and to examine the sources of support and stress which impinge upon the parent's ability to establish an affectionate bond with the infant. In addition, the capacity of the infant to respond to the parent's attachment behaviors exerts a powerful influence on the parent's development of affectional ties and on the parent's belief that there may be a happy outcome from the life threatening illness which the infant has suffered. These issues will be discussed in greater detail below.

It is possible to interpret the increased incidence of significant parenting disorders (failure-to-thrive, child abuse and neglect) seen in infants who have required neonatal hospitalization as being due to a variety of factors, of which separation is only one aspect. The development of the parent-infant relationship, in which the parent nurtures the physical, affective, cognitive, and social development of the child as well as experiences a sense of reward and enduring affection, is influenced by the life experiences of the parent as well as by the parent's current life stresses and supports. Further, characteristics of the newborn such as consolability, self-quieting, "cuteness," cuddliness, and others affect caregiver behavior and feelings about the infant.

A review of child abuse and neglect literature by Hunter et al. (1978) identified the following stressful life circumstances of parents as being related to instances of later parenting disorder:

> adolescent parent or inexperienced in child care;
> prior neonatal morbidity or mortality;
> inadequate child spacing;
> abortion of current pregnancy seriously considered;
> failure to accept pregnancy after first trimester;
> lack of needed infant equipment;
> social isolation and poor support system;
> marital maladjustment, separation, divorce;
> precarious financial situation;
> inadequate child care arrangements;
> family history of abuse or neglect;
> lack of confidence in parenting skills;
> disappoinment over sex of infant;
> retarded or illiterate;
> drug dependency.

Hill (1978) states that "If there is . . . stress in the mother's life that causes her to be insensitive to her infant's cues . . . then the interaction can break down" (Class 3, p. 11). It may be concluded that any factor which the prospective parent experiences as a stressor may influence the parent's ability to successfully progress through pregnancy, labor and delivery, initial interaction with the newborn, and assumption of caregiving. The parenting role requires mastery of behavioral and psychological tasks in which the parent accepts impending parenthood and perceives the infant as a separate individual with affective responses and physical and psychological needs. Anything which threatens family relationships or integrity during these developmental periods may inhibit adequate accomplishment of the role of parent.

When the family is confronted with evidence that the pregnancy is not "going well," in terms of their own definition of what "going well" means, coping mechanisms are mobilized. The family whose internal and external sources of support are great will have enhanced ability to deal constructively and realistically with the problems encountered. The family whose supports are weak has a high probability of failure in coping realistically with problems. For such a family, denial or distortion of the reality of pregnancy complications and serious illness in the newborn may impair realistic problem-solving approaches.

Even for the well-supported family, premature birth or the birth of an infant who is critically ill is a crisis situation because of the parent's guilt in having produced a non-normal infant, the fear that the infant may not survive, and the fear that the infant may sustain permanent damage. There are many clinical descriptions of shock, anger, and other emotional reactions of parents whose infants require neonatal hospitalization (Caplan, Mason, and Kaplan, 1965; Prugh, 1953; Kopf and McFadden, 1974; Slade et al., 1977; and Kennedy, 1973). The crisis of serious illness in the neonate produces psychological disequilibrium which is temporary but which may be necessary in order to provide sufficient resources so that the parent and infant under stress will be able to make a satisfactory adjustment. During the period in which the infant is critically ill, parents may experience a sense of distance from the infant, a lack of emotional involvement with him. If the infant's condition remains critical for an extended period, with consequent hindrance to usual parent-infant interaction, the risk for disordered relationship increases (Hunter et al., 1978). Financial stress, family discord, chronic fatigue, and multiple other factors may impinge on the parent to further impair ability to relate to the infant.

Characteristics of the infant are another potent influencer of parent-infant interaction and, thus, parent-infant attachment. The infant who does not give clear cues as to his needs or when his needs have been satisfied is a challenge to the most secure and competent caregiver. It has been shown that the small-for-gestational-age infant, very low birth-weight infant, or very premature infant is more likely to be a "difficult" baby than is the normal full-term infant (Brazelton et al., 1974; Field, 1977a and this volume). The premature infant is limited in his ability to handle stimuli due to his neurological immaturity and often manifests this difficulty through gaze aversion in interaction. Difficulties in rhythmicity of patterns of eating, sleeping, and quiet alert states are also more common in premature, low birthweight, or inappropriate-for-gestational-age infants (Drillien, 1964; Lubchenco et al., 1963; Brazelton et al., 1974). Barnard (1978) found that the nonalert, nonresponsive infant shows less readiness to learn when observed in a learning situation throughout the first year of life. Mothers of these infants reported a decreasing amount of involvement with the infant over the year, and at 12 months of age there was less optimal communication between mother and infant when the infant was not alert and responsive as a newborn.

Kennedy (1973) concluded that "mothers tend to believe that their newborn likes them and appreciates their ministrations when the infant's behavior is characterized by nursing eagerly, cuddling, smiling after feeding, focusing in the direction of the mother's face, listening to her voice, quieting when touched, and sleeping for relatively long periods after a feeding. Behavior that leads mothers to believe that their infants have a critical, rejecting attitude toward them includes refusal to suck, vomiting, crying during or after a feeding, angry crying, or closing the mouth firmly" (p. 551).

In summary, it can be said that many factors impinge on the development of parent-infant attachment. These include characteristics of the parents such as readiness for parenthood and resources for coping with stress, as well as characteristics of the infant such as extent of deviation from the expected or hoped-for "ideal" infant, seriousness of illness in the neonatal period, sequelae of neonatal illness which interfere with giving of clear cues, and factors such as cuddliness, consolability, response decrement, and general appearance. Further, the circumstances surrounding the initial interactions of parent and infant either facilitate parent-infant attachment or hinder this process.

If the process by which parents develop enduring affectional ties to the infant requires, as T. G. R. Bower posits, "the development of a set of communicational routines involving specific meanings and specific interchanges" (p. 158), then in situations such as high risk nurseries in which early and extended separation of parent and infant occurs, the early forms of these communicational routines have little or no opportunity to develop. For the infant whose hospital course is stormy, who requires prolonged stay within the intensive care unit with its beeping monitors and hurried staff, the possibility for disruption of the initial interactions between parent and infant becomes great indeed.

Scanlon (1978), addressing the National Perinatal Association, pointed out that although, with the application of medical technology, neonatal mortality rates have been reduced by 30 percent since 1970, there has been no corresponding drop in infant mortality rates. Thus, the critically ill newborn may survive his first month of life, only to succumb within the first year due to inadequate or abusive parenting. Klaus and Kennell note that "In this century both birth and death, the two most important events in the life of an individual, have been moved into the hospital and away from the family and centuries of traditions and cultural patterns of behavior. Practices surrounding both events have been almost wholly determined by the psychological needs, the convenience, the limited perspective and the bias of the dominant members of the hospital culture (nurse, physician, administrator)" (1970, p. 1026).

In taking a more comprehensive view of the issues of separation, family preparation for parenthood, coping mechanisms, and the effects of serious illness on the infant's ability to respond to parental attachment behavior, it is important to realize that restructuring of hospital neonatal facilities, policies, practices, and preparation of staff is required if parents are not to suffer interactional deprivation during their infant's stay in the hospital. At a time when parental stress and infant stress are at a peak, it is essential that health professionals and facilities enhance rather than inhibit the parent's early contact with the seriously ill infant.

8

Fathers and Risk: A Hospital-Based Model of Intervention

ROSS D. PARKE,
SHELLEY HYMEL,
THOMAS G. POWER, and
BARBARA R. TINSLEY
University of Illinois at Champaign-Urbana

In recent years, there has been increasing recognition that the quality of caretaking, as well as the infant's biological status, plays an important role in determining later infant development. Sameroff's (1975a) conceptualization of continua of reproductive as well as caretaking casualty has captured the dual nature of the influence process and provided a useful framework for guiding research in infant development. According to this model, the subsequent development of the infant who may be at risk for later developmental anomalies due to reproductive factors (e.g., birth complications, anoxia, prematurity, etc.) can only be understood by a consideration of the caretaking environment. The aim of the present chapter is to show that our usual conceptualization of the caretaking environment is too narrowly defined by an exclusive focus on the mother-infant relationship. It will be argued that the father's role as a participant in the development of the infant merits consideration. Second, the necessity of providing more adequate support systems for fathers

Preparation of this chapter and the research reported here was supported by the following grants: NICHD Training Grant, HD-00244, Office of Child Development Grant, OHD 90-C-900, and a grant from the Grant Foundation. Thanks are extended to Brenda Congdon for her preparation of the manuscript.

174

n their role as caretakers will be discussed. To illustrate the feasibility
f father-oriented programs, a recently implemented hospital-based train-
ng program for fathers will be described.

RE-CASTING THE EARLY SOCIAL ENVIRONMENT:
FATHERS AS CARETAKERS

The infant's social environment has usually been recognized as a
"mother" environment and thus most theoretical and investigative at-
ention has been paid to mother-infant interaction under the assumption
hat variations in early mother-infant interactions could potentially place
n infant at risk (Sameroff & Chandler, 1975; Yarrow, Rubinstein, &
'edersen, 1975). However, increasingly, fathers are becoming recognized
s playing an important role in early development (Lamb, 1976b; Parke,
1978). Evaluation of the significance of the father has taken two direc-
ions. First, fathers have a *direct* impact on their infant's social and cognitive development through caretaking and play. However, the father
an also *indirectly* affect the infant's development by his mediating impact on the mother and mother-infant interaction (Parke, Power, &
Gottman, 1978). For example, Feiring and Taylor (1978) found a posi-
ive relationship between mother's perception of support from a secondary parent and the degree of maternal involvement. Sixty-seven percent
of the secondary parents in this study were fathers.

At the same time that the father is being recognized as an important
contributor to infant development, cultural trends are increasing the
pressure on fathers to assume a more active role in early infant care
and development. This is evidenced in several ways. First, there are an
increasing number of mothers who work full-time, either for economic
or other reasons (Bronfenbrenner, 1975). In turn, this often results in
the father's assuming a greater proportion of the responsibility for infant
caretaking. Studies of the division of labor in households of working
mothers show that the husbands in these families tend to offer support
primarily through child-rearing assistance (Geiken, 1964; Hoffman,
1960). A second emerging phenomenon which results in a larger role for
the father in child-rearing is the greater frequency with which fathers
are assuming custody for children as a result of divorce or other legal
action (Orthner, Brown, & Ferguson, 1976). In most of these custody
cases, fathers are required to provide all the physical and psychological
child-care skills which had previously been at least partly the responsibility of the child's mother. Thirdly, physicians are permitting shorter

postpartum hospital stays for mothers and newborn infants. Mothers may arrive home not yet fully recovered from childbirth which, in turn, places increased demands on the father in terms of housekeeping and infant caregiving. Lopata (1971) found that husbands readily took on a greater proportion of household tasks in similar emergencies. Mothers are also returning to work much sooner after birth than in previous years (Bronfenbrenner, 1975). This effectively serves as an added caregiving burden on the father, as discussed above. Finally, the father has become the main supportive "other" in families due to greater mobility of U.S. families and the resulting reduction in the probability that the extended family can function as a primary support system. There is an increasing shift from the existence of extended family support networks to self-contained nuclear families. For example, 50 years ago, 50 percent of the households of Massachusetts included at least one other adult besides the parents. In 1974, this figure had been reduced to 4 percent (Bronfenbrenner, 1975).

These pressures toward greater father participation in early child care are not restricted to normal full-term infants. In fact, the father's role may be more important in cases of high-risk infants, such as the premature or low-birthweight infant. Both direct and indirect effects need to be considered. In a direct sense, fathers may be required to assume a larger share of responsibility for care and stimulation of the premature infant. Since premature infants are often transported to a central neonatal unit—often without the mother—fathers frequently have more contact and more responsibility for early feeding during the period of hospitalization than mothers. It is ironic that advances in the medical technology of newborn care have resulted in reduced mother-infant contact.

The father may affect the infant indirectly through the quality and quantity of support that he provides his wife in her caretaking role. Pedersen et al. (1977) have found that maternal feeding skill is positively related to paternal attitudes concerning her caretaking competence, which might be particularly relevant with a premature infant. (It is recognized, of course, that the direction of causation could be reversed in this case, whereby the mother's competence may alter paternal attitudes.) Similarly, Minde et al. (1977) recently reported that the frequency with which mothers visited their hospitalized premature infants was related to the quality of the husband-wife relationship; visitation was less frequent in distressed marriages than in nondistressed families. In light of the relationship between visitation patterns and parenting disorders such as child abuse (Fanaroff, Kennell, & Klaus, 1972), these findings assume more significance. While low frequencies of visitation by mothers may contribute to later problems due to the lack of opportunity for the development of a strong mother-infant relationship, it is possible that the poor husband-wife relationship may be the cause of *both* low involvement (visitation) and subsequent parenting disorders. For example, infant or child abuse can be an outcome of husband-wife quarrels. Alternatively, the husband in a poor marriage may not share in the caretaking activities, which may increase the likelihood of stress-related abuse of infants by mothers (Parke, 1978; Parke & Collmer, 1975).

In view of the potential role that fathers can play in early infant development and in light of the secular trends toward greater father involvement, it is important to examine the adequacy of current support systems for fathers. With the exception of popular advice in books for fathers, which are seldom used by parents as guides for child care (Clarke-Stewart, 1978b), there are very few programs that are specifically designed to teach fathers the skills necessary for adequate parenting. The vast majority of programs are mother-oriented, while fathers are virtually ignored.

What kinds of support programs should be designed for fathers?

INTERVENTION AS A SUPPORT SYSTEM FOR FATHERS

Supportive intervention for fathers could occur at a variety of time points and need not take place only after the advent of fathering responsibilities. Three major points of intervention merit consideration: (1) preparenthood, (2) pregnancy and (3) postpartum. These time points for intervention are not viewed as mutually exclusive alternatives, but as a complementary and sequential set of intervention points that can guide the implementation of programs at different phases of development toward parenthood. Each period may require different types of programs, different content emphases, different intervention sites and agents.

In assessing the feasibility and potential impact of parent training programs at each of these periods, two important issues will be considered: the accessibility and the motivation of the participants. It is assumed that even the most carefully designed program will have little impact if it reaches only a limited number of potential participants or if it reaches the audience at a time when there is little interest or motivation to learn parenting skills. In the following sections, we will briefly describe and evaluate the types of programs that could be implemented at each of the three major time points (preparenthood, pregnancy and postpartum).

Preparenthood

Parent education often begins well before individuals require parenting skills. Parent education programs have been developed for implementation in high schools. The aims of these programs are to educate future parents concerning a variety of aspects associated with parenting including: (1) the economics of raising a family; (2) the impact of children on the recreational and social activities of a couple; (3) basic principles of child development; and (4) basic parenting skills and behavioral management techniques. It is likely that these types of courses are particularly important for males, as most adolescent males have much less contact with children than their female peers (babysitting, etc.). Such courses would provide an opportunity for males to acquire caretaking skills and realistic expectations concerning parenting. However, attendance records show that a very low proportion of males take advantage of this opportunity for parent education. This suggests low motivation on the part of male students, and although mandatory attendance could provide for high accessibility, motivation would still be low.

Thus, during this period of preparenthood, males can be made accessible in large numbers for parent education, but do not appear motivated to learn parenting skills at this point. This is not to argue against the existence of such programs, but to suggest that such programs may not be very effective since most males during this period probably see little relevance in learning parenting skills and are thus not motivated to do so.

Pregnancy

Pregnancy is a common intervention period and programs in this period usually take the form of childbirth preparation classes. Special attention is often devoted to the father's role as a support figure during labor and delivery. While preparation for the labor and delivery experience is important (Tanzer & Block, 1972; Kitzinger, 1972), there is little evidence that this type of preparation affects the father's interaction with his infant (Parke, O'Leary, & West, 1972) or the father's postpartum adjustment to his fatherhood role (Wente & Crockenberg, 1976). In assessing the impact of Lamaze childbirth classes, these latter investigators stated, "many men said they were pleased with their training for childbirth but felt totally unprepared for what comes after" (p. 356). In part, this is due to the fact that these preparation classes do not usually focus on postpartum caretaking skills. Combined with the fact that only a small percentage of fathers participate in prenatal classes, it is clear that pregnancy cannot be a sole point of intervention.

Thus, in contrast to high school programs, pregnancy is a period where motivation is high, but accessibility is low. Although programs initiated during this time can be very effective for those involved (given the high level of motivation), the need for intervention to occur at a time when both motivation and accessibility are high becomes increasingly more evident.

Postpartum

Immediately following birth, during the mother's postpartum hospital stay, both the father's accessibility and motivation to learn parenting skills may be high. Many programs take advantage of this fact. Most hospitals now permit fathers in both the labor and delivery room and recent research (Anderson & Standley, 1976) indicates that fathers can provide important support for the mother during the birth process. Similarly, many hospitals are modifying visiting arrangements to permit fathers regular and extended contact with their infants during the early postpartum period.

Other types of modification in institutional practices could be made to facilitate father involvement in the care of infants, which, in turn, would provide a supportive environment for mothers as well. For example, paternity leaves would permit fathers to fully participate in the birth process and permit them to be available for infant care in the early postpartum period.

However, the opportunity to have contact with their infants and participate in their early caretaking may not be sufficient to acquire the knowledge and skills necessary for competent caretaking of their infants. Specific training programs designed to provide guidelines for father care of infants is an important but neglected form of early support. To illustrate the feasibility and value of a father-oriented intervention program in the hospital during the early postpartum period was the aim of our recent project.

A HOSPITAL-BASED INTERVENTION PROGRAM FOR FATHERS

In light of the increasing pressure on fathers to take an active role in early infant care and in light of the lack of support offered those fathers who want to take an active role, an intervention program was designed to provide early postpartum training for fathers. The early postpartum period was chosen as an intervention point as fathers were thought to be most motivated to learn infant-care skills during this period and most fathers are accessible at this time.

Overview

The project involves an assessment of the effect of exposure to a specially designed intervention during the postpartum hospital period on the attitudes and behavior of fathers. Briefly, one group of fathers saw a 15-minute videotape, "Fathers and Infants," while a control group of fathers followed the usual hospital routine and saw no videotape presentation. To assess the impact of the intervention, a variety of attitudinal measures and observational measures of father-infant interaction were secured in the hospital in the early postpartum period and in the home at three weeks and three months for both intervention and control groups. At three months, the typical level of father participation in routine caretaking activities in the home was assessed. The purpose of the project was to assess the effectiveness of this limited intervention on paternal attitudes, interaction patterns and levels of participation in infant care.

Sample and Design

A total of 32 Caucasian fathers and their infants participated in this study. The fathers ranged in age from 19 to 31. All fathers had completed high school, and several had obtained advanced professional training.

The father-infant pairs were assigned to a $2 \times 2 \times 2$ factorial design involving sex of infant (males and females), ordinal position (first versus later born) and treatment (videotape intervention versus no intervention). There were four father-infant dyads in each cell of the design.

The videotape presentation: "Fathers and Infants." The videotape was designed to serve three purposes. The first aim was to modify father's sex role attitudes concerning the appropriateness of infant caretaking for adult males. A second aim was to provide specific demonstration of feeding and diapering to increase the skill level of the fathers in the intervention program. A third aim was to increase fathers' knowledge concerning the infant's perceptual and cognitive capacities. It was assumed that modifying fathers' knowledge about infant capacities would, in turn, modify their patterns of interaction with their infants. This is based on the assumption that a low level of parental involvement with their infants, may be, in part, due to an underestimation of their infants' cognitive-perceptual capacities (Parke, 1978).

The videotape presentation consisted of the following sections. First, the narrator introduced the videotape by describing infants with an emphasis on the infant's capacity for social interaction. Second, three different fathers were shown interacting with their infants. These models demonstrated the visual and auditory tracking capacities of the infant, using both a toy and face and hands as tracking objects. Third, the film emphasized other ways of stimulating infants by touching, vocalizing and smiling, as well as imitation as a form of early caretaker-infant play. Fourth, each father fed the infant for a few minutes. During the feeding sequences, the narrator described the correct position for holding the infant and described techniques for stimulating the infant to feed. At the end of the feeding sequence, two different positions for burping the infant were demonstrated by all three fathers. Next, a diapering sequence was presented. At the end of this sequence, each of the father models briefly played with his infant in order to emphasize that the caretaking context was a good time for play. In the final scenes, the narrator restated the central themes of the presentation: (1) fathers can play an active role in play and caretaking; and (2) babies—even from the newborn period— are more perceptually, cognitively, and socially competent than we had previously believed. The film was well received by both hospital personnel and the fathers themselves.

Procedure

Parents were recruited into the study during the postpartum hospital period. The study was presented as a project concerning "how parents interact with their infants in different settings and ages." In addition, parents were informed that some fathers would view a short videotape in order to assess its usefulness for inclusion as part of a future hospital program. Fathers were randomly assigned to a film or no-film control condition.

Fathers in the film condition were shown the videotape in a room on the maternity floor one or two days after the birth of their infant. Fathers in both film and control conditions followed a similar schedule of assessments. Briefly, the fathers filled out an attitude questionnaire and were observed during a 20-minute period with their infant in the hospital and again at three weeks and three months in the home. At three months, a parental diary of caretaking activity was completed. All assessments for the film group were completed after viewing the film.

Assessments

Attitudes. Attitudes were assessed using a 50-item questionnaire, originally developed by Parke and Sawin (1975). Fathers rated their agreement/disagreement to each item on a seven-point scale. Based on earlier factor analyses, the questionnaire was found to tap the following general areas: (1) parental knowledge of infant perceptual capacities (sample items include, "newborn infants can follow an object; infants can discriminate parts of faces"); (2) parent's perceptions concerning the infant's need for affection and stimulation (sample items: "It's good to cuddle babies; diapering is a good time for play; it's important to talk to babies"); (3) parent's concern for infant happiness (sample item: "It makes young babies happy when you smile at them"); (4) parental resentment of the infant (sample item: "Having a baby forces you to give up many of your favorite activities"); (5) parental perception of their caretaking competence (sample item: "I would be nervous about holding a baby when alone with him"); and (6) parental sex role attitudes concerning their attitudes regarding degree of paternal responsibility for infant care (sample item: "It is not a father's role to share in the caretaking of a young baby").

Observational meaures of parent-infant interaction. The structured observation sessions of parent-infant interaction consisted of two phases: (1) ten minutes of feeding and (2) ten minutes of nonfeeding, play interaction. The father-infant observations are made immediately after the film presentation (for the experimental group fathers), or at a similar time without the film manipulation for the control fathers. All hospital observations began at the start of a regular feeding period. At the end of the feeding session the 10-minute observation of nonfeeding play interaction was made. For the play session, the parent was given a standard toy, a commercially available "Flower Rattle" which (1) is brightly colored, (2) has one mirrored side and a second face-like side, (3) makes a pleasant rattle sound, and (4) is easily held by the parent. Both infants and parents enjoyed the toy and, at the end of the play session, the toy was presented to the family as a gift. All father-infant observations took place in a separate quiet room on the maternity floor. A Datamyte recorder was used to record the observational data. This device yielded both frequencies and durations of father and infant behavior.

Home observations. During visits to the home at three weeks and three months, the following observation was made: father-infant interaction was observed in play and feeding contexts. As in the hospital, these structured interaction sessions consisted of 10 minutes of feeding and 10 minutes of play.

As a further means of assessing "typical" levels of responsibility for (1) play and (2) routine caretaking, a *daily diary* of parental activity was kept for the week prior to the home visit. Based on earlier work by Richards and Bernal (1972), the instrument consists of a time-marked form with instructions for recording the time that the infant is in the crib, cries and is bathed. The caretakers (mother, father or other) that perform the activity are recorded. To illustrate the utility of this hospital-based intervention program, some representative results from each type of assessment will be presented.

Results

Father's attitudes. First we turn to an examination of the impact of the film on the father's attitudes and knowledge. An analysis employing previously derived factors scores (Parke & Sawin, 1975) based on the questionnaire data revealed that the fathers' attitudes and knowledge were significantly altered by exposure to the film. First, parental knowledge of infant perceptual capacities (e.g., newborn infants can follow an object; infants can discriminate parts of faces, etc.) was significantly modified. Fathers who viewed the film received higher scores on this factor than control fathers. The difference was statistically significant at all three time points. Second, in comparison to controls, fathers who viewed the film were higher on the factor, "parent's perceptions concerning the infant's need for affection and stimulation" at the hospital period. There was no difference at three weeks and three months. This factor included items such as, "It's good to cuddle babies"; "Diapering is a good time for play" and "It's important to talk to babies." Third, fathers who viewed the film were higher on the factor labeled "concern for infant happiness," than fathers who did not watch the film, which includes such items as, "It makes young babies happy when you smile at them." Again, the effect was present in the hospital, but was not significant at three weeks and three months.

Although the parental role factor did not yield film vs. control differences, analyses of individual items revealed that some aspects of parental role attitudes were modified. For example, fathers who viewed the film were less likely to agree with the statement, "I am not interested in sharing in caretaking," than fathers who did not view the film. However, this difference was present only for fathers of boys; fathers of girls who saw the film were just as likely to agree as fathers of girls who saw no film.

Fathers' interactive behaviors. Some general findings that were present for both film and control fathers will be noted first. Overall, fathers vocalize, smile, touch and kiss their infants more during play than during feeding. Generally, the frequency of these behaviors increased across the first three months—especially during play sessions. Our results are consistent with earlier research (Parke & Sawin, 1980) and underline the important role of *context* in determining the quality of early parent-infant interaction.

The film modified selective aspects of father behavior in both feeding and play contexts. One of the techniques that was presented in the film was "stimulate to feed," a technique that can be used to maintain infant sucking during feeding (e.g., stroking the infant's lips and cheeks, moving the bottle in the baby's mouth, etc.). Fathers who viewed the film used this stimulation technique more often at all three observation points (hospital, three weeks, three months) than fathers who had not viewed the film. During the play sessions, fathers who saw the film directed more vocalizations to their boys than control or no-film fathers, but only if the infants were first-borns. Again the effect was present at all three time points. There were no film vs. control differences for girls or later born boys.

In summary, the observational data indicated that fathers who saw the film modified their behavior in the feeding session by more frequently stimulating their infants to eat (stimulate feeding) and by vocalizing more to their first-born male infants during play sessions.

Paternal involvement in infant care at three months. To assess the impact of observing the film on the extent to which fathers participate in various types of activities, parents' diaries of activity in the home at three months were used. As noted above, a daily diary of parental activity was kept by the parents for the week prior to the three-month home visit. Each individual diary was scored in the following way. Frequencies of playing, feeding, diapering, and bathing were calculated for three caretaker categories. These were father alone, mother alone and mother and father together. Overall caregiving scores for each task (diapering, feed, bathe, and play) were calculated across the seven days that the diary was

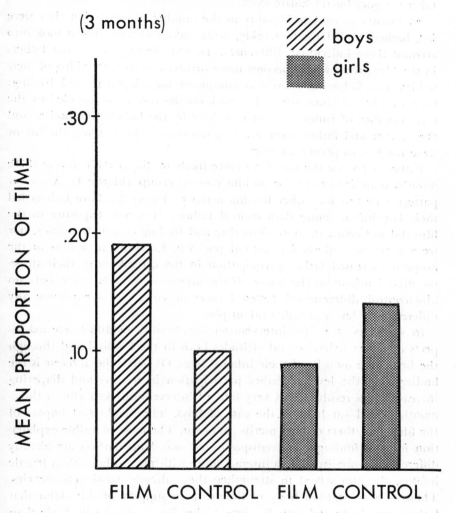

FIG. 1

kept. These scores represented the total number of times a particular task was done by those individuals (or that individual) making up each care-taker category for the entire week.

As infants varied considerably in the number of times that they were fed, bathed, and diapered weekly, ratios were constructed that took into account these individual differences. To test the hypothesis that fathers in the film group would become more involved in the caretaking of their babies, the following ratio was computed for diapering and feeding: total number of times the father took on the task alone divided by the total number of times the task was done by the father, the mother and the mother and father together. The frequencies for bathing the infant were too low to permit analyses.

Fathers who saw the film were more likely to diaper their sons at three months than fathers in the no-film control group (Figure 1). A similar pattern emerged for father feeding activity (Figure 2): Film fathers fed their boy infants more than control fathers. However, exposure to the film did *not* result in more diapering and feeding of female infants, nor were there any effects for ordinal position. Exposure to a film in the hospital increased father participation in the caretaking of their three-month-old infants in the home—if the infants were male; there were no film/control differences between fathers of girls. Nor were there any differences in levels of father-infant play.

In summary, the film intervention significantly modified selected aspects of father behavior and attitudes both in the hospital and through the first three months of their infants' lives. Of particular interest is the finding that the level of father participation in feeding and diapering increased as a result of this very limited intervention even after a three-month period—at least in the case of boys. The heightened impact of the film for fathers of boys merits comment. The most plausible explanation for this finding is a predispositional one. Since fathers are already differentially predisposed to interact more with male infants than female infants, the film served to strengthen these already existing tendencies. There is a substantial body of literature in support of this claim that fathers anticipate and actually show higher involvement with male than with female infants (see Parke, 1978 for a review). Similarly, previous social influence research is consistent with the view that further change in a direction that is already favored is easier to produce than change in a nonfavored direction (McGuire, 1968).

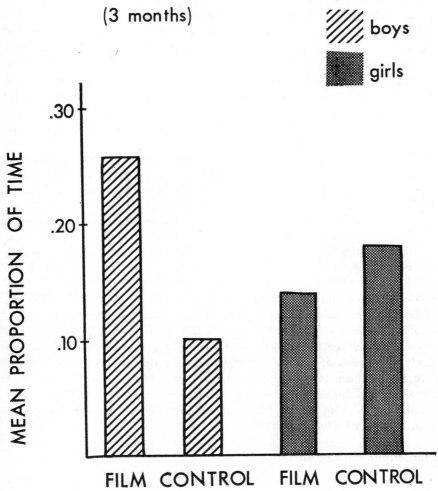

FATHER FEEDING PARTICIPATION
(3 months)

boys

girls

MEAN PROPORTION OF TIME

.30

.20

.10

FILM CONTROL   FILM CONTROL

FIG. 2

DISCUSSION

It is assumed that the relatively enduring impact of the film on father involvement is, in part, mediated by changes in attitudes and values concerning the propriety of male involvement in early child care activities. The results of this program illustrate the feasibility and effectiveness of using the hospital period as a point of intervention for fathers. Further research is necessary both to determine which aspects of the film presentation were most effective in producing these changes and to determine ways in which the involvement of fathers of girls can be successfully increased.

The role that the mother plays in mediating these effects also merits detailed examination in future research. Does the knowledge that their husbands participated in our film program modify wives' expectations concerning the level of caretaking that they anticipate from their husbands? Unfortunately, we do not have any relevant data on this issue. Although our film intervention was restricted to fathers, it is likely that mothers' behaviors were modified as well. An analysis of the mothers who participated in this study is currently underway and should yield some information on the secondary effects of the father film on the mother's behavior. Just as Klaus and Gray (1968) found that the siblings of the child who participated in a cognitive intervention program also benefited, it is not unlikely that the mother would be affected by the type of father intervention program that we have described. Perhaps the quality of the mother's involvement with the infant is modified as a consequence of either the direct imitation of the father's behavior or more likely as a result of the relief that increased father involvement in child care allows the mother. Implicit in this discussion is an endorsement of the view that the family should be conceptualized as a social system in which the roles of all of the members are viewed as interdependent (Parke, Power & Gottman, 1978).

Limitations and Considerations

Any intervention program must be sensitive to the value system of the target population. This is especially true in dealing with the distribution of infant caregiving responsibilities. In spite of the characteristically American slogan that "more is always better," it is inappropriate to attempt to increase father's involvement without considering the *family's* views on the division of family responsibilities for each member. Although cultural and social norms and values are changing, we cannot assume *arbitrarily* that fathers and mothers in all types of families should share all tasks equally in early caregiving and early social interaction. Our task is to facilitate and legitimize father involvement so that fathers are capable of engaging in early caretaking to the extent that families feel is most optimal.

In families where a great deal of direct involvement is unrealistic, the father can be involved in numerous indirect ways—by being supportive of the mother. As discussed earlier, Pedersen, Anderson and Cain (1977) recently demonstrated that the quality of the husband-wife relationship is positively correlated with the quality of mother-infant relations. In families where the father was more supportive of the mother (e.g., evaluated her maternal skills more positively), the mother was more effective in caretaking activities such as feeding. The reverse holds true for marital discord. High tension and conflict in the marriage were associated with less competent feeding on the part of the mother. Thus, increased, direct involvement by fathers in infant care may not necessarily be better if more involvement is threatening to the mother and contributes to tension between the parents. We should, therefore, make cultural support systems available to fathers, but permit fathers to determine their own level of involvement in routine caretaking activities. However, by legitimizing father participation in caretaking, fathers will be more likely to participate and execute these tasks effectively and view these behaviors as role consistent.

Expansion of parent-support programs such as ours should include special parenting problems associated with premature or handicapped infants for whom an optimal caretaking environment is especially important. As suggested above, the father's assistance in the feeding, diapering, and stimulation of a premature or handicapped infant may have a significant impact on the mother's ability to cope following the stress involved with the birth of such an infant. This, in turn, will increase the rate with which the family regains equilibrium.

Fathers can and will share infant caretaking and play with mothers. By treating the father as a legitimate member of the family and by encouraging and expecting him to contribute positively to the infant's caretaking environment, risks for infants should be reduced. In the final analysis, reducing psychosocial risk is our goal.

9

Pain-Filled Fruit of the Tree of Knowledge: Problems and Paradoxes in the Sanctity of Life

BERNARD Z. FRIEDLANDER

University of Hartford

Most professional people subscribe to prevailing views on appropriate roles for the mothers and fathers of high risk infants and severely disabled children. These views are based on popular assumptions about the characteristics of good parental behavior. But these popular views are, in fact, limited to a very narrow range of contemporary values. This narrow range of approved values places high demands on the parents of severely disabled babies and children to follow a strict behavior code that stresses attachment, sacrifice, repression, and self-denial.

This code denies that the parents of severely disabled children might have intense and fundamental feelings of anger, resentment, and desire for escape from problems for which there are no easy solutions. Further, this code ignores exceptionally powerful and pervasive forces in our culture that broadly encourage self-indulgence, superficial happiness, and belief in easy solutions to complex difficulties. It also denies access to problem solving measures that are deeply embedded in phylogenetic and human history.

As helping professionals, we must confront the fact that the agonies and perplexities of dealing with severely impaired infants are inescapably bound-up in our work. These agonies and perplexities should force us to question our basic values about the sanctity and quality of human life.

This article is based on the transcription of a verbal presentation delivered *ex tempore* from notes. I am very grateful to Joy Penticuff and Mary Anne Winston for their editorial assistance.

190

As professionals, we have come to accept the myth that the close, constructive, supportive, self-actualizing family network is a commonplace in contemporary society. We assume it has always been the operating model for effective family life and we regard it as a norm to which all should subscribe. I assert that we must reexamine that proposition.

In the last few decades we have erected an idealized structure as to what constitutes the skeleton, the ligaments, and the integument that hold families together. We count on *love* as the exclusive bonding agent of family connectedness. Yet, until very modern times attitudes about other values such as property, loyalty, obedience, discipline, authority, and dynasty were the fibers that made up the fabric of family bonding. It is only since the later 19th century in American life that love has become idealized as the fundamental frequency in the chords of family living. It is only recently that children have gained an emotional role to play as individuals in family life that goes beyond their significance as economic units and agents for satisfying the parents' personal wishes.

With this short history in mind, we should consider very carefully whether or not it is fair to expect or demand a family style based on self-actualizing love bonds from parents of a severely impaired baby or young child. In fact, when we make this demand or project this expectation, we may make a significant error of underlying assumptions.

The narrow range of approved values—self-actualizing love, family solidarity, and togetherness and sharing—places high demands on parents to be supportive and to develop a fulfilling love bond between parent and child. In fact, the preexisting styles of interpersonal and family relationships before the birth of the impaired child may offer little or no room for that kind of bonding to flourish in the way we professionals idealize it. The behavior code of the "stiff upper lip" courage we expect from parents of severely disabled children denies the validity of powerful and fundamental feelings parents may have of anger, resentment, rejection, and longing for escape from permanent problems. These are the feelings that parents actually express when their guard is down, or that the sensitive observer detects.

In my experience, it is a very rare parent counselor who has the knowledge of inner psychic life and the security of his or her own value system to be able to allow parents to express their intense negative feelings about the harshly limiting effect on their child's and their own lives that stem from their child's impairment. It is rare for parents to acknowledge or express the haunting, constant wrath that will not go away when every act, decision, or emotion is filtered through the intrapsychic sieve of demands, responsibilities, and guilts associated with the continued existence of the endlessly needful child. It is not unnatural or inhumane for such parents occasionally to experience the wish for the death of their severely impaired child. Yet because the death wish is taboo, as well as being so poorly understood, its legitimacy is denied to most parents who seek help. Consequently, the wish and the guilts arising from it are additional burdens they must cope with without genuine assistance.

With a normal baby there are many compensations available in the present, and in prospects for the future, that ease the burden associated with the infant's need for constant care. These compensations seldom exist when a baby is severely disabled. The parents often feel that they are perpetually imprisoned by their child's unrelenting needs. The continuing, unending dependence of the severely impaired child obliges the parents to adapt to an almost total revision of their sense of self and of the outside world.

Visions of a decent life for ordinary people in modern America revolve about images of ease and convenience. But life cannot be easy and convenient for parents who are totally bound to feeding a severely cerebral palsied baby whose feeding takes hours out of every day. Life cannot be easy and convenient for the parents of an innocently destructive autistic child who can pull a room to pieces in an unwatched minute. Life cannot be easy and convenient for the parents of a multiply handicapped deaf-blind child who can never be expected to perform the simplest acts of self-care. These parents must endure a constant struggle between fantasies of an easy life they feel might otherwise be theirs and the reality of the hard life they take every day with its endless burdens and special requirements of child care.

Current value systems for imposing expectations of attachment, sacrifice, and self-denial upon the parents of severely disabled babies also deny these parents access to problem solving measures that are deeply embedded in human history. At other times and in other places it has been legitimate for individuals to confront the crisis of severe disability directly by acting upon the impulse to terminate life. Our present value structure with its many pretensions about reverence for life and sanctity of life, and especially of infant life, represents what is at best only an incomplete sample of the great variety of ways in which people have dealt with the manifold complexities which arise from the birth and existence of the seriously impaired infant.

It is impossible to draw a clear, hard line between points that define levels of disability, probabilities of recovery, capacities for adaptation, and values surrounding normality and the quality of life. It is equally impossible to specify who should be empowered to make life and death decisions in the absence of clear definitions. Yet, for every child's life that is extended happily by our impressive modern technologies, there may be another child's life that is extended in agony—the agony either of the child itself or the agony of those who must care for and pay for the child's marginal state of being that doesn't quite flicker out. Such extended lifetimes of physical suffering and mental anguish may result in neglect, blame, marital disruption, exhaustion, abuse, and financial catastrophe.

Only people who have experienced child disability in their own families or who have some special sensitivity and capacity for empathy have an awareness of the kind of pain that occurs in having to deal with perpetual disability. The pain has several levels. In part it is a matter of sheer physical pain that cannot be controlled by medication. In part it is a matter of coping with the demands of everyday life and the wholly justifiable anxiety about the ability to do so. In part it is a matter of unfulfilled hopes associated with parenthood. In part it is profound anxiety, shame, guilt, sorrow, and magical fears that the child's condition is punishment for the parents' own misbehavior. In part it is fear of and resentment against the effects of the child's status on marital life and parental sexuality. In part it is deeply embedded fear and rage that God or Creation can impose such a brutal act as to destroy both the infant's and the parents' potential for a normal life.

An interesting sidelight on the phenomenon of parental rage is now becoming visible in the research on relationships between child disability and child abuse. There are indications that a disproportionately large number of abused children are children with disabilities (Parke & Collmer, 1975). It appears that in many cases the children who need the most in terms of love and support and assistance with their adaptive coping are the ones who receive anger, rage, and resentment from parents who boil over explosively in frustration at their own helplessness, and in reaction against what life has done in giving them a disabled child.

One of the most instructive contacts I ever had with the parent of a disabled child was with the perpetually angry father of a severely involved cerebral palsied girl who was terrified of every adult in the clinic until she discovered by repeated experience that some adults would be kind to her. This father said bitterly on one occasion, "This God of yours has lousy quality control in his kid factory. If I got a car from Detroit that worked as badly as my girl's arms, I'd raise hell until they fixed it.

And if they didn't fix it, I'd raise more hell and burn down the god-damned plant where it was made."

I was outraged by his crudeness at the time, but the more I think about that man the more I suspect there may be a share of his anger lurking and waiting to come out in many of the seemingly calmer parents whom we expect to meet their children's needs with a spirit of acceptance, sacrifice, and nobility.

It is especially objectionable to ordinary people trying to cope with their difficult lives when noble stereotypes of saintly parental virtue that only a few can attain are generalized and held forth as desirable models for all. It seems to be the custom in some child care facilities to find parents who are particularly successful in dealing with their disabled child—parents who are especially rich in the capacity to give love and support—and idealize them as models other parents are implicitly expected to emulate. It is certainly inspirational and beautiful to behold when an elevated level of dealing with misfortune rises naturally from people's characterological endowment, their way of dealing with what life has to offer, both good and bad. But when these inspirational models are laid on others—more ordinary people—as an expectation, as a template or stencil for how they *should* feel and how they *should* react to what may be the most distressing of life experiences, then they are traps that deny people the validity of their real and inescapable feelings.

This problem is compounded when differences in social class and prestige expand the gulf between stricken parents struggling to cope with disaster and professional helpers who are bystanders to the catastrophe. It is an especially ugly form of social class imperialism when upscale professionals impose their own class-bound value norms in judging both the behavior and the emotional responses of downscale clients. The behavioral and emotional value norms of social classes and ethnic groups different from their own may be far more adaptive to the realities of actual life circumstances in the clients' world than the professional workers can readily imagine.

I don't like to be reminded of some of the case conferences I've attended where the full roster of an eminent treatment team made judgments about the apparently negligent mother who had not visited her salvaged, institutionalized, vegetative child in many months or many years. In my reflections now, I think the absent mother, struggling with other life demands, may have shown more life wisdom in seeking to bury the helpless past in the best way she knew how than the professionals who criticized her for doing so.

Newspaper accounts of the Karen Ann Quinlan case and recent interest on the part of medical ethicists point to the fact that there is increasing openness in discussions of terminating life as an alternative to the prolonging of life without dignity or meaning. However, it can be the most painful agony that professional child nurturers must deal with when the downward trajectory of the child's inevitable death is imposed upon doctors, nurses, and attendants who feel that it is their highest mission to provide healing and to support life. Once it has been decided not to support life—to adopt a strategy of passive euthanasia—it is rare to find situations in which the end of life occurs with dignity and purpose. It is more often the case that the end of life occurs with a sense of evasion, furtiveness, pain, and distress. In some cases, the parents' wishes to withdraw or not to initiate life-sustaining procedures are overruled by the community through court action. It may well be that the society which imposes a marginal existence upon the child, who is thus "saved," and upon the family, which must provide for its care, is ultimately unconcerned about its responsibilities for the pain of these individual lives that it has dictated must be lived. Does our society feel that we collectively have fulfilled our responsibility simply by activating and implementing the legal powers of the state?

Aside from the disturbing realities of the emotional pain and effort expended by the severely disabled child's family, there comes the realization that vast amounts of money are required for the maintenance of life of children in institutions for the seriously impaired. At a conservative estimate of $10,000 per child per year, the cost of sustaining life for the quarter to half a million children with serious disabilities approaches five billion dollars annually. One of the galling facts in caring for the seriously disabled is that there is seldom enough money available to do all the worthwhile things for the children's benefit that might be done or that ought to be done. We see that the home care of the grossly impaired child imposes exceptional stresses on family life and frequently disrupts marriages and the lives of siblings, yet it is also clear that institutional care often does not improve the quality of life for the child, but merely extends existence, and at enormous cost.

When we deal with these topics, we must recognize that we are engaged in conscious negotiation of termination of the seriously impaired infant's life, as an act of choice. It is difficult to imagine any other topic that is so heavily cloaked in taboo, especially among the general public and among people who find the meaning in their own lives in nurturing and supporting the lives of others. Professional workers can go home after a day's work to live their own lives of family, recreation, or further study, while the client goes home from the clinic still having to cope with a broken baby, who will *always* be there.

Within the constraints of present laws and values, it is possible to offer greater comfort and wider alternatives than are generally available to help the stricken parents of severely disabled infants and children. It is not enough just to develop new studies and new technologies to attempt to maintain and repair the children themselves. More compassion, greater understanding, and wider life options must be mobilized to give suffering parents the help they really need to cope with their agonizing plight. This help can take many forms—from depth psychology to the deep waters of local, state, and national politics where public funds are apportioned as proof or disproof of society's real commitment to the sanctity of life.

Finally, and fundamentally, we must be prepared to deal with death as a negotiable option. We must stand face to face with the issues of living and dying. We must look with courage upon the honesty of decent death, just as we cultivate our faith in the sanctity of hopeful life.

Commentaries on Chapter 9

Infanticide, Parental Crisis, and the Double-Edged Sword: A Commentary

LARRY A. BUGEN

St. Edwards University

Friedlander's observations offer us a reasonable perspective regarding some significant stressors and concomitant strains which accompany the birth of a severely disabled child. In particular: (1) Enculturated role stereotypes often do dictate parental behaviors such as "attachment, sacrifice, repression and self-denial"; (2) negative feeling states such as anger are typically considered unacceptable human responses—even in response to unwanted, decremental transitions (Bugen, 1979a) such as defective births or infanticide; and (3) the development of psychosocial resources may mollify the traumatic effects of coping with severely disabled children.

Friedlander, as well as Fletcher (this volume), Diamond (this volume), and Hawkins (this volume) all argue for more compassion, greater understanding, greater comfort and wider options for the agonized parents of disabled infants. The clear implication is that increased primary and secondary preventive efforts may reduce the incidence and severity of emotional duress associated with infant trauma. As a counseling/community psychologist, I would certainly be an anomaly if I were not in favor of such humanistic proposals. In addition to supporting such essential mental health efforts as these, however, it is also important to provide a somewhat pessimistic backdrop to this scene of parents of high-risk infants.

One of the apparent alternatives for parents in the Friedlander viewpoint is passive euthanasia. Since the infants would themselves not be capable of participating in the decision, the responsibility obviously lies with the medical support staff and/or parents. By participating in the

197

decision for elective death, parents would be spared the prolonged stress of maintaining a defective child and may even experience a more rapid resolution of the grief process (Benfield, Lieb, & Vollman, 1978). Numerous examples of increased control and participation in the death-related decision-making by lay persons can be seen in regard to living wills, Laetrile debates, funeral prearrangement, and right-to-die legislation. These issues have been elaborated on in regard to quality of life issues elsewhere (Bugen, 1979b).

As important as parental involvement appears to be in regard to infant elective death, the very process of participating in the decision may complicate grief and actually prolong the response. Bugen (1977) has hypothesized that two dimensions—closeness of relationship and griever's belief in the preventability of death—interact to predict both intensity and duration of bereavement.

(1) An intense and prolonged grief process may be expected when a central relationship exists and a belief that the death could have been prevented is maintained.

(2) An intense but brief mourning period would be expected when a central relationship exists in the absence of a belief in preventability.

(3) A mild but prolonged grief response would be expected of a peripheral relationship where a belief in preventability existed.

(4) A mild but brief mourning process would be expected in peripheral relations where a belief in preventability did not exist.

Parents involved in decisions regarding infanticide would be expected to experience intense and prolonged grief since their relationships with their infants are close and their participation with the process of euthanasia is related to preventability. A double-edged sword for these parents therefore seems to exist. Their choice is one of prolonged stress (that is, preserving life) or prolonged grief (that is, electing death).

Primary and secondary prevention programs might be helpful in dealing with this predictable stress and/or grief; however, one NIMH spokesperson (Goldston, 1976) has warned that numerous barriers must be overcome for such efforts to be effective:

(1) Sufficient scientific evidence must be obtained which documents the efficacy of primary prevention.

(2) Prevention has little political clout in that its constituency is small in number.

(3) Professional mental health workers are typically trained with traditional clinical concerns in mind.

(4) Fiscal allocations for primary prevention activities are usually inadequate at best; at worst, nonexistent.

(5) Public health values continue to be held as inferior to clinical values.

Assuming that the above barriers could be surmounted, we must still be realistic about the severity of such a loss as infanticide. The birth and subsequent death of an infant represent significant life events. Much evidence (Holmes & Rahe, 1967; Dohrenwend & Dohrenwend, 1974) suggests that recent life events relate to the precipitation of illness episodes if significant readjustment is necessary. Using the Social Readjustment Rating Scale (Holmes & Rahe, 1967), we can readily see that parents of high-risk infants would experience the following life events in a very brief period of time: (1) pregnancy, (2) gain of a new family member, (3) change of financial state, (4) change in living conditions, (5) change in personal habits, (6) change in social activities, (7) change in sleeping habits, (8) change in eating habits, (9) change in health of family member, and (10) death of close family member. The Social Readjustment Rating Scale assigns point values to these life events which reflect the amount of readjustment a person has to make in life as a result of the changes. The magnitude of the readjustment required by these ten life events alone totals over 300 points and constitutes a major life crisis with a 79% likelihood of concomitant physical illness (Holmes & Rahe, 1967).

Parents of high-risk infants will need to marshall all available resources to endure such a momentous life crisis. There is a clear need for increased primary and secondary prevention efforts to provide support for these parents. However, we must also be cautious with our expectations for positive resolutions. Parents who enter the arena of choice must understand the implications of their decision, i.e., the dilemma of the "double-edged sword." Neither the choice to preserve life nor that to elect death is likely to bring about a swift resolution to the parents' crisis and assuage their suffering. Instead, parents and professionals are faced with deciding the "least painful resolution" for each case. Parents giving birth to high-risk infants, therefore, (1) should have a realistic understanding of the magnitude of their life crisis, (2) should understand the risks of their involvement in the decision-making process, and (3) should be linked with a viable environmental support network throughout their ordeal, no matter which painful choice they make.

A Physician's Perspective on the Problems and Paradoxes in the Sanctity of Life

ANNE B. FLETCHER

George Washington University
and Children's Hospital National Medical Center,
Washington

Although one may basically agree with the Friedlander's premises, it is appropriate to take with a "grain of salt" his representation of the prevailing views of professional people and their thoughts on appropriate parental roles, parental emotions, and contemporary values of severely disabled infants. In point of fact, professionals', parents', and society's views of what should or should not be done in the perpetuation of certain infants' lives have been changing. In many institutions, life and death decisions are being made by parents and professionals. It is unfortunate that changes in contemporary values regarding the quality and the sanctity of life have been addressed more in theory in the literature than by citing what is actually practiced when a damaged infant's life is in question (Fost, 1976; Report on the 65th Ross Conference on Pediatric Research, October 1973; Jansen & Garland, 1976). The stresses and benefits for parents of defective or dying children have been documented, as have the grief responses and follow-up of parents who experience a perinatal death (Benfield et al., 1978; Rowe et al., 1978; Kennell et al., 1970).

There is no doubt that, with the advent of neonatal intensive care in the early 1960s, there has been an increase in survival of smaller premature infants and those with hyaline membrane disease. A number of studies suggest that there has been a concomitant decrease in the morbidity on follow-up (Fitzhardinge, 1976; Pape et al., 1978; Stewart and Reynolds, 1974). It is obvious, however, that with the modern technology of today some "unfit" infants are still being kept alive that would once have died. Thus, ethical and moral decisions of "how far to go" have begun to receive considerable attention in the literature, newspapers and journals. A recent conference on Ethical Issues in Newborn Care attended by a multidisciplinary group in California attempted to deal with four issues (Jansen & Garland, 1976):

   (1) Would it ever be right not to resuscitate an infant at birth?

   (2) Would it ever be right to withdraw life support from a clearly diagnosed poor prognosis infant?

   (3) Would it ever be right to intervene directly to kill a self-sustaining infant?

   (4) Would it ever be right to displace poor prognosis infant A in order to provide intensive care to better prognosis infant B?

All participants responded yes to numbers 1 and 2. Most said yes to 3 and 4. Examples and criteria were given for each issue. A few responded by saying that their answers were based on belief and theory rather than on what they could do in actuality. While this is a beginning, it is far from a solution.

Infanticide, while widely practiced both actively and passively until the 20th century, is no longer acceptable at least in its active form. Thus, an alternative plan must be found and practiced by modern neonatologists. To date, individual infants with Down's syndrome and those with severe meningomyeloceles have by far received the most attention as possible candidates for passive euthanasia (Lebaiqz, 1972; *Pediatric News*, December, 1973; Colen, 1974; Lorber, 1973; Stein et al., 1974). Differences in opinions continue to exist (Ames & Schut, 1972). There are those who would still give medical and nursing care no matter what the outcome. Only two pediatricians, Duff and Campbell (1976), have actually put into print that 14% of their infant mortality was due to cessation of treatment that was no longer helpful. Others would tell us that the withholding or termination of treatment may have criminal liability and that following the legal process and changing inappropriate laws are preferable to establishing criteria for those classes of infants who should be allowed to die (Robertson & Fost, 1976). It is unlikely that either changing the laws or setting up classifications will be sufficient. Each infant has to be considered individually, in his own parental environment and social and economic situation. Therefore, it would appear that while decisions about infant lives are being made and will continue they will have to be thought through in a more organized fashion and with better parental guidance and support.

How then should decisions be made and how is one to change the philosophy of those who refuse to make them? With the exception of certain infants who definitely should not be resuscitated at birth (i.e., the anencephalics, those grossly hydrocephalic or the stillborn, just to name a few), there must be sufficient time for observation. This time may vary from a few hours to weeks depending on the infant's condition. This observation time will allow mature, objective assessment, appropriate testing, and time for neurologic evaluation which is often difficult in the premature infant. Decisions are usually ultimately made by the physician in charge with agreement and understanding of the parents, although much input comes from nursing, resident physicians, social service, and the clergy. All of the concerned individuals, but particularly the parents, must be allowed to pass through the stages of shock, denial, and depression, until they can accept the decision. This preparation can often be integrated with the time of observation if communications are open and ongoing. On occasion, infanticide would seem easier, with less suffering of the infant and others involved. This, however, is illegal; thus, withdrawing therapy is preferable.

How to change the philosophy of some of those giving care to ill infants is a more difficult subject. It is not easy to change a basic or subconscious feeling. Certainly changes in health sciences curricula with at least some emphasis on ethical and moral issues would help. Dealing with and discussing these issues in professional residency and fellowship programs have been useful. Society has become more aware of the possibility for life-death decisions through newspaper accounts of the Karen Ann Quinlan case. Test cases in the courts have and will continue to arise. Yet, that these can or should lead to new laws or change old ones, particularly on such controversial ethical issues, is probably inappropriate and impossible. Despite cessation of therapy for severely damaged newborns, some infants exit from the nursery with extremely poor developmental prognosis because there has been no opportunity for choice. Thus physicians and others must push for better development of follow-up and supportive facilities, institutions, and financial support to aid the parent and their defective child.

Though sometimes overquoted for exactly the opposite reasons, it would still be wise to remember that part of the Hippocratic Oath which says:

I will follow that method of treatment which according to my ability and judgment I consider for the benefit of my patients and abstain from what is deleterious and mischievous.

We as physicians need to remind ourselves of the *quality of life,* that which is so hard to define and measure, and not just the *quantity* of life. In answer to Dr. Friedlander, we are headed in the direction he suggests but he should remember that the possibility of error always exists in decision-making. Yet this possibility for error must be lived with in spite of its finality.

Perspectives on Decisions for Nontreatment of Damaged Newborns

JAMES M. DIAMOND

Kaiser Permanente Medical Center
South San Francisco, California

To see infants born with profound damage or deformity, whether these infants live or die, surely brings pain to all of us, and particularly to the parents of these infants. Yet the increasing ability which medicine now has to prolong such lives certainly has brought with it an increment in the pain, because it has added an entirely new sort of torture which centers around the making of moral decisions. Medical technology forces upon us acts of judgment for which we must now take responsibility, rather than blaming nature or God. In what follows, I will give the thoughts of one who has participated in the making of some of these uncomfortable decisions to treat or to withhold treatment, and who has tried to understand the values and constraints which surround such decisions. I want to emphasize that my focus is not on right and wrong, but on the process of medical decision making.

Most of us realize that there is no scientific basis upon which to decide matters such as whether to do everything possible in order to save the life of a severely neurologically damaged child. In Great Britain, a myelomeningocele at the L2 level will generally not be repaired, whereas in this country physicians with very similar training, expertise, and personal value systems will operate (to prevent meningitis) within 24 hours (Ellis, 1974; Stein et al., 1974; Freeman, 1973; Lorber, 1971, 1972). We may adduce all sort of arguments having to do with mental constructs such as mortality, ethics, religion, responsibility, but decisions like this are not likely to become any easier as our technical knowledge increases.

Crucial elements about any ethical decision are who makes it, and for whose benefit. In these cases, the decision is always supposed to be for the benefit of the infant (patient), yet interpreting this benefit and translating it into action are the responsibility of the parents and physicians. Parents should act not for their own benefit, not for the benefit of their family unit, but for the benefit of the particular infant for whom a decision is being made. This is, I believe, the heaviest demand made upon them. Yet when parents are asked whether a respirator should be stopped, whether death should be allowed a victory, the very fact that they are being consulted, rather than having the decision announced by the physician, tells them that they are expected to speak in the child's interest. All of us must recognize that this is so, just as parents must feel the responsibility to live up to a code of "attachment, sacrifice . . . self-denial" (Friedlander, this volume), for if they say something such as "I don't want her to live if she may need to go to special schools," we all feel very uncomfortable, realizing that we have no license to kill those who may need special schooling. In such cases the parents have really forfeited their small right to input into medical decisions because they have not understood and lived up to the narrow rules which, though unwritten, circumscribe these delicate negotiations of life and death.

Those who can find a way to escape pain generally do so, and physicians are no exception. We have, I believe, three main escapes. The first and probably the most used is to keep doing everything within our powers to prolong life, so that in fact we take responsibility only for our competence, not for our ultimate judgment that it would be better if our patient were to die. If the patient dies, it is a defeat for us, but we are able to avoid the *decision* for the death until there is virtually no decision left, until there is no chance for survival. Second, and complementing this first means of escape, we have what we call our professional ethics. This is at one and the same time a code of conduct which others expect of us, which we impose on ourselves, and which we suppose to be rooted in important religious or moral values. However, as I and others have argued elsewhere (Rachels, 1975; Fletcher, 1975), a most significant thing about medical ethics is that even though it is all these things, it is not consistent, and cannot be used as the basis for logical decision making when the issue is whether to allow or hasten death. Third is the escape by which we give responsibility for such a painful decision to the family of our patient. This escape is actually an expression of our professional ethics. To quote the AMA House of Delegates (December, 1973):

> The cessation of the employment of extraordinary means to prolong the life of the body when there is irrefutable evidence that biological

death is imminent is the decision of the patient and/or his immediate family. The advice and judgment of the physician should be freely available. . . .

We thus claim that even the inevitable should be the responsibility of others—if not God, then patient or family. To the psychologist, sociologist, or anthropologist, these devices are undoubtedly transparent. Speaking as a physician, I can attest that it has taken me great effort to put these mechanisms in a social perspective, and that despite my hard-won psychological insights, I use these devices almost as second nature when I am confronted with the prospect of infant euthanasia. Indeed, physicians who act otherwise may run grave legal risks (Robertson & Fost, 1976).

Now what of the rights of parents? The role we leave to them is little more than to relieve the physician of pain. We physicians take their expressed desires into account only as far as is comfortable. This may vary with the physician, but it is an interesting fact that those who become neonatal specialists become treatment enthusiasts almost without exception. I suspect this is a question of the physician increasingly using the first pain escape mechanism mentioned above to deal with the steadily increasing amounts of pain they would otherwise be required to face. To a certain extent, it may also be that those who go into this field are those with a special desire to seek technological solutions to difficult problems. No matter, in any case they are among the forefront of those who are "denying the release of death and healing grief to the parents of children with shattered lives" (Friedlander, this volume).

As the grief-stricken parents of these shattered children negotiate with individual physicians, too many times every day, too many times every week, let us realize that there is a problem which goes beyond the sum of all the individual tragedies involved, massive as that is. There is a problem in decision making. To place this latter problem in context, one need but recall that in this world of ours, human potential is everywhere held in check in thonsands of ways by poverty, prejudice, and the structure of institutions. The decision to try to prevent the death of one defective newborn restricts decisions we might wish to make for the benefit of other children. The equivalent of the monthly salary for a public health nurse is spent on one hopeless infant during one day—and this example is multiplied in most intensive care nurseries so often that one soon stops mentioning the irony of it. There you have the true nature of the problem. If you would solve it, I urge you to help bring about decision making by those who will be in the best position to benefit from the alternatives: thus a community could decide that instead of a new infant warmer and respirator being purchased, auto safety seats should be provided free on loan to the parents of every newborn. Note that this is a decision in favor of saving lives! I think society and medical practice will both be served if they can ally themselves to form more decisions of this sort. If we don't, the monumental diversion of resources must be counted a far smaller price than the perversion of priorities which results.

Alternatives to Passive Euthanasia for Ameliorating the Psychosocial Burdens of Parents Giving Birth to Severely Damaged Infants

RAYMOND C. HAWKINS, II

The University of Texas at Austin

This volume has been concerned with identifying psychosocial risk factors which may place certain infants and their parents at a disadvantage for optimal cognitive and social development. Friedlander (this volume) presents a provocative emotional and ethical argument that recent medical technological advances enabling extraordinary life sustaining efforts for severely damaged infants may impose substantial psychosocial burdens upon the parents. The prevailing professional ethical code emphasizing the "sanctity of life" is alleged to encourage excessive parenting efforts and self-sacrifice which may exceed the tolerance levels of some parents who give birth to defective infants. Indeed, the negative psychosocial impact of having a damaged infant may be substantial (for a review, see Gorham et al. 1975; Suran & Rizzo, 1979). Violation of parental expectations for a healthy, responsive infant may pose difficulties for the formation of optimal caregiver-infant bonding (Zaslow & Breger, 1969), which in turn may compound the effects of biophysical disabilities and increase the likelihood of impaired infant development (Hawkins, this volume). More importantly, however, are the detrimental effects upon the parents and the family of having a severely damaged infant: depression, hostility, sexual dysfunctions, increased risk for marital discord and divorce, as well as relative neglect of the developmental needs of healthy siblings (Benfield, Leib, & Vollman, 1978; Mcintyre, 1977; Rowe, Clyman, Green, Mikkelsen, Haight, & Ataide, 1978; Suran & Rizzo, 1979). Friedlander also argues that disadvantaged families from lower social class backgrounds may be particularly oppressed by these prevailing values.

Two remedies are offered for alleviating the suffering of parents of severely defective infants. The first is a substantial increase in supportive services and financial aid at the local, state, and federal levels for the affected parents. The second remedy, by far the more provocative and controversial, would be to allow parents, with sufficient counsel from professional personnel, to opt for letting a severely defective infant die, i.e. passive euthanasia. Preceding commentaries by Fletcher (this volume) and by Diamond (this volume) have acknowledged the importance of the Friedlander viewpoint. Fletcher agrees that professionals are moving in the direction that Friedlander proposes, and Diamond is concerned with improving the decision-making process through which life sustaining efforts are provided or withheld from damaged infants. The thorny question, alluded to by Diamond, is "Who decides (medical personnel, parents, and/or legal authorities), and on the basis of what criteria?"

With regard to the first remedy, it is very probably true that successful life sustaining efforts may present considerable psychosocial burdens to parents having severely defective infants. Furthermore, it would seem prudent to consider mechanisms for providing additional support systems for primary and secondary prevention efforts for assisting such parents. Admittedly, increased usage of the option of passive euthanasia might somewhat reduce the numbers of defective infants and children receiving custodial care in state institutions with a resultant savings that could be passed on to prevention/intervention programs for the affected families. But are there "viable" alternatives to passive euthanasia for ameliorating the reality-based and intrapsychic psychosocial burdens imposed upon parents of these defective infants?

This question brings us to the first *caveat* for Friedlander's viewpoint: Medical, legal, ethical decision-making is obviously culture bound. Persons from certain ethnic, racial, and socioeconomic backgrounds would not even entertain the thought of infanticide. For example, a defective infant may be regarded as a "visitation from God" justifying self-sacrifice on the part of the parents (Suran & Rizzo, 1979). Certainly, such differences in cultural value orientations (Papajohn & Spiegel, 1975) need to be recognized in this policy making. Indeed, one study has shown that the presence of certain religious beliefs, educational background, and availability of indigenous social support networks may enable some parents to accept relatively comfortably even the most severe infant disabilities (Zuk, Miller, Bartram, & Kling, 1961, as cited by Suran & Rizzo, 1979). It would be a serious error to substitute a new set of cultural values emphasizing the importance of parental self-interest and of the infant's potential for "beauty, brains, and productivity" as a standard for determining whether life sustaining efforts should be administered for infants with severe defects, in place of more traditional values emphasizing the sanctity of life.

Given this cultural-ethical *caveat*, we need to consider carefully the question of whether mobilization of social/financial supports can ameliorate the negative psychosocial burdens of sustaining the life of a severely defective infant. More research is needed to determine if this remedy will work. Such as perspective, if feasible, would allow us to bypass the emotionally charged and philosophically unanswerable question of whether the parents' anguish outweighs the suffering of a severely damaged infant who is allowed to slowly die. Furthermore, provision of financial and social supports for parents concurrent with maintaining every effort to sustain the life of their damaged infant would permit continued medical research that may yield invaluable knowledge about the natural course of genetically or congenitally based defects, as well as possible biochemical and/or psychosocial interventions that may improve the quality of life for such infants.

What, then, might be some specific alternatives to passive euthanasia? It is beyond the scope of this commentary to elaborate ways in which financial aid might be offered to families and communities for assistance in coping with the psychosocial burdens of rearing defective infants. However, some specific ways of providing information and support to parents in such circumstances should be considered. The first possibility would be the increased use of procedures for diagnosing genetic risks prior to conception (e.g. screening persons of Jewish ancestry for the presence of heterozygote carriers of the genetic recessive Tay-Sachs disease, Kaback, 1977). After conception, but prior to birth, amniocentesis and other techniques may be used to detect congenital anomalies (Lubs & de la Cruz, 1977). Such an increased emphasis upon primary prevention and detection might reduce the incidence of severely defective offspring. Admittedly, this solution would raise other ethical, moral, and legal issues about contraception and abortion, but at least the best available scientific information could be provided to prospective parents. This would perhaps ameliorate the violation of overly optimistic parental expectations and permit a more realistic awareness of the liabilities of producing and caring for a defective infant.

The second alternative, and perhaps the most important one from the standpoint of minimizing parental psychosocial burdens, would be provision of postnatal genetic counseling and adjunctive psychotherapy (Gorham et al. 1975; Lubs & de la Cruz, 1977; Suran & Rizzo, 1979). Recent reviews of genetic counseling (cf. Lubs & de la Cruz, 1977) have shown it to be a promising, effective means of providing accurate, assimilable information to parents with severely defective offspring. This information serves two related goals: (1) assisting parents in evaluating the recurrence risk for defects in subsequent children, and (2) minimizing the reactive guilt, hostility, depression, and other negative outcomes. In many cases it is possible for the genetic counselor to restore the parents' hope that future pregnancies will yield viable, healthy offspring. Provision of accurate information, repeatedly and sensitively presented, may thus lessen the intrapsychic burdens associated with having a defective infant, particularly when this is combined with supportive psychotherapy (McIntyre, 1977*). Providing information about the nature of the genetic or congenitally based defect, and specific suggestions for parenting the defective infant, would not conflict with parental cultural values.

In sum, it can be argued that at the present time the least detrimental alternative for minimizing the suffering of the defective infant and its affected family members would be to increase support via prenatal and postnatal intervention. Further research is desperately needed to document the intensity and longevity of the psychosocial burdens associated with having a severely damaged child, as well as to determine the most effective means for intervening to minimize the negative outcomes of these burdens. As Friedlander suggests, passive euthanasia may be the best option in some select cases. With our present knowledge, however, it is arguable that passive euthanasia may actually increase parents' intrapsychic burdens, relative to the alternative procedures described above. Parents' participation in the decision-making process leading to their infant's death may enhance their guilt and prolong their grief reaction (Bugen, this volume). Therefore, a supportive approach which minimizes conflicts with parental cultural values and personal wishes and provides information for the parents to permit their participation in the decision-making process, without their assuming primary responsibility for determining the fate of their severely damaged infant, seems most appropriate.

---

* McIntyre (1977) defines the goals of such a genetic counseling supportive therapy approach as "(a) helping the couple accept the reality of the situation and giving them an opportunity to ventilate their feelings about it freely and completely without fear of recriminations, (b) strengthening the weakened self-image of each partner, (c) teaching the couple techniques for practicing and achieving more open and honest communication, and (d) helping the couple overcome the sexual dysfunction which is so often present and promoting the development of a full and gratifying sexual relationship" (p. 569).

Part IV

PARENTAL ATTITUDES ABOUT INFANTS: ISSUES IN ASSESSMENT AND IMPLICATIONS FOR PARENTING BEHAVIOR

In the preceding section, several papers deal with situations in which parental expectations for a normal, term infant are violated. Further, the Parke, Hymel, Power, and Tinsley chapter postulates that parental attitudes may be a significant phenomenon in mediating parental behaviors. While research directed to parental attitudes is not new, the field lacks a clearly delineated model of the relationship between parental attitudes and parental behavior. Such a model would be helpful in understanding the interplay of parental attitudes and behaviors which directly lead to psychosocial risk for the infant. In cases such as premature birth or birth of a physically or behaviorally impaired infant, there is the added need for understanding how violation of parental expectations for a normal, term infant may affect parental attitudes and behaviors.

The Pharis and Manosevitz chapter presents a fresh perspective for research on parental attitudes in the concept of parental models, although the question of continuity in parental attitudes across developmental phases is not addressed. As delineated by these authors, parental models encompass models of the infant, the parenting role, and life changes following the birth of the baby. Though the Pharis and Manosevitz chapter only describes parental models during pregnancy, the chapter may lay the ground for longitudinal research which explores the significance of prenatal models for postnatal risk. Parental models may be significant where certain models are associated with risk fostering parental behavior as well as where parental models are violated by infant outcomes, e.g.,

213

congenitally malformed infants or behavioral deviations of small-for-gestational-age (Als, Tronick, Adamson, & Brazelton, 1976) and premature infants (Field, this volume).

The study of parental attitudes is clouded by the ambiguity of the concept of attitudes and other related concepts, such as expectations, beliefs, and affect. In the Walker paper the work of Fishbein is reviewed in an effort to delineate more precisely the concepts of attitudes and beliefs and their relationship to behaviors. Using an unidimensional notion of attitude as affective in nature, the cumulative role of beliefs in shaping attitudes is described. Further, behavior is seen as a function of attitudes as well as societal and personal norms and motivation to comply with these norms. Additional factors (e.g., infant individuality) pertinent to the developing parent-infant relationship are proposed as affecting parental attitudes and behaviors. Methods for both directly and inferentially measuring attitudes are presented in the discussion of the semantic differential and belief statement techniques. The chapter ends with a description of a preliminary research design which incorporates a multivariable orientation to parental attitude research. Reliability data are presented on several instruments measuring early parental attitudes, and continuities and shifts in patterns of attitudes during the neonatal period are described.

While the conceptual orientations adopted by Pharis and Manosevitz and Walker differ, both chapters provide more refined perspectives for the study of parental attitudes. Convergence of such research efforts offers a base for more meaningful assessment of prenatal parental models as well as for postnatal predictive and intervention research programs. While it is not possible to judge the ultimate significance of parental attitudes as a field of study for assessment and intervention in psychosocial risk, these chapters indicate that field holds promise.

10

Parental Models: A Means for Evaluating Different Prenatal Contexts

MARY E. PHARIS and
MARTIN MANOSEVITZ
University of Texas at Austin

Studies of parent-infant interaction during the neonatal period constitute one of the most active areas of developmental research at the present time. Behavioral scientists are observing and recording parent-infant gaze interactions, vocal exchanges, holding styles, and activity "dialogues" in minute detail in the first minutes, days and weeks of an infant's life, even including delivery room observations (Macfarlane, 1977). Elegant designs and methodologies have been developed to chart the typical and atypical developmental patterns of such interactions (see chapters by Bakeman, Sackett, Thoman, & Tronick, this volume; Lewis & Rosenblum, 1974). Individual differences in infants and parents have been studied to determine what they may contribute to the development of parent-infant interaction patterns (Brazelton, 1973c; Carey, 1973; Korner, 1973b; Osofsky, 1976; Thomas & Chess, 1977).

However, there has been little systematic study of the psychosocial aspects of the environment into which a baby is born. By psychosocial aspects of the environment, we mean such variables as socioeconomic status, age of parents, racial and ethnic factors, parental personality, education and prior contact with babies. These variables are associated

We would like to express our thanks to the parents and students who participated in the study, to the staffs of St. David's Hospital and Seton Hospital, Austin, Texas, and to the other professionals who aided in recruitment. This research received funding from the University of Texas Institute of Human Development and a National Science Foundation grant #BNS 76 - 10703, both to Martin Manosevitz, and a predoctoral research fellowship award from NIMH, #MH 05494 to Mary E. Pharis.

with each other and interact in a dynamic manner throughout the life cycle to affect attitudes, expectations, beliefs and behaviors in the realm of parenting. However, in the terminology of systems theory, there is much more study of the components of the system (the infant and the parent) and the dynamics of the system (the patterns of exchange in different modalities) than of the psychosocial environment of the system.

Yet Sameroff (this volume) contends that the major continuities in development may be more closely associated with the contextual differences in which development occurs, such as socioeconomic, racial, or cultural differences, than with specifics of individual behavior. He would argue that, if we hope to predict anything at all about a child's development, it may be more important to know the race and socioeconomic level of that child's parents than the amount of time the mother spent with the infant on its first day of life, the temperament of the infant, or the Bayley scores the child obtained at six months of age. In a fascinating volume edited by Leiderman, Tulkin and Rosenfeld (1977), researchers present papers on cross-cultural and intra-cultural studies of environmental variables which support this contention.

Caldwell's studies with the Home Observation for Measurement of the Environment (HOME) inventory (Bradley & Caldwell, 1976; Elardo, Bradley, & Caldwell, 1975) lend some support to Sameroff's contention. This instrument taps the environment of a home in six specific areas. Variables assessed include the play materials available to the child, the organization of physical and temporal aspects of the environment, and specific aspects of the maternal and paternal interaction with the child. The HOME inventory successfully discriminates between samples of various educational and economic backgrounds (Hollenbeck, 1978) and to some degree may be viewed as a means for operationalizing those socioeconomic contextual differences to which Sameroff calls our attention. It is, therefore, of particular interest that scores on the HOME inventory correlate more highly with a child's score at age three on the Stanford-Binet Intelligence Scale than does the child's own score on the Bayley Scales of Infant Development given at six months (Elardo et al., 1975).

Moreover, in an analysis of data from a large subsample of the Collaborative Perinatal Research Project, Willerman, Broman and Fiedler (1970) have also shown that parental socioeconomic status may affect the child's intellectual development. For a child from a lower socioeconomic status home, as classified by paternal education, occupation and income, a score in the lowest quartile on the Bayley Scales at eight months is associated with lower scores on the Stanford-Binet at four years. But in a higher socioeconomic status home, a child's poor scores on the Bayley Scales at eight months do not carry the same dire prognostic implication.

Despite such clear indications that the environment into which a baby is born may have powerful impact on development, there has been surprisingly little study of pertinent aspects of the prenatal environment and few attempts to identify differences in environmental context in a manner similar to that of Caldwell and her collaborators.

EVALUATING CONTEXT: PARENTAL MODELS

At the University of Texas at Austin, we have begun a research program to evaluate various aspects of the prenatal environmental context. Our thesis is that in order to grasp the meaning of the various parent-infant interactions that child development researchers are now charting, and to determine what is, indeed, typical and atypical, we need to understand more fully the variations in the parental context or environment which exist prior to a baby's birth. Thus, the research program is aimed at developing means for assessing the ecological milieu into which an infant is born.

Our effort to understand the psychosocial context into which children are born led us to postulate the concept of parental models. As an important aspect of parental adaptation prior to and during pregnancy, we assumed that expectant parents were building models, or conglomerates of images, fantasies, attitudes and ideas regarding the meaning of the pregnancy and parenthood in relation to their own lives. The concept of parental models was viewed as manifesting at least three distinct aspects: models of the infant, models of the parenting role, and models of how life changes following the birth of a baby.

Each of these aspects was assumed to be complex and multifaceted in nature. That is, a parent's model of the infant might include a model of a normative or average infant, its abilities at birth, its pace of development, the degree of difficulty it might have with various bodily functions, and the like. At the same time, a parent might entertain a model of a "good" and a "bad" infant; in addition, as a distinct subcategory of the parent's model of infancy, there might exist a fantasy model of what the parent's own coming baby will be like.

In a similar fashion, the model of the parenting role might include expectations and attitudes about what the average parent is like, and what a "good" or a "bad" parent might be like. Moreover, the model of parenting held by any particular expectant mother or father might well include some estimate of what he or she will actually be like in the role.

Likewise, the model of how life changes following the birth of a baby might include ideas about the number of areas in one's life that change as a result of becoming a parent, as well as the degree to which those changes are seen as major or minimal; in addition, parents might hold a model of how life changes that reflects expectations for changes in either a positive or negative direction.

Individuals' parental models were expected to reveal themselves not only through direct statements of expectations for infants and the parental role, but also via behavior such as the timing and type of concrete preparations for a baby, selections of names, preparations of living space, purchases, reading, and the like. Parental reports of subjective responses such as dreaming and daily thoughts of the coming infant, pleasure with the pregnancy, and confidence in regard to specific child care tasks were also seen as important in an evaluation of the psychosocial aspects of preparation for a baby.

Our hope is that the concept of parental models, as one means for operationalizing particular aspects of the environmental and emotional contexts which exist prior to a baby's birth, will provide a versatile and useful set of "descriptors" of psychosocial adaptation in pregnancy.

PARENTAL MODELS RESEARCH

To date, we have completed three studies of parental models. In this chapter we will briefly summarize the first study, and present some selected results from the second and third studies.

In our first study, a pilot project with 25 married couples who were expecting a first-born child, we recorded and analyzed responses to a series of broad and open-ended questions. The questions were formulated after review of previous studies of expectant couples, after evaluation of the areas of concern and content that appeared in popular literature for expectant parents, such as books and magazine articles addressed to expectant parents, and in collaboration with nurses who taught prenatal courses and served on labor and delivery services in local hospitals. The instrument which we tested in this first pilot project was designed to inform us about the kinds of questions and information parents had about infants, their concerns during pregnancy, their fantasies, and the concrete preparations they had undertaken in preparing for their babies.

We found in the pilot study that men and women did not appear to have identical expectations for infants; in particular, there were indications that women expected a more rapid pace of development from babies than did men. There were also some indications that men and women both held an image of their own forthcoming baby which was different in their minds from their image of an average baby. We viewed the results of the pilot project as tentative, and of use primarily for the development of a tighter instrument and set of procedures for a more formal study of parental models.

In our second study, we compared the parental models of 20 younger couples expecting a first baby with those of 20 older couples who were also expecting a first-born. In our third study, we evaluated the parental models of 25 male and 25 female undergraduates who were not married and not parents. Thus, parental models as they are influenced by age, sex, and pregnancy status were assessed.

Since each study was lengthy and complex, the results are too extensive to thoroughly review in this chapter. Only those data pertaining to differences between the 80 expectant parents in our second study and the 50 unmarried college students in our third study will be presented here.

Relevant demographic characteristics of these 80 expectant parents and 50 students are presented in Table 1. All the subjects in these two studies were white, had educational attainment of at least the median number of years in school for U.S. whites, and were of primarily middle-

TABLE 1

Characteristics of Samples in Study Two and Study Three of
the Parental Models Research

STUDY TWO: 80 EXPECTANT PARENTS	Age Years M SD	Days Pregnant M SD	Educ to Present M SD	Years Married M SD	SES Level, S's Father
Younger Couples					
20 Females	22.4 .9	235 19.5	13.6 1.5		III
				2.26 1.0	
20 Males	23.9 1.6		13.8 1.6		III
Older Couples					
20 Females	30.7 1.2	238 15.1	15.8 2.6		III
				5.85 3.0	
20 Males	31.8 2.5		16.8 2.0		III
STUDY THREE: 50 SINGLE STUDENTS					
20 Females	19.1 .9		12.6 .9		II
20 Males	19.7 1.0		13.0 1.0		II

class and upper-middle-class socioeconomic status, as classified by Hollingshead's (1957) occupational index applied to the occupation of each subject's father. No subject had previously been a parent. All expectant couples were married.

The procedure with expectant parents combined administration of a questionnaire which required an average of 75 minutes to complete with an interview which required an additional 75 minutes. The questionnaire and interview covered parental models' variables such as: prior contact with infants, knowledge about infant abilities at birth, preparations and expectations regarding one's own child care abilities, prediction of characteristics of the coming baby, knowledge of the pace of an infant's development, expectations for change in the year following a baby's birth, gender preferences and predictions, and self-ratings of confidence on specific child care tasks. The procedure with students eliminated questions which had to do with concrete preparations for a baby, pregnancy symptomatology, and reaction to confirmation of the pregnancy, since these were irrelevant to that sample. In addition, the interview was eliminated and students responded to all questions in written form.

The students who participated in the research had for the most part already decided that they wished someday to have children; only one male and one female student reported that they did not think they would have children someday in the future. Expectant parents and students were all asked to report the number of children they wished to have. Students reported wanting families with a mean of 2.56 children, while expectant couples planned a mean of 2.06 children; this difference was not significant.

Moreover, students and expectant parents had previous contacts with infants which were equivalent. All subjects reported on 36 items of previous contact with infants in three time periods (to age 12, from 13 to 16, and within the last two years). From these 36 items, a scale was devised on which a high score reflected a high degree of previous contact with infants. An analysis of variance indicated that females, in both the student and expectant parent groups, had more previous experience with infants than did males, F (3, 126) $= 27.49$, $p < .001$. There was no significant difference, however, between students and expectant parents in reported amount of previous contact with infants, F (3, 126) $= .71$, $p < .40$.

However, despite equivalent prior contact with infants, and despite an apparently positive orientation toward babies and parenthood, find-

IN THE FIRST YEAR AFTER THE BABY IS BORN . . .

-3 = Very Much Less than before
-2 = Somewhat Less than before
-1 = A Bit Less than before
0 = No change from before
+1 = A Bit More than before
+2 = Somewhat More than before
+3 = Very Much More than before

	Less (Decrease)			No Change			More (Increase)
cc. Will the amount of food you will eat each day increase or decrease?	−3	−2	−1	0	+1	+2	+3
dd. Will the amount of alcoholic beverages you will consume increase or decrease?	−3	−2	−1	0	+1	+2	+3
ee. Will the number of fights you will have with spouse increase or decrease?	−3	−2	−1	0	+1	+2	+3
ff. Will you feel more physically attractive than before or less attractive?	−3	−2	−1	0	+1	+2	+3
gg. Will you feel more clear about who you are and where you are going in life, or less clear?	−3	−2	−1	0	+1	+2	+3
hh. Will the amount of money you will be able to put in savings increase or decrease?	−3	−2	−1	0	+1	+2	+3
ii. Will the amount of satisfaction you feel in the sexual relationship with your spouse increase or decrease?	−3	−2	−1	0	+1	+2	+3

FIGURE 1. Sample Change Items

ings from our research indicated that students and expectant parents have consistently different parental models, or expectations for infants and the parenting role.

Nowhere is this more clear than in analysis of data on expectations for the life changes parents will experience following a baby's birth. Students and parents were asked 35 specific questions regarding changes which might occur in the year following a baby's birth; Figure 1 shows the format and a portion of the 35 items. Data analysis of student and expectant parent responses to these 35 items of change yielded a discriminant function which indicated that students and expectant parents differed significantly in their perceptions of how life changes after a baby is born (Wilk's lamda, .499, $p < .001$). Using the function generated by this analysis, 84% of the cases were correctly classified, $\chi^2 = 54.24$, $p < .001$. The canonical correlation associated with the discriminant function was .708; this indicates that the majority of the variability of scores on the discriminant function is explained by marital and pregnancy status, i.e. by the student (unmarried, nonpregnant) and expectant parent (married, pregnant) classification.

Additional analyses of variance were undertaken to determine which of the 35 variables were contributing most heavily to differences in perceptions of parents and students. The areas of difference proved interesting.

On nine of the 35 items, students and expectant parents differed in their expectations for change at the 5% level of significance or less. Specifically, students expected that time for hobbies and sports would be reduced by a baby's birth significantly more than expectant parents did, $F (1, 128) = 23.14$, $p < .0001$; students felt that time with their friends in the company of the spouse would be reduced more than did expectant parents, $F (1, 127) = 8.24$, $p < .005$, and they also felt that time with friends when spouse is not around would be reduced more than did expectant parents, $F (1, 125) = 6.52$, $p < .01$; students thought a baby would increase the time they spent worrying about things in general more than did parents, $F (1, 126) = 5.24$, $p < .02$; students believed that fathers have to increase time on the job significantly more in the year after a baby is born than parents believed, $F (1, 126) = 15.01$, $p < .0002$; students thought that a baby would mean a couple would have their vacation time reduced significantly more than did parents, $F (1, 127) = 9.23$, $p < .003$; students thought that the number of phone calls they would make each day would increase less than expectant parents thought, $F (1, 128) = 4.20$, $p < .04$; students expected that their alcohol consumption would be reduced significantly more in the year following a baby's birth than did expectant parents, F (1, 127) $=$ 12.53, $p < .0006$; and perhaps most interesting of all, students expected a baby would make them feel less physically attractive, while expectant parents looked forward to feeling more attractive physically in the year following a baby's birth, F (1, 127) $=$ 18.89, $p < .0001$.

In general, the differences between students and expectant parents in perception of changes in life following the birth of a baby appeared to be of two types. First, students expected that there would be more change. An analysis of variance in the number of times "no change" was endorsed yielded no main effect for sex of respondent, but students expected some change on an average of 23 out of the 35 items. On the average, expectant parents thought only 19 out of the 35 items would change in the first year after a baby's birth, F (3, 126) $=$ 25.4, $p < .001$. Secondly, students expected that changes would be in a more negative direction. A scoring procedure was devised to combine responses which indicated expectations for a high degree of change in an undesirable direction in the year following the baby's birth. An analysis of variance on scores generated by this procedure indicated that men and women did not differ in their perceptions of the nature of the changes which follow a baby's birth, but there was a main effect for pregnancy status. Students expected the birth of a baby to generate more negative changes in the first year than did the expectant parents, F (3, 126) $=$ 10.21, $p < .002$.

Thus, when students' and expectant parents' responses are compared, students see life as changing more, and in a more negative direction following a baby's birth. The baby's arrival is seen by students as an event which would intrude more on social life and activities, and would be associated with less leisure time, more worry, and decreased feelings of attractiveness. The parental model of how life changes is, therefore, considerably different for students and expectant parents. That is, students may see a baby as more disruptive to their life-style and this may be consonant with their life circumstances. The expectant parents, who on the basis of our research appear to be low-risk parents, view a baby as entering their family system with considerably less disruption to their life patterns. On this basis, we can speculate that an optimal first pregnancy is characterized by expectations for a moderate and manageable degree of change. In contrast, the high-risk family may expect no change at all or overwhelming change as a result of adding an additional member to the family system.

Another area in which students and expectant parents differed markedly involved gender preferences and predictions. All expectant parents had been asked, as part of the research interview in the eighth month of pregnancy, "Do you hope this baby will be a boy, a girl, or either is okay?" and later they were asked, "What do you think the baby actually is—a boy, a girl, or don't you know?" On their written questionnaire students reported their preferences for the gender of the first baby they might someday have, and also they were asked if they had any idea of what gender their first baby might actually be.

Results are presented in Figures 2 and 3. Of all of the expectant parents, 60% would not state a preference for the gender of the coming baby. Of the 32 individuals who did express a preference, 25 wanted a male first-born. Expectant parents freely predicted the gender of the

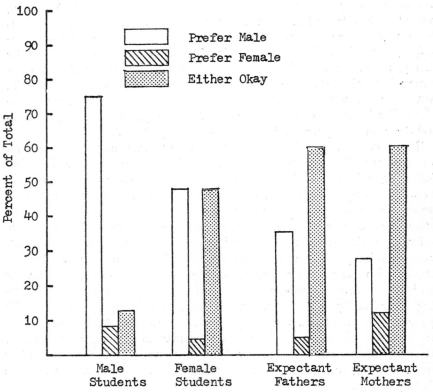

FIGURE 2. Preference for Gender of First-born, By Sex and Status of Respondents.

coming baby: 78% expressed a belief about the sex of the fetus, and of those again the majority (57%) predicted a boy.

In contrast, students often showed preferences about the gender of the first-born: Almost 70% of these young men and women expressed a prefer-ence, and most (over 90% of those who gave a preference) wanted a son as a first-born child. However, students would not chance a prediction as to the gender of a child they might someday have; 42 out of 50 stated they had no idea of what gender their first child would be.

Thus, young unmarried students tend to report they would prefer a male first-born, but they do not predict the gender of the first baby. Couples actually expecting a first child have taken an almost opposite stance. They no longer will state a preference, yet apparently they often

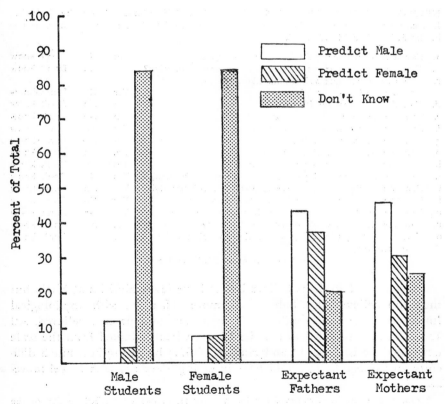

FIGURE 3. Prediction of Gender of First-born, By Sex and Status of Respondents.

have a sufficiently well developed model of the fetus to chance a prediction as to its gender.

Another area in which the expectant parents and students differed in a systematic manner involved the abilities which they were willing to attribute to newborns. Subjects were asked to report on newborn abilities in 18 specific areas of functioning, such as those illustrated in Figure 4. For each subject, a total was generated for the number of abilities which the respondents thought newborns possessed, the number they thought newborns did not possess, and the number of items on which they responded that they did not know. An analysis of variance for main effects of marital status and sex indicated that students viewed newborns as having significantly fewer abilities at birth than did expectant parents, F (3, 126) = 12.04, p < .001.

NEWBORN INFANT ABILITIES AND ACTIVITIES. Please fill out the following list, circling your answers. Consider a "newborn baby" to be an average child that is in the FIRST WEEK OF LIFE.

a.	Can a newborn see a toy held up in front of it?	Yes	No	Don't know
b.	Can a newborn hear loud sounds like a door slamming?	Yes	No	Don't know
c.	Can a newborn hear soft sounds like quiet talk in the next room?	Yes	No	Don't know
d.	Can the newborn see in color?	Yes	No	Don't know
e.	Can the newborn smell odors?	Yes	No	Don't know
f.	Can the newborn taste different flavors?	Yes	No	Don't know
g.	Can the newborn feel heat?	Yes	No	Don't know
h.	Can the newborn feel cold?	Yes	No	Don't know
i.	Can the newborn feel pain on his skin?	Yes	No	Don't know
j.	Can the newborn feel pain inside, like stomach pain?	Yes	No	Don't know
k.	Can the newborn look where it wants to, voluntarily?	Yes	No	Don't know
l.	Can the newborn turn its head where it wants to?	Yes	No	Don't know
m.	Can the newborn suck by himself without learning?	Yes	No	Don't know
n.	Can the newborn grasp objects in its hand?	Yes	No	Don't know
o.	If it is holding something, can it let go voluntarily?	Yes	No	Don't know

(continued)

FIGURE 4. Sample Abilities Items.

Not only did students believe babies have fewer abilities at birth, but they also believed that babies have more difficulties with physiological function in the first month of life than expectant parents believed. All 130 subjects responded to a series of seven items adapted from the scale developed by Broussard* and Hartner (1971) by rating how much difficulty an average baby would have in eating, sleeping, with bowel move-

---

* Our thanks to Dr. Broussard for her permission to use a modified version of the Neonatal Perception Inventory.

ments, setting a regular schedule, etc., on a five-point scale. The proce-dures were such that each subject gave a separate estimate for difficulties his/her own baby would have on the same functions. These latter ratings were given independently, at a point when the subjects could not review their earlier ratings for the average baby. These data are shown in Table 2. On ratings given for both the average and own baby, analyses of variance for main effects of pregnancy status and sex yielded significant differences between students and expectant parents, with students rating both average and own baby as having more difficulty, F for average baby total ratings (3, 125) $= 44.09$, $p < .001$; F for own baby total ratings (3, 123) $= 69.34$, $p < .001$.

In addition, all subjects were asked to give estimates for the age at which babies achieve certain developmental milestones. Again, procedures were arranged so that two separate sets of estimates were solicited, one for the pace of development of an average baby, and another for the pace of development of the subject's own baby. Fourteen of the items relating to developmental pace were drawn from the manual of the Bayley Scales of Infant Development (Bayley, 1969).

To approach the question of different perceptions that students and expectant parents might have for infants, scales were developed to com-pare each subject's estimates on the 14 items drawn from the Bayley Scales with the norms given by Bayley for the standardization sample on which her testing procedure was developed. For example, when a student or an expectant parent estimated that the average baby (or his/her own future baby) would be able to stack three blocks into a tower at 52 weeks, the Bayley norm for this item, 71.81 weeks, was subtracted from 52 weeks, yielding -19.81 weeks. For this single item, therefore, the subject expected a baby to achieve the ability to stack three blocks some 20 weeks earlier than Bayley norms.

In this same way, all 14 estimates given by a subject were used to calculate 14 deviations from Bayley norms, and the 14 deviation scores were summed together. When the deviations were calculated from esti-mates given for an average baby, the summary score was named DEVN-AVG, or deviations from Bayley norms drawn from estimates for the average baby; when the deviations were calculated from estimates for one's own baby in the future, the summary score was named DEVN-OWN. On both of these scales, a score of $+14$ might mean that a subject had estimated development on each item at one week later than Bayley norms, while a -14 might mean the subject had given 14 estimates which were each one week earlier than Bayley norms.

TABLE 2

Difficulty Ratings for Average and Own Baby, Given by Expectant Parents and Students

| | AVERAGE BABY | | | | | | OWN BABY | | | | | |
| | Expectant Parents | | | Students | | | Expectant Parents | | | Students | | |
	N	M	SD	N	M	SD	N	M	SD	N	M	SD
How much crying	80	3.24	.56	49	3.65	.66	80	2.99	.56	48	3.48	.77
How much trouble in feeding	80	2.36	.66	49	2.96	.71	79	2.23	.60	48	2.81	.53
How much spitting up and vomiting	80	2.95	.57	49	3.02	.66	79	2.65	.66	48	3.00	.62
How much trouble in sleeping	80	2.16	.68	49	2.41	.79	80	2.13	.64	49	2.61	.67
How much trouble with bms	80	2.19	.58	49	2.59	.76	79	2.10	.59	49	2.61	.61
How much trouble setting schedule	80	2.75	.68	50	3.08	.80	80	2.44	.65	49	3.02	.69
How much care needed in handling (fragile)	80	3.16	.85	50	4.04	.88	80	3.06	.93	49	3.86	.96

Ratings were as follows:

1 = None
2 = Very Little
3 = Moderate Amount
4 = A Good Bit
5 = A Great Deal

Modified from Broussard & Hartner (1971)

In Figure 5, the distribution of scores on DEVN-AVG and DEVN-OWN by group and sex are displayed. Analyses of variance indicated that on each of the two summary variables, there was a main effect for sex, with women estimating the pace of development on these 14 items as earlier than men, F for DEVN-AVG (3, 85) = 9.73, $p < .002$; F for DEVN-OWN (3, 92) = 15.95, $p < .001$. In addition, there was a significant main effect for pregnancy status on both summary variables, with students expecting slower development for an average baby, F (3, 85) = 25.45, $p < .001$, and for a baby of their own in the future as well, F (3, 92) = 12.71, $p < .001$. On both DEVN-AVG and DEVN-OWN, male students gave significantly later estimates for the pace of development. The reason for this difference is not explained by our data. However, it may be that young women begin to develop more accurate estimates of infants even before they marry or become pregnant.

Thus, the parental model of the infant was different for students and expectant couples. We found a similar disparity in their model of the parenting role. Despite their equivalence to expectant couples in terms of prior contact with infants, students did not have similar confidence that they could handle specific child care tasks. Each subject rated his or her own confidence regarding 12 tasks including confidence in ability to give a bath to an infant, change a wet diaper skillfully, care for a newborn's navel, take the temperature of an infant, and similar child care tasks. Rating were made on a five-point scale. On the total score obtained from summing confidence self-ratings on the 12 variables, students rated themselves as significantly less confident than expectant parents, F (3, 124) = 20.47, $p < .001$.

Thus, compared to expectant parents, students were less confident that they could handle specific child care tasks; they viewed babies as having more difficulties and fewer abilities at birth; they expected babies' development to progress at a slower pace; and they thought that babies changed a parent's life more and in a less favorable direction.

Since students were younger than the expectant parents, the question remained as to whether it was merely the difference in age which accounted for the systematic differences found in the parental models of students and expectant couples. To assess this possibility, a series of multiple regressions was performed using four important independent variables, age, sex, prior baby care experience score, and status (which may be seen as pregnancy or marital status, both of which separated students from expectant parents) to predict scores on selected dependent variables.

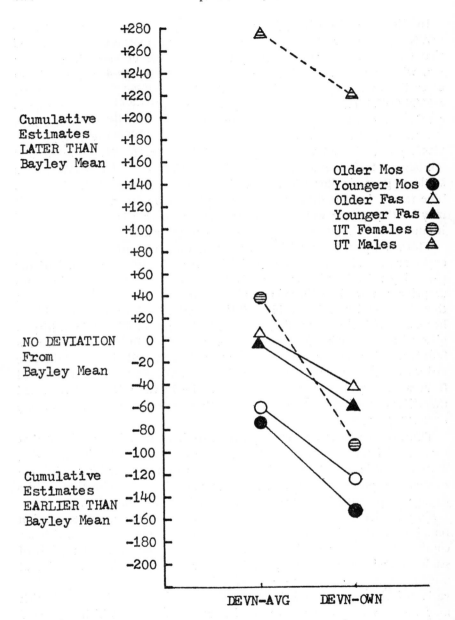

FIGURE 5. Deviations of Estimates on 14 Pace of Development Items, Calculated from Bayley Scale Norms.

The selected dependent variables are those already reported: (1) confidence totals for 12 specific child care tasks; (2) total rating of difficulty on seven items for an average baby (on the modified Broussard and Hartner scale); (3) total rating of difficulty on seven items as given for own baby; (4) number of items scored as "no change" in the first year following a baby's birth; (5) scores on the scale of expected changes for the worse in the year following a baby's birth; (6) DEVN-AVG scores, from 14 estimates for the pace of an average baby's development; (7) DEVN-OWN scores, from 14 pace estimates for own baby.

Each of the multiple regressions performed on these seven dependent variables yielded significant overall F values, indicating that in each case the four independent variables of age, sex, prior experience with infants, and status worked together to account for a significant portion of variability in scores on the seven dependent variables. But in not one of the multiple regressions did age serve as a significant predictor.

Sex of respondent served as the best predictor of scores on the confidence items, and sex was also the best predictor of scores on the pace of development items; women were more confident of their abilities on child care tasks, and they predicted earlier development for an average and their own baby. Status of respondent (student or expectant parent) was also a significant predictor of scores on these three variables, and the *only* significant predictor of scores on the other five dependent variables as well. Thus, it seems that age of subject did not contribute nearly so decisively to differences in scores on a number of parental models variables as did differences in pregnancy status. The students apparently gave different responses not because they were younger, but because they were not married and not pregnant.

CONTEXTUAL DIFFERENCES

Viewed from a broad perspective, then, these studies demonstrate that middle- and upper-middle-class, white, well educated students do not have expectations for babies, for the parental role, or for how life is affected by the birth of a baby which are similar to those of expectant parents of the same racial and socioeconomic background. While there is no doubt that pregnancy itself can influence parental models, it is conceivable that many babies are born to parents who have ideas about infants and parenthood similar to those of the students we studied, rather than those of the expectant parents in our research. And a baby born to a mother or father whose parental models were similar to those of the students in our study would begin life in an entirely different psychosocial environment, and perhaps would be at greater risk than would a baby born to parents like the ones who participated in our research.

Additional data from our studies indicate that the parental models of men and women differ in specific and significant ways as well. This evidence suggests that the psychosocial context in which the first *mother*-infant interactions take place may not necessarily be the same as the context in which early *father*-infant interactions occur.

Therefore, it is evident that students and expectant parents who share similar racial and socioeconomic backgrounds can hold sharply different parental models. Moreover, men and women can differ in their expectations for babies and the parental role as well. Therefore, it seems likely that those aspects of prenatal psychosocial context which are tapped by the parental models studies differ also among racial and cultural lines and between social class groups as well.

PROSPECTUS

We believe that assessment of parental models provides a good beginning in the search for methods which can quantify different prenatal contexts. Our next step in the program of research will be to assess parental models in independent samples from socioeconomic and racial populations which are different from those we have already studied. Thereafter, having laid the groundwork by developing the method and evaluating the contributions of age, sex, socioeconomic status, race and pregnancy status to parental models, we will return to the essential question which has motivated the research all along: "How do parental models relate to a child's development?"

Insofar as the parental models procedure is indeed a method for assessing differential prenatal context, the question is actually "How does prenatal context—the parents' psychosocial status prior to the baby's birth—contribute to the child's status at birth and development through infancy and childhood?" In emphasizing the prenatal context, we are not proposing that the psychosocial situation which exists prior to the baby's arrival is the most important variable in determining the course of parent-infant interaction as it unfolds. We suggest only that the prenatal context be considered as one relevant factor in the marvelously complex equation which seeks to describe dynamics of human development.

Mothers differ from one another; fathers differ; babies differ. Psychologists need to know much about each of the individuals in the family system, and about the interactions among them. But we must also learn more about the environment in which, at the beginning, the system operates. This means knowing more about where parents are, psychologically and sociologically, on the day the baby is born. We agree with Sameroff (this volume) that a clearer understanding of the prenatal context will bring us closer to a clear understanding of all which follows.

11

Early Parental Attitudes and the Parent-Infant Relationship

LORRAINE OLSZEWSKI WALKER

Associate Professor, University of Texas at Austin

The influence of early parental attitudes* on parenting behavior and infant development finds strong support among clinicians, such as doctors, nurses, and clinical psychologists. For example, a "negative parental attitude" as intuitively sensed by a clinician may be an important factor in determining the frequency of clinic appointments or in allocating supportive services to a parent. In the research context there is also evidence that researchers are attracted to the notion that attitudes in the early parenting years influence or actually predict subsequent parental behavior. This notion is currently reflected in predictive research studies relating parental attitudes to child abuse behavior (Schneider, Hoffmeister & Helfer, 1976)** The work of Moss (1967) and Broussard and Hartner (1970, 1971) supports the intuitive appeal of the notion that there are measurable psychological antecedents of later parenting behavior. Moss, for example, found that prepregnancy attitudes were related to later ma-

I wish to thank H. Paul Kelly for his review of an earlier draft of this chapter and Claudia Anderson and Barbara Poley for assistance in data collection and analysis. This research was supported, in part, by grants from the Institute of Human Development of the University of Texas at Austin and the Center for Health Care Research and Evaluation of the University of Texas System School of Nursing.

* While the term "parental attitudes" not "maternal attitudes" is used here, it is important to note that existing research has not treated the attitudes of both maternal and paternal parents with equal attention. "Parental attitudes" was selected, however, to signal the potential contribution of research concerning early attitudes of both mothers and fathers.

** The interpretation of Schneider-Hoffmeister-Helfer tool as largely attitudinal is this writer's interpretation. The authors describe it as a questionnaire which assesses parental attitudes, perceptions, and experiences related to childrearing (1976, p. 393).

ternal parenting behavior. In turn, Broussard and Hartner reported that maternal perceptions of one-month-old infants predicted the later psychological adjustment of the same children at four and a half years of age. From a different point of view, psychoanalysts such as Deutsch (1945) reinforce the belief that there is continuity between psychological attitudes and perceptions and the later relationship between mother and infant.

Effectively demonstrating the causal chain assumed by clinicians between parental attitudes and parental behaviors or infant outcomes, however, may present significant difficulties to empirical investigators. In the general field of attitudinal research there is a vast body of evidence related to attitude-behavior consistency. No conclusive evidence has been found, however, to indicate that attitudes and behaviors are related in a systematic and reliable way. In fact, the inconsistency between attitudes and behavior has been documented repeatedly since LaPiere (1934), and more recent reviews (e.g., Deutscher, 1966; Wicker, 1969) continue to come to the same conclusion. So compelling has been the evidence against a clear relationship between attitudes and behavior that Deutscher has said:

> It seems to me that we have sufficient grounds to reject any evaluation of an action program which employs attitudinal change as a criterion of "success" except in the unlikely event that the goal of the program is solely to change attitudes without concern for subsequent behavioral changes (1966, p. 250).

Reactions among investigators in the attitude field to the evidence of inconsistency between attitudes and behavior seem to have taken three directions: first, abandonment of attitude-behavior consistency research; second, greater attention to methodological concerns, particularly measurement methods used for both attitudes and behavior; and third, reexamination and reformulation of conceptual models, definitions and assumptions related to attitudes.

Being a dogged optimist, I will refrain from recommending that investigators close up shop on attitude-behavior consistency research. Especially in the area of parental attitudes and behavior, there seems to be something so intuitively true and powerful about the proposition that attitudes and behavior are related that it seems worthy of further investigation. As a cautionary note, however, I must report Wicker's comment that few investigators who have studied the attitude-behavior relationship have published more than one study (1969, p. 67). While Wicker's observation is open to multiple inferences, certainly it suggests that attitude-behavior research may be an area where only the naive tread, and the experienced researcher withdraws.

Having thus rejected abandoning attitude-behavior research, I would like to focus on the second, and then, third, directions that might be taken, i.e., attention to theoretical and methodological, especially measurement, concerns. In so doing, I would like to attend to socio-psychological processes in the early parent-child relationship from the perspective of attitudinal theory and methods.

THEORETICAL CONSIDERATIONS

In reviewing research on early parental attitudes, it becomes apparent that research in this area has not been conducted from a clear and explicit conceptual framework of attitudes. Attitudes may be viewed as either multidimensional or unidimensional. In the multidimensional framework, attitudes are broadly defined to include cognitive, conative and affective components (Himmelfarb & Eagly, 1974; Fishbein, 1967b). The multidimensional concept of attitudes leads to the methodological assumptions that attitudes are empirically reflected in all three of these components, and that any one component studied alone does not necessarily reflect the totality of attitude toward an object. Despite these assumptions, proponents of the multidimensional framework typically operationalized attitudes in terms of unidimensional measures (Fishbein, 1967b). In contrast, others have argued for an unidimensional concept of attitude identified with only the affective dimension. The unidimensional notion was espoused by Thurstone (1931) and has a present day proponent in Fishbein (Fishbein, 1967a, 1967b; Fishbein & Ajzen, 1975). Fishbein has argued cogently that attitudes should be considered as a phenomenon conceptually distinct from, but related to, such concepts as beliefs and behavioral intentions, as well as overt behavior. In Fishbein and Ajzen's (1975) unidimensional framework, attitudes are defined as "the amount of affect for or against some object" (p. 11). In contrast, beliefs represent a person's information about an object, i.e., "the subjective probability of a relationship between the object of belief and some other object, value, concept or attribute" (Fishbein & Ajzen, 1975, p. 131). Beliefs deal with discriminable aspects of a person's world and may include diverse content such as a person's cognitions about himself as well as about the physical and social environment in which he lives.

In Fishbein's (1967a) framework, attitudes reflect the summation of beliefs a person holds about an attitudinal object and the evaluative content of those beliefs. The evaluative content of beliefs may vary from favorable to neutral to unfavorable.* Thus, from a summation of beliefs and the evaluative aspects of those beliefs, one may infer attitude toward an object. Given Fishbein's framework in which attitude is a function of the many beliefs a person may hold relative to an attitudinal object, any one belief taken in isolation may be an unreliable indicator of attitude. In turn, measuring a wide range of beliefs related to an object is a much more reliable indicator of attitude (Fishbein, 1967a). This framework of attitudes has implications for measurement of attitudes which will be addressed in the methodological section of the paper.

Fishbein has also delineated a model of the relationship of attitudes to behavior in which behavioral intentions serve as the connective between attitudes and behavior. Further, behavior is not predicted solely from attitude, but also from personal and social norms governing behavior and motivation to comply with these norms. In the model the respective influence of attitudes, norms, and motivation on behavioral intentions, and subsequently behavior, is not constant, but subject to fluctuation. These relationships are expressed symbolically as follows:

$$B \approx BI = [A_{act}]w_0 + [(NB_p)(Mc_p)]w_1 + [(NB_s)(Mc_s)]w_2$$

where

B   stands for overt behavior
BI   stands for behavioral intention
A_{act} for attitude toward an act
NB_p for personal norms
Mc   for motivation to comply
NB_s for social norms and
w_0, w_1, w_2 for weights applied the respective components of
        the equation (Fishbein, 1967a).

While Fishbein's model of the relationship of attitudes to behavior has undergone some modification (Ajzen & Fishbein, 1970), the model continues to represent the multiple inputs of both psychological phenomena and social phenomena in predicting behavior. The model further suggests that predicting behavior from attitudes alone can at best be only partially successful. In applying the model to the prediction of early parenting behavior, and ultimately the parent-infant relationship,

---

* Standard attitudinal measurement procedures only measure the subject's belief strength and assume evaluative aspects of those beliefs to be the same for all subjects (Fishbein & Ajzen, 1975, p. 61).

several extrapolations may be hypothesized: (1) The totality of beliefs about oneself as a parent and about one's infant may be expected to directly influence attitudes toward parenting and, secondarily, to varying degrees to influence actual parenting behavior. (2) The social environment may be expected to varying degrees to have an impact on behavior as the environment affects norms held, or perceived, by parents and parental motivation to comply with these norms. For example, a mother may behave differently in terms of publicly breastfeeding when her disapproving mother-in-law is present rather than supportive friends, despite her positive attitude toward breastfeeding. (3) As parental inputs and infant inputs (Lewis & Rosenblum, 1974; Korner, 1970; Chess, 1967) and the interactions between these two (Thoman, 1974; Brazelton, 1973a; Korner, 1973b; Coleman, Kris, & Provence, 1953; Sander, 1962, 1964, 1969) alter behaviors in the parent-infant relationship, parental beliefs, and consequently attitudes, may change. The complexity of the relationship between attitudes and behavior presented here, particularly as the attitudes and behavior of interest are nested within a context of rapid developmental change, suggests a need to reformulate questions addressed in parental attitude-behavior research. In place of isolated two factor questions—e.g., the relationship of parental attitudes to infant development, multivariable orientations* are needed which reflect, with suitable specificity, the complex relationships believed to obtain among parental beliefs, attitudes, and behaviors; infant behaviors; and salient environmental influences. Proposed examples of such research will be presented later in this chapter.

Finally, it is of special importance to place benchmarks within the infinite array of attitudinal objects toward which parents hold attitudes so that those of greatest possible salience to an understanding of the dynamics of the early parent-infant relationship may be identified. The domain of parental attitudes and beliefs about oneself, both as parent and as person, and attitudes and beliefs relative to the infant are of special interest in this regard. Each of these is briefly discussed below.

In the study of beliefs about oneself, Leifer (1977) has provided an illuminating descriptive account of the attitudinal and emotional dynamics of pregnancy and motherhood. Threaded throughout her article are descriptions of beliefs and attitudes which mothers express about themselves. Particularly during the postpartum period, beliefs about

---

* Within the attitude field several writers have identified "other variables" that interact with attitudes to influence behavior (see Wicker, 1969; Rokeach, 1968; Cook & Selltiz, 1964; Liska, 1975; Fishbein & Ajzen, 1975).

one's adequacy are tied to such events as ability to nurse successfully. Rubin (1961, 1967) has also elaborated the continuing self-appraisals inherent in the mother's early experiences in the role of mother. Separation of mothers from their prematurely born infants has been shown negatively to affect mothers' beliefs about their caregiving competence compared to other caregivers (Seashore, Leifer, Barnett, & Leiderman, 1973). Interestingly, an attitude toward the self entitled, "I'm No Damn Good," has been identified as one of the clusters useful in predictive research with child abusers (Schneider, Hoffmeister, & Helfer, 1976).

The second set of beliefs and attitudes that appears to be especially meaningful is that related to the infant. Brazelton (1973a) has spoken of the positive role that maternal expectations (beliefs about desired behaviors) may play on infant development even among newborns who have experienced malnourishment during the gestational period. Tulkin and Kagan (1972) have suggested that maternal beliefs about certain incapacities of infants—e.g., the infant's inability to express adult-like emotions or communicate with others—underlie social class differences in mothers' interactive behaviors with infants. Interestingly, subsequent research has demonstrated a relationship between beliefs about infants and mothers' behavior among middle-class mothers, but not among working class mothers (Tulkin & Cohler, 1973; Moss & Jones, 1977).

Perhaps the most intriguing findings about maternal beliefs about the infant are found in the work of Broussard and Hartner (1970, 1971). From an initial sample of 318 primiparous mothers completing the Neonatal Perception Inventories (NPI) at one to two days postpartum and again at one month postpartum, 85 were included in a longitudinal study. On the NPI mothers rated both the "average baby" and their own babies in terms of the amount of difficulty experienced in six behavioral areas: crying, spitting up, feeding, elimination, sleeping, and predictability. Babies whose mothers rated them as "better than average" were classified as low risk. Babies whose mothers failed to rate them as better than average were in turn classified as high risk. At approximately four and a half years of age the offspring of the 85 mothers were examined and classified according to their "need for therapeutic intervention" using diagnostic categories from the G.A.P. Committee on Child Psychiatry. While NPI risk classifications from the first or second postpartum days were not predictive of need for intervention, those taken at one month postpartum were. Of the 49 offsprings classified as low risk based on NPI scores at one month of age, 20.4 percent were judged to need therapeutic intervention in contrast to 66 percent of the 36 high risk offspring. While the Broussard and Hartner study leaves open the question of the factors operative in shaping both the mothers' one-month perceptions of their infants as well as the later adjustment of their offspring, the findings do underscore the significance of maternal beliefs about their infants as reflected on the NPI.

METHODOLOGICAL CONSIDERATIONS

Further data from the Broussard and Hartner research (1970, 1971) provide an interesting point from which to address methodological considerations related to attitudinal research in the early parenting period. From the first administration of the NPI to the second, 54 percent of the 85 mothers changed their perceptions of their infants (32 from negative to positive and 14 from positive to negative) and 46 percent maintained their original perception (17 remained positive and 22 remained negative). The Broussard-Hartner data suggest that maternal beliefs about their infants do change after experience with the infant. These findings are interesting when juxtaposed with attitudinal findings reported by Goldstein, Taub, Caputo and Silberstein (1976) which did not reveal changes in maternal beliefs after experience with the infant. Using the control and hostility factors from the Parent Attitude Research Instrument (PARI) administered to mothers at one to two days postpartum and again when the infants were approximately 12 months old, Goldstein and others found a large measure of stability in maternal childrearing attitudes. The test-retest correlations for the control and hostility factors were .76 and .63 respectively. Further, when infant status characteristics at birth—e.g., birth weight, Apgar score, activity rating—were used to predict the respective childrearing attitudes at 12 months, neither of the multiple regressions was statistically significant.

While these two studies are not comparable in many ways—e.g., Broussard and Hartner studied primiparae delivering normal, term infants while Goldstein and others studied both primiparae and multiparae delivering both term and preterm infants—for illustrative purposes I believe it is useful to contrast the measures of maternal beliefs used. The NPI used by Broussard and Hartner measures each mother's perception of, i.e., beliefs about her infant relative to her perception of the average infant on specific items such as crying, sleeping patterns, and spitting up. In contrast, the PARI measures subject agreement or disagreement with statements about childrearing phrased in the generalized third person

(Becker & Krug, 1965). For example, the first three items on the PARI are stated as follows (Schaefer & Bell, 1958):

(1) Children should be allowed to disagree with their parents if they feel their own ideas are better.
(2) A good mother should shelter her child from life's little difficulties.
(3) The home is the only thing that matters to a good mother.

The object of the mother's beliefs as measured on the NPI is not only more specific than that of the PARI, but also more relevant to the developmental issues confronting the mother of an infant. For this reason, maternal perceptions assessed by the NPI may be more reactive to experience in infant caregiving. In this line Tulkin and Cohler (1973) have argued for the importance of using parent attitudinal measures which are congruent with the developmental levels of the children of the parents being studied.

It is interesting to speculate about results Goldstein and others might have obtained had they used a measure in which the attitudinal object was each mother's own infant and in which the item content was relevant specifically to infant care and behavior. Still further, substituting a measure of infant status at birth which directly taps infant interactive capacities—e.g., the Brazelton Neonatal Behavioral Assessment Scale (Brazelton, 1973b)—for the original infant status index would offer a more precise test of the effects of infant characteristics upon maternal attitudes. While the results of the study conducted by Goldstein and others appear inconclusive given the design limitations mentioned above, the study is of importance in that it represents the multivariable orientation to parental attitude research argued for in this chapter.

Before moving further into consideration of research designs in parental attitude research, two major attitudinal measurement approaches will be presented as part of the psychometric concerns pertinent to the design of parental attitude research. These two approaches include the semantic differential technique and the belief statement approach exemplified by the Likert method.

Fishbein (1967; Fishbein & Ajzen, 1975) has identified the semantic differential technique (Osgood, Suci, & Tannenbaum, 1957), as one of the direct measures of attitude toward an object. Using bipolar adjective pairs, e.g., good-bad, sweet-sour, which have evaluative content relative to the concept under study, one may obtain a direct measure of the affective response to the stimulus concept. Using the semantic differential technique as an attitudinal measure is complicated by the fact that adjective pairs vary in their evaluative content when applied to different stimulus concepts, i.e., attitude objects (Fishbein & Ajzen, 1975). Thus, for each concept under study one must determine by factor analysis the relevant evaluative adjective pairs. Keeping in mind this prerequisite to the use of the semantic differential technique, the method offers a means of directly tapping parental attitudes toward concepts of interest.

In the Likert technique, an indirect measure of attitude is obtained by examining persons' belief strength relative to a set of statements (Fishbein & Ajzen, 1975). For example, persons might respond to the statement, "Babies are a lot of fun to care for," on a seven-point scale ranging from "strongly agree" to "strongly disagree." From a summation of responses to belief statements, attitude is inferred. In constructing or selecting attitude scales based on belief statements, it is important to sample a number of beliefs related to the attitude object under study to be able to accurately infer attitude toward the object. (While the NPI is not constructed in the standard Likert manner, it does appear to capture a range of belief content relative to infants and in this regard may also be considered as a measure of beliefs.)

While semantic differential and Likert-type instruments are relatively easy to construct, addressing the psychometric properties of such tools may be thorny. Attention to instrument reliability and validity (Nunnally, 1967) is especially pertinent where the state of parental attitude measurement lacks tools for attitudinal measurement which have met accepted psychometric standards (Becker & Krug, 1965; Freese & Thoman, 1978; Cohler, Weiss & Grunebaum, Note 1). While it is beyond the scope of this chapter to review the psychometric evidence relative to commonly used measures of early parental attitudes or to discuss reliability and validity in general, one especially perplexing dimension of psychometric evaluation of instruments will be addressed, construct validity. According to Nunnally (1967), construct validity, in contrast to predictive and content validity, is concerned with the measurement of psychological traits. In sum, construct validity entails demonstrating a correspondence between a construct under study and the operational procedure and instrument used for its measurement. Where there is an accepted standard for the measurement of a construct, then arguing for the construct validity of new measures of that same construct is easily done if the new measures can be shown to be highly related to results obtained with the standard method. For example, new methods of measuring temperature will be accepted as valid to the degree to which results correspond to an accepted method of measuring temperature. (It is of course possible that new methods may overthrow an accepted standard of measurement if the new methods are shown to have greater precision than the standard.)

Providing evidence for the construct validity of tools measuring ill-defined constructs such as "parental attitudes" where the specific attitudinal object is unclear, or of tools measuring constructs which lack an accepted measurement standard, presents investigators with special problems. An inductive strategy proposed by Campbell and Fiske (1959), the multitrait-multimethod approach, and adapted for use with attitudinal instruments (Fishbein, 1967; Fishbein & Ajzen, 1975) is one method for coping with the problem of construct validity in the measurement of early parental attitudes. Since the multitrait-multimethod approach is widely known, it will not be discussed in general. Rather, the requirements for the use of this approach in measuring early parental attitudes will be addressed. Carrying out the multitrait-multimethod approach in parental attitudes requires: (1) that instruments measuring several theoretically unrelated concepts or constructs be included in the design and (2) that each of these concepts or constructs be measured by several tools which reflect differing measurement methods. By comparing correlation coefficients generated from among instruments, discriminant and convergent validity may be examined.

Many of the measurement procedures used in measuring attitudes may also be applied to measuring parental behaviors which are expected to be influenced by given attitudes. Sampling not one, but several behaviors to form a multi-act index related to the attitudinal object increases the reliability and validity of the behavioral measures (Fishbein & Ajzen, 1975). Fishbein has made a strong argument that behaviors as indicators may lack reliability and validity in the same manner as items on an attitude scale. Following this analogy, Fishbein and Ajzen (1975) have argued for the systematic assessment of the measurement properties of behavioral as well as attitudinal measures. Fishbein and Ajzen (1975) have presented evidence to indicate that when multi-item attitudinal scales are used with multi-item behavioral indices substantially higher attitude-behavior consistencies are found than with single-item behavioral measures.

Both this section on methodological considerations and the preceding one on theoretical concerns have pointed to multi-variable orientations in early parental attitudinal research. In the next section illustrative data leading to this end are presented and further research aimed at multi-variable orientations is proposed.

PRELIMINARY DESIGN FOR EARLY PARENTAL
ATTITUDE RESEARCH

The study reported below was conducted to gather preliminary data for a larger study designed to investigate the relationship of maternal attitudes and perceptions and infant characteristics to subsequent mother-infant interaction. Given the constraints of sample size and the pilot nature of the work, the study is presented primarily to illustrate some directions for early parental attitude research. While the entire design of the study is reported, only data on the attitudinal measures will be reported.

Method

Subjects in the study consisted of 30 mother-infant pairs selected from a private hospital. Mothers were all initially breastfeeding and experienced pregnancies and labors without major medical complications. Infants were all first-born females with no major neonatal illnesses or anomalies. All deliveries were conducted under regional or local anesthesia. Infants were assessed in the newborn nursery using the Brazelton Neonatal Behavioral Assessment Scale. The Brazelton Scale is purported to assess infants' interactive capacities in relation to the environment (Brazelton, 1973b).

During the hospital stay following delivery mothers completed a battery of attitudinal and perception scales including: maternal self-confidence paired comparisons (Seashore, Leifer, Barnett, & Leiderman, 1973), semantic differential scales (Osgood, Suci, & Tannenbaum, 1957) related to the concepts MY BABY and MYSELF AS A MOTHER (Walker, Note 2), the Neonatal Perception Inventory (Broussard & Hartner, 1970, 1971), and the Parent-Child Relationships Subscale of the Traditional Family Ideology Scale (Levinson & Huffman, 1955). With the exception of the subscale from the Traditional Family Ideology Scale, all the instruments were completed again by the mothers at 4-6 weeks post-delivery.

The maternal self-confidence paired comparisons (MSC) measure the mother's self-confidence in contrast to that of four other care providers on seven caretaking or interactive tasks with their infants: showing affection to the baby, holding the baby, calming the baby, diapering the baby, understanding what the baby wants, bathing the baby, and feeding the baby.

The semantic differential scales contained two factors related to the concept MY BABY: "Infant Ideals" and "Infant Size," and two factors related to the concept MYSELF AS A MOTHER: "Maternal Ideals" and "Maternal Security-Maturity." Adjective pairs on Infant Ideals (II) included: sick-healthy, sweet-sour, good-bad, pleasant-unpleasant, difficult-easy, and belligerent-peaceful; those for Infant Size (IS) were small-large and light-heavy. Adjective pairs on Maternal Ideals (MI) included: fast-slow, graceful-awkward, weak-strong, kind-cruel, good-bad, successful-unsuccessful, and calm-excitable; those on Maternal Security-Maturity (MSM) included: unwilling-willing; dangerous-safe, complete-incomplete, and mature-inmature.

As discussed earlier in this chapter, the Neonatal Perception Inventory (NPI) measures mothers' perceptions of their own infants and their perception of the average baby on six behavioral items. Typically, a difference score is calculated on these two components of the NPI.

The Traditional Family Ideology Scale is reported to be a measure of authoritarianism in family relations. The Parent-Child Relationships Subscale contains 15 items to which subjects respond on a Likert scale of agreement-disagreement.

Brief interviews were conducted with the mothers during the hospitalization period and four to six weeks later. The first interview included data on the mother's age, education, labor ratings, pregnancy ratings, time at which the baby was first held by the mother, time at which the mother first saw the baby's eyes, and type of prenatal classes attended. The second interview included data on the mother's feelings during separation from the baby, previous child care experience, estimate of her preparedness for parenthood and whether she was still breastfeeding the baby. Mothers were also videotaped in the home at four to six weeks post-delivery in two situations: a diaper change and a play interaction.

Results

Since there was limited or no previous reliability data available on the maternal attitudinal and perceptual instruments, internal consistency of the instruments was assessed. Examination of the coefficient alpha values (Cronbach, 1951) indicated that several of the instruments presented low internal consistency within this sample. Thus, one item was deleted from the Neonatal Perception Inventory (NPI) and three from the Traditional Family Ideology Subscale (TFIS). After these adjustments the coefficient alpha values presented in Table 1 were obtained. Because of the low internal consistency on parts of the NPI, scoring was modified and the difference score between mothers' perception of their baby compared to the average baby was not computed. Instead, the rating of the average baby and your baby portions were treated as separate scales for all the data analyses reported below.

TABLE 1

Coefficient Alpha Values for Attitude and
Perception Scales at t_1* and t_2*

Scale	t_1	t_2
Neonatal Perception Inventory (NPI)		
Average Baby	.6084	.6367
Neonatal Perception Inventory (NPI)		
Your Baby	.5526	.7681
Maternal Self-Confidence (MSC)	.7808	.7974
Traditional Family Ideology Subscale (TFIS)	.7157	
Infant Ideals (II)	.7726	.7239
Infant Size (IS)	.9356	.8048
Maternal Ideals (MI)	.6598	.7457
Maternal Security-Maturity (MSM)	.7758	.6474

*t_1 refers to the hospitalization period and t_2 to the 4-6 week follow-up period.

The Maternal Ideals (MI), Maternal Security-Maturity (MSM), and Infants Ideals (II) scales were significantly intercorrelated at both administrations. Also the average baby rating on the NPI and the II were significantly correlated with the Your Baby portion of the NPI at both administrations. Two shifts in correlational patterns occurred for the

TABLE 2

Intercorrelation of Attitude/Perception
Scales at 1-3 Days Postpartum

	TFIS	MI	MSM	II	IS	NPI-AVERAGE	NPI-YOUR
MI[a]	—						
MSM	—	.658**					
II	—	.658**	.534**				
IS	—	—	—	—			
NPI-Average Baby[b]	—	—.375*	—	—.366*	—		
NPI-Your Baby[b]	—	—.489**	—.449*	—.597**	—	.413*	—
MSC	—	—	—	—	.428*	—	—

* p < .05
** p < .01

[a] TFIS = Traditional Family Ideology Subscale, MI = Maternal Ideals, MSM = Maternal Security-Maturity, II = Infant Ideals, IS = Infant Size, NPI = Neonatal Perception Inventory, MSC = Maternal Self-Confidence.

[b] The Negative sign on correlation coefficients for NPI is an artifact of the direction of scoring and not a genuine inverse relationship.

TABLE 3

Intercorrelation of Attitude/Perception
Scales at 4-6 Weeks Postpartum

	MI	MSM	II	IS	NPI-AVER-AGE	NPI-MY
MSMa	.677**					
II	.569*	.415*				
IS	—	—	—.416*			
NPI-Average Babyb	—	—	—	—		
NPI-Your Babyb	—	—	—.492**	—	.424*	
MSC	.405*	.619**	—	—	—	—

* p < .05
** p < .01

a MI = Maternal Ideals, MSM = Maternal Security-Maturity, II = Infant Ideals, IS = Infant Size, NPI = Neonatal Perception Inventory, MSC = Maternal Self-Confidence.
b The negative sign on correlation coefficients for NPI is an artifact of the direction of scoring and not a genuine inverse relationship.

MI-MSM complex: while YOUR BABY scores on the NPI were signifi-cantly correlated with this complex at the first administration, this rela-tionship was not significant at the second. In contrast, maternal self-confidence (MSC) was correlated with the MI-MSM complex at the second administration, but not the first.

Each of the seven scales which was administered at both time intervals was significantly correlated with itself. These correlations ranged from $r = .400$ for the Neonatal Perception Inventory—average baby portion—to $r = .798$ for Infant Size.

Discussion

The data presented provide some preliminary evidence for both in-ternal consistency reliability and the patterning of maternal attitudes and perceptions during the neonatal period. While coefficient alpha values were generally within minimal acceptable levels, modifying instruments in an attempt to improve these values would be desirable.

Examining the patterns of correlations between attitudinal and percep-tion measures both within and across time intervals provides a beginning point for assessing construct validity of certain instruments as well as describing some of the attitudinal and belief dynamics of the neonatal period. Unfortunately, the lack of a precise and clear conceptual defini-tion of the traits or domains measured by each attitudinal or perception tool, along with the lack of parallel tools using alternate measurement methods, precludes a clear application of the multitrait-multimethod approach. Future research design should definitely aim at meeting these requirements for the inductive assessment of construct validity.

Keeping in mind these psychometric limitations, several preliminary generalizations may be made. Each of the seven instruments administered at both time intervals was significantly correlated with itself. This finding suggests some degree of stability in specific maternal attitudes and perceptions. In contrast, only some of the correlational patterns between the seven instruments were maintained over both testing periods. Among these enduring correlational patterns was a set related to evaluative aspects of the mother and infant, viz. Maternal Ideals, Maternal Security-Maturity, and Infant Ideals, and a set related to attitudes and beliefs about infants, viz. Your Baby and "the average baby" on the NPI and Infant Ideals. The former set may represent idealizations or projected hopes rather than actual reality based evaluations of self and infant. This conclusion seems plausible because the MI-MSM complex was unrelated to maternal self-confidence in caregiving on the MSC during hospitalization. This is a time when mothers would be expected to be less adept in infant care and thus less self-confident. At the four to six week follow-up, however, the MI-MSM complex and MSC were significantly correlated. This is a time when one would expect projected hopes and actual maternal skill to be more congruent.

This tentative interpretation of the MI-MSM complex may also explain the second complex of attitudes and beliefs about the infant, especially those measured by the Your Baby portion of the NPI. This scale correlated positively with the MI-MSM complex at hospitalization, but not at follow-up. This shift in correlational pattern may reflect initial "mother centered" beliefs about the infant's behavior, i.e. maternal beliefs untempered by the actual infant characteristics, which then undergo a transition during the post-hospitalization period so that the beliefs become more reflective of infant inputs into the maternal belief structure, i.e. more infant centered. These tentative interpretations of the pilot data suggest that infant characteristics should be included in the longitudinal prediction of maternal attitudes and beliefs to more directly test the predictions made.

Application of multi-variable theoretical orientations to the data generated from the type of design presented here requires the use of statistical methods such as multiple regression using models of linear as well as perhaps non-linear relationships (Ward & Jennings, 1973). While these methods were not justified given the sample size of this preliminary study, application of such methods in future research would permit an examination of questions such as (1) the joint impact of initial maternal attitudes and infant characteristics on subsequent maternal interactive behavior, and (2) the influence of initial maternal attitudes and infant characteristics on subsequent maternal attitudes. The latter question is of special interest with such tools as the NPI because of its reported value in predicting later child adjustment. Not included in the design above, but of interest in future research, is the inclusion of instruments which are aimed at measurement of parental norms and motivation to comply with these norms. Inclusion of such measures in the design would permit a fuller application of the Fishbein framework to early parental attitude research as well as test the validity of the Fishbein model.

CONCLUSION

In this chapter an argument has been made for the continuation of research in early parental attitudes and beliefs. While recognizing the generally negative history of attitude-behavior research, several means were presented for more successfully attacking questions related to early parental attitudes and accompanying beliefs. These included clarification of the concept of attitude and its relationship to behavior, as well as strengthening methods of attitudinal research. As Causey (1969) has noted, nothing fails in research like the repetition of past failures; however, introduction of new methods or understandings can lead to rich and productive research efforts.

Part V

METHODOLOGICAL ISSUES IN ASSESSING INFANT CHARACTERISTICS AND THE QUALITY OF PARENT-INFANT INTERACTIONS

This section is devoted to discussions of methodological strategies for characterizing the quality of parent-infant interaction and of the behavioral characteristics of the individual participants. Of particular interest is the assessment of disturbed patterns of parent-infant interaction which are a function of psychosocial risk factors in the infant and/or parent and which may contribute to psychosocial risk in the infant's development.

The measurement and evaluation of these processes in the past have been difficult tasks because of limitations in theory and in research methodologies. Theories about the infant's contribution to the nature of parent interactions are themselves in the infancy stage. Theories about the specific qualities of parent interactive styles that are significant determinants of infant development are also in their early stages. Finally, there is no well formulated theory about the qualitative aspects of the infant-environment transaction that is most relevant to optimal infant development. These problems make the decisions about the specific individual characteristics and interactional, behavioral variables to measure a difficult one.

In addition to these limitations of current theory, there are also limited empirical data pertaining to these issues. Until recently, the research literature has provided inadequate bases for selecting empirically derived, manageable sets of global or summary behavioral variables (e.g., cluster or factor scores) to serve as indices of the quality of interactional patterns

251

and as predictors of later interactional patterns and infant development.

Consequently, recent research of qualitative differences in parent-infant interaction and the factors that contribute to these differences has involved multivariate strategies in which large numbers of individual characteristics and large numbers of behavioral variables for both infant and parent have been included. The two problems of these large scale assessment strategies are: (1) how to deal with apparently unmanageable, large numbers of variables in the analyses of the data, and (2) how to characterize the individual participants in interactions as well as the qualitative aspects of the interactional process with a more limited number of "best" variables—best in the sense of reliability and validity, especially predictive validity for subsequent infant development.

The three papers in this section deal with these problems directly. Each chapter describes a strategy for reducing large numbers of specific and molecular variables into a set of summary variables that serve to characterize the infants and parents along dimensions that are relevant to the quality of parent-infant interaction as well as dimensions that characterize the quality of the interactional process itself.

The chapter by Yang is a description of a methodological strategy for characterizing infants in terms of temperamental and behavioral qualities and includes a discussion of the superiority of this strategy to earlier ones. Specifically, Yang proposes the use of factor scores to characterize infants and, especially, in the determination of the stability of infant characteristics over time. This discussion includes a demonstration of the superiority of factor stability over single item test-retest stability and also demonstrates impressive predictive validity of factor scores for later infant and child characteristics.

A conceptually similar goal—reducing large numbers of variables into a fewer number of more global indices—is described in the chapter by Bakeman and Brown. However, in this chapter, the focus is on characterizing qualitative aspects of interactions in parent-infant dyads—specifically, the sequential dependencies between parent behaviors and infant behaviors in the stream of behavioral dialogues. The especially unique contribution of this paper is the "levels of analysis" strategy wherein data reduction is accomplished in steps moving from molecular analyses to global analyses with each level providing different, but compatible and consistent, information about the quality of parent-infant interactions. Finally, the validity and utility of these procedures are demonstrated by their ability to meaningfully discriminate between patterns of interaction involving preterm infants as opposed to full-term infants.

The last chapter in this section goes a step further toward deriving techniques to characterize qualitative aspects of behavioral interactions. In a highly sophisticated advance in the use of sequential probabilities among behaviors in a stream of behavior, Sackett describes analytical techniques for deriving indices of the types of roles played by each of the interactors and the impact that each interactor has on the other interactors over time. Thus he provides us with ways to characterize the interactors as well as the quality of the interaction itself. By using these analyses, large quantities of sequential probabilities for large numbers of variables can be reduced to a few global indices that accurately capture the qualitative character of the interaction, the nature of the role played by each interactor, the influence of this role on the role played by the other interactors, and the changing character of these transactions over time and as a function of earlier interactions.

12

Dimensional Analyses of Newborn Behavior and Their Significance for Later Behavior: The Example of the Bethesda Longitudinal Study

RAYMOND K. YANG

University of Georgia

Although publications in most areas of psychological research have increased, the growing research focus on infancy is of special significance for it reflects an important presumption: Development is marked by continuity. Presumably, early predictors of later development can be found. This presumption is best exemplified by the large number of standardized infant assessments developed over the years (for reviews see Thomas, 1970; Yang & Bell, 1975; Brooks & Weinraub, 1976), whose major interest was not to describe concurrent individual differences, but to predict emergent differences in ability.

However, the prediction of ensuing differences in ability and the description of concurrent individual differences are not completely separable. The prediction of later differences in ability requires that differences in early behavior be found. That requirement is not substantive, but logical; early differences must exist in order for prediction to be possible. Nevertheless, only a portion of the research describing early differences in behavior has prediction as a direct and ultimate goal. Considerable research is oriented not directly at prediction, but at describing the human infant as a "sensory surface" and perceptual processor (for reviews, see Cohen and Salapatek, 1975, 1976). This paper does not deal with that literature, but focuses on the assessment of early individual differences and their longitudinal relationships. It also does not deal with studies assessing longitudinal continuities in intelligence (that is, IQ, developmental status, developmental quotient, etc.). These studies form a group of their own.

THREE CONSIDERATIONS IN STUDYING INFANTS

It is often remarked that the increased study of human infants is as much a result of theoretical motivation as their "discovery" as an available population. Notwithstanding, their availability is a mixed blessing, for their availability does not insure their participation and cooperation. Left to their own devices, infants (newborns included) easily terminate procedures by falling asleep or becoming irritable. Indeed, subject loss is a frequent and significant, if little discussed, problem in infant research (Graham & Jackson, 1970; Lewis & Johnson, 1971). Attempts to cope with these problems have included the development of state/lability measures, e.g., Brazelton Neonatal Behavioral Assessment Scale (Brazelton, 1973c), a type of measure unique to infancy, as well as the development of brief procedures lessening the likelihood that an infant will change states during testing. And by no means is the skill of the tester unimportant; the ability of the tester to establish rapport and elicit (e.g., cajole) the "best" performance from the subject has sometimes been seen as a valid predictor of later outcome (Escalona, 1950).

The second difficulty in working with infants involves communication. The lack of a common communicative mode (language) between subject and researcher creates unique difficulties and misperceptions. Often, the infant is presumed to be a more simple organism, relative to the adult; more appropriate would be the assumption that the infant is *different*, but certainly no less complex. Lacking language, the infant is also seen as being less psychologically freighted—somehow lacking in personality, but not so devoid of it as to impair our ability to anthropomorphize. The effect is twofold: First, measures that have face validity become problematic when examined from a psychological perspective (What is the real meaning of crying?). Thus, over time, can the identical measure reflect the same underlying dimension? Kagan (1971) and Bell (1972) have proposed specific mediating constructs to deal with these issues. Second, lacking a psychology, is the infant, *de facto*, a physiological entity? This question, reflecting if nothing else the remnants of dualism, often prevented infants from being studied as social creatures. Infants, as sensory surfaces, responded to largely auditory, visual, and tactile stimuli under experimental conditions. Their lot was deemed psychophysical long before it was social.

The third consideration deals with the presumption that infancy is the place to start searching for longitudinal continuities; or essentially, that birth represents the beginning of life. Most studies of early infancy have lacked either the interdisciplinary perspective or the technology to study their subject in the uterine environment. Nevertheless, it is well known that the relative rate of growth is most rapid during the first trimester and decelerates thereafter. It is also well known that the environmental interventions (iatrogenic or teratogenic) occurring during this period have massive effects upon the organism. It is not so much that as behavioral scientists we ignore these facts, but that, as obsessive observers, we choose to study only those things that we can observe directly. Thus there are many studies of the pregnant mother, more studies of the neonate and infant, and very few studies of the fetus *in utero* (i.e., Spelt, 1948; Walters, 1965).

The overall effect of these considerations is to reveal the focus on the human infant as somewhat arbitrary, if understandable. In addition, these considerations place the popularity of measures such as heart rate change, sucking and sensory thresholds in perspective: At the same time that the measures reflect the presumption of the "simpler" organism (linguistically incompetent, smaller), they also serve as proxies for what will later emerge as "psychological." Thus heart rate change, for example, as a measure of autonomic arousal, will later become fear, attentiveness, or affective lability.

Longitudinal studies of neonatal and infant development confront these considerations directly. This chapter describes a recently conducted longitudinal study, a portion of which included data from early infancy. The study was designed to yield sizeable amounts of longitudinal data on a relatively small sample. The study was also designed so that assessments at each stage were conducted by independent teams of researchers. The data analytic techniques engendered by these factors and some of their initial substantive results are the focus of this chapter.

THE BETHESDA LONGITUDINAL STUDY

Newborn Data Collection and Analyses

Under the direction of Wells Goodrich (between 1959 and 1963) and Richard Bell (from 1963 to 1973), the National Institute of Mental Health Intramural Research Program conducted a longitudinal study of early family development. A part of that study consisted of a newborn assessment.*

In 1971, Bell, Weller, and Waldrop reported a major analysis of a pilot cohort in the longitudinal study. They studied 75 white, second- or later-born neonates delivered in the metropolitan Washington, D.C. area. Each infant was studied for two three-and-a-half-hour sessions; each session contained one sleeping and waking period. Of a total of 31 measures, 12 were of sufficient test-retest stability to retain for further analyses. During sleep, the stable measures described mouthing movements, closed eye movements, respiration, and tactile threshold. During waking, the stable measures described gross muscle strength (the prone head response) non-nutritive sucking, formula consumption (controlling for body weight), crying, and response latencies.

Principal component analyses of these measures yielded three interpretable factors. The first factor described nonnutritive and nutritive sucking; Bell et al. (1971) labeled this factor "feeding." The second factor was labeled "sleep" and described respiratory movements and tactile threshold. The third factor described crying and response latencies. A fourth factor describing movements in sleep was obtained for males only. These factors were used to construct composite scores which, in addition to the 12 single measures, served as the basis for examining longitudinal relations. In all, there were 16 measures for males and 15 measures for females that were used in Bell et al.'s longitudinal analyses.

In 1976, Yang, Federman, and Douthitt reported an analysis of a larger newborn sample (n = 137) from the Bethesda Longitudinal Study. Although these infants were first-borns (unlike those in the Bell et al., 1971 study), they were also from the metropolitan Washington, D.C. area. These infants were studied for two three-hour sessions during which sleep and waking behaviors were assessed. Four levels of state, heart and respiratory rates, and observations of gross motor activity were used to create 15 measures characterizing sleep. Eight behaviors were assessed while the infant was awake. These behaviors included nonnutritive sucking and responses to interruption of sucking, the prone head response, and responses to aversive stimulation with and without comforting.

---

* Preparation for the entire study began in 1959. The overall plan included an assessment of the newlywed couple, an assessment of the expectant mother, and later, her newborn. At three, 11, and 30 months, the child was tested again. Several pilot cohorts were tested at each stage. Data for the study were collected between 1965 and 1973. Richard Q. Bell, Thomas Douthitt, Charles F. Halverson, Jr., Sandra Jones-Kearns, Howard Moss, David H. Olson, Robert G. Ryder, Mary Waldrop, and myself conducted the study.

(These measures are described in detail in Yang, Federman, & Douthitt, 1976.) Gestational age and a composite score representing body size completed the set of newborn measures.

Unlike the procedure adopted by Bell et al. in which single measures not exhibiting adequate test-retest stability were omitted from further analyses, Yang et al. submitted their entire set of variables to factor analyses. Yang's belief was that inadequate test-retest stability was not appropriate as the *sole* criterion for discarding measures of newborn behavior. The very nature of newborns included frequent changes in state. To discard measures on the basis of a characteristic of the organism from which those measures were obtained was self-defeating (e.g., Lewis & Johnson, 1971).

Yang et al. factored the measures obtained from each of the two testing sessions separately. The data from one session were used to explore various factor analytic solutions; data from the other session were used to assess the stability of the final solution. Using this procedure, three stable factors were formed that replicated across both sessions.

The first factor, *reactivity-irritability*, grouped all variables measuring some aspect of crying and appeared to be the most interpretable and consistent of the three factors. The factor described a high-scoring neonate as responding rapidly to the withdrawal of a nipple and crying many times in response to that withdrawal and to other aversive stimulation. Grouping all measures that could be construed as aversive, this factor was similar to one obtained by Bakow et al. (1973) in their analysis of the Neonatal Behavioral Assessment Scale (Brazelton, 1973c). Bakow et al. (1973) described an "irritability" factor that included measures assessing activity, excitability, tonus, and rapidity of buildup. The importance of the factor is clear when its function is examined. The factor groups measures of overt distress, which are not only responses to stimulation, but also signals for caregiving. Maternal responses to the neonate, therefore, might be directly related to this dimension.

The second factor, *maturity*, described a high-scoring infant as large (weight and size), of long gestation, rapid respiratory rate, and of low autonomic variability during sleep. This factor combined data obtained from medical records as well as from the assessment procedure. The clustering of variables suggested that gestation-related distinctions could be made between neonates during sleep. During these periods, low autonomic variability could be interpreted as reflecting homeostatic efficiency, that is, maintaining resting autonomic functions within relatively narrow boundaries. This could be an energy-conserving device, functional during periods of relative nonstimulation when behavioral responses were at minimal levels.

The third factor, *reflexive and discriminative sucking*, described a high-scoring infant as having high levels of reflexive and discriminative sucking, accompanied by a high percentage of active sleep and a low percentage of quiet sleep. The sucking stimuli were the only ones in the entire procedure which could be construed as being of moderate intensity. Moreover, the behavior elicited was the only one in the procedure that could be construed as stimulus enhancing (accepting, seeking). Such an infant, sensitive to stimulation optimally elicitive of responses, spent a lower percentage of time in quiet sleep.

Thus two major efforts to describe two samples of newborns produced results that were somewhat similar. Bell et al.'s (1971) factors describing response to nipple removal (crying) was similar to Yang et al.'s (1976) reactivity-irritability factor. The grouping of measures on the reactivity-irritability factor more clearly defined that dimension as being associated with *aversive* stimulation. The feeding factor described by Bell et al. was similar to Yang et al.'s reflexive and discriminative sucking. Nonetheless, the feeding factor actually contained a measure of nutritive intake while Yang et al.'s factor did not. Finally, two factors were noncomparable: Bell et al.'s sleep factor and Yang et al.'s maturity factor had no counterparts. Summarizing over both analyses, two dimensions had been located: One dealt with crying in response to aversive stimulation; the other dealt with feeding and sucking.

Both Bell et al.'s and Yang et al.'s efforts had occurred in the context of the Bethesda Longitudinal Study. There was, therefore, considerable overlap in the approach to both data sets. Indeed, to the extent that co-ordination and similarity in procedures can occur in any large data collection, these efforts were probably near the maximum. Nonetheless, there were several differences between the efforts. Bell's sample was comprised of second- and later-borns. Yang's was comprised of first-borns exclusively. Bell's sample, being a pilot sample, was considerably smaller than Yang's. Yang's assessment involved considerably more measures than Bell's. These three differences were less elective than they were required: The changes were viewed as improvements in technique, technology, or breadth of assessment. The final difference occurred in the data analysis. Bell discarded measures not exhibiting adequate individual stability and conducted principal components analyses separately for males and females. Yang retained all individual measures, conducted principal component and varimax rotation analyses of the entire sample (males and females), and replicated the final factor solution.

These different data-analytic approaches may have been a function of the flexibility associated with increased sample size. Bell reduced an original set of 31 measures to a final set of 12 measures for factoring. Given that his sample of females numbered only 35, the retention of all 31 measures for factoring would have been inappropriate. Yang's sample, being larger, had the option of factoring its entire set of measures. Thus, Yang was able to examine the effect of using a criterion other than single-measure stability in developing reliable descriptive dimensions. That criterion, factor stability, was more flexible than the requirement of single-measure stability because it was equally satisfied by *concurrent* stability. While single-measure stability traditionally deals with the relation between a variable measured at time-1 and measured again at time-2, concurrent stability deals with the relation between two different variables at the same moment. If two variables are correlated with each other at time-1, and exhibit that same correlation at time-2, then they will load on the same factor (i.e., exhibit concurrent stability), irrespective of what their individual test-retest stabilities are. The dimensions developed by Yang et al. capitalized on this.

Longitudinal Relations

In the Bethesda Longitudinal Study, independent assessments were conducted at five points in the family's life cycle: the newlywed couple; the pregnant mother; the newborn infant; the mother and infant at three months; and the young child at two-and-one-half years of age. Two-and-one-half years was selected as the criterion age.

In their analysis of the pilot cohort, Bell et al. reported an important relation between their newborn assessment and behavior at two-and-one-half years:

> High speed, frequency, and magnitude of newborn behavior were associated with less vigor and responsiveness to the nursery school play settings and social context, while low levels of functioning in the newborn period were associated with higher involvement and activity later (Bell et al., 1971, p. 122).

This "inversion of intensity" characterized males primarily and suggested that there might be a ". . . need to revise the notion that high vigor and responsiveness in the newborn period indicate (d) an optimal status" (Bell et al., 1971. p. 132).

These relations emerged from selected individual measures and factor composites that Bell et al. had generated from their principal component analyses. These newborn variables were correlated with various *individual* variables at two-and-one-half years. (The two-and-one-half year measures had been factored. However, relations between these two-and-one-half year factors and all newborn measures did not exceed chance levels.)

Specifically, the longitudinal correlations described an "inverted" relation of the individual newborn measures representing the crying/response latency composite and sleep composite for males with selected individual measures at two-and-one-half years. Remarking on the lack of relation to two-and-one-half year factors, Bell et al. observed that ". . . it is apparent that latency and cries 'selected' later correlates without regard to their organization in terms of shared variance at the preschool period" and added, "This fact does not make them any less (sic) difficult to interpret; however, since variations on a common thread of interest and active involvement in the games and routines of the nursery school is readily apparent . . ." (Bell et al., 1971, p. 85). Two components of the newborn sleep factor were correlated with a large activity factor ("intensity-barrier-peer") at two-and-one-half years. Measures of rapid and slow respiratory rates during sleep were negatively correlated with activity.

In 1976, Yang and Halverson attempted to replicate the inversion of intensity in the large sample of the Bethesda Longitudinal Study. The replication was comprised of two parts, a replication and an extension. Part One was an attempt to recreate, on a measure by measure basis, each of the variables contributing to the inversion for males. Of 19 statistically significant relations of newborn crying and response latency with behaviors at two-and-one-half that were located by Bell et al., Yang and Halverson were able to reconstruct 11 of the relationships. None of the reconstructed relationships was statistically significant, although most were in a direction consistent with Bell's original findings.

The relations between the newborn respiratory measures during sleep and the two-and-one-half year activity composite and its components were also reconstructed. Bell had found respiratory rates to be negatively correlated with preschool activity. Yang and Halverson reconstructed six of the nine components of the activity composite that exhibited statistically significant relations to either of the respiratory measures in Bell's analysis. Of the reconstructed relations, 11 were statistically significant in Bell's analysis. Only one was statistically significant in Yang and Halverson's analysis. In summary, 20 relationships found to be statistically significant in Bell's analysis were reconstructed in the second sample of the Bethesda Longitudinal Study. Only one statistically significant relation was replicated.

The second part of Yang and Halverson's study was an attempt to test the inversion in a conceptually broader fashion. This involved using measures that were relevant to intensity but were not used in the Bell et al. analysis. Intensity was conceptualized as high-magnitude, energy-expending activity.

At the newborn period, ten measures were drawn from periods of sleep and waking. These measures were factored (principal components analysis, varimax rotation), yielding two orthogonal dimensions. The first factor, describing crying responses to aversive stimulation, was labeled *Reactive*. This factor was similar to Bell's composite representing crying and response latency. The second factor, containing measures of heart and respiratory rate during sleep, and spontaneous arousal, was labeled *Basal*.

At the preschool period, a rating of intense, vigorous play was used as a criterion for defining intensity. Twenty-five measures for males and 34 measures for females that were highly correlated with vigorous play were factored; the first principal component was labeled *Intensity*. This principal component (for each sex) was further divided into socially positive and negative components. These components were constructed so that the "inversion" concept could be better represented; suboptimal behavior at any period could be represented by a lack of "valued" behavior as well as the presence of objectionable behavior. The positive and negative components were constructed so that the inversion could be examined relative to each type of behavior. The negative component contained measures of negative peer interaction, impatient and frenetic behavior, and behaviors requiring teacher intervention. The positive component contained the measures that had not been used to define the negative components. Thus, three sets of measures had been constructed: one principal component representing vigorous play; and two composites derived from the principal component, one representing positive and the other representing negative social behavior. These three measures were correlated with the orthogonal factors representing newborn reactive and basal intensity. The correlations are presented in Table 1. Four of 12 correlations were statistically significant, one of which supported Bell et al.'s inversion interpretation: Male reactive intensity was negatively correlated with vigorous play in nursery school.

Table 1

Correlations Between Newborn and Nursery School Intensity Factors

	Vigorous Play		Preschool Intensity Socially Positive		Socially Negative	
	Male[a]	Female[b]	Male	Female	Male	Female
Newborn intensity						
Reactive	—.27*	—.10	—.22	—.06	—.32**	—.15
Basal	—.15	—.23*	—.06	—.25	—.39***	—.16

[a] $n = 30—39$
[b] $n = 38—39$
  * $p < .10$, one-tailed
 ** $p < .10$, two-tailed
*** $p < .02$, two-tailed

Two other relations, however, clarified this inverse relationship: Male reactive and basal intensity was negatively correlated with socially negative intensity at nursery school and uncorrelated with socially positive intensity. These relations indicated that only the socially negative aspects of intensity at nursery school were related to newborn intensity.

These correlations, while negative, did not constitute an "inversion." The inversion of intensity was based on the presumption that optimal and socially valued behavior was indexed at the newborn and nursery phases in some unitary way. The Bell et al. inversion was a negative association between optimal newborn behavior and nursery school behavior that presumably was socially valued (and vice versa). The data in the Yang and Halverson analysis indicated that optimal behavior at the newborn phase was negatively associated with *negative* nursery school behaviors. To the extent that the specific absence of negative behavior could be viewed positively, optimal newborn behavior was associated with positive behavior at nursery school.

In summary, Bell et al.'s initial finding of an inverse relation between newborn and preschool behaviors led them to propose an inversion of intensity hypothesis. Yang and Halverson attempted to reconstruct the original relationship upon which the inversion interpretation was based. Although able to reconstruct most of the relations, they were unable to replicate Bell's statistically significant findings. A broader and more conceptually based attempt to test the inversion hypothesis generated results similar to Bell's original finding, but also revealed that the inversion was oversimplified: The longitudinal relation was not on a unidimensional continuum of intensity, but on dimensions that involved, at least in preschool, socially negative behaviors.

HOW LONG IS LONGITUDINAL?

Many of the complex issues in planning longitudinal research can be captured in the single question above. Theoretical, methodological, and substantive matters are directly concerned with the selection of a beginning and criterion-point in the study. Cultural, economic, and administrative considerations also enter in, perhaps not so directly, but with equally powerful effects. Baltes, Bell, Eichorn, McCall, Schaie, and Wohlwill have discussed these issues at length (Baltes & Schaie, 1973; Bell, 1953; Eichorn, 1976; McCall, 1977; Schaie, 1965; Wohlwill, 1970) and the interested reader is referred to them.

In the analyses conducted by Bell et al. and Yang and Halverson, "longitudinal" was two and one half years. The preschool period was selected for two reasons: It was chronologically distant enough to allow for major organizational changes in behavior and physical setting, but not so removed as to be seriously affected by subject loss. The main sample of the Bethesda Longitudinal Study was assessed at three months postpartum in expectation of those major changes; at three months, the infant was presumed to have reached a developmental plateau from which he or she would soon depart (Moss, 1974).

Thus, the possibility that the "length" of longitudinal could indirectly affect relations was raised. Reorganizations in behavior patterns and settings could affect the interpretation of criterion measures. For example, vociferation indoors during quiet individual activity could be interpreted as poor impulse control. Outdoors, it might reflect vigorous involvement in group activities. Similarly, fleeting visual contact with an object could be interpreted as familiarity (versus novelty) or distractibility, depending upon the events that preceded it and the contemporaneous setting.

The factoring procedures used in the Bethesda Longitudinal Study, as much as they provided a convenient method by which variables could be summarized, were also attempts to represent these behavioral reorganizations. In summarizing the data describing the infants at three months of age, Moss (1977) obtained three factors describing males and four factors describing females. The first factor described an infant that was vocal, alert, had high muscle tonus, and was physically active (*Tonic-*

Active). The second factor described an infant that smiled, vocalized, and engaged in vis-à-vis behavior (*Social*). The third factor was characterized by a single rating: clarity of cues (*Clarity*). For females, four factors were obtained. The first factor described an infant who was vocal, smiled, kicked and thrashed, and engaged in vis-à-vis behavior (*Active-Social*). The second factor described an infant with high muscle tonus, who was visually alert, and infrequently drowsy (*Tonic*). The third factor described an infant engaging in high amounts of vocal behavior and low amounts of protesting (*Positive Vocalization*). The fourth factor, comparable to the male last factor, was characterized by a single rating: clarity of cues (*Clarity*).

Correlations between the three newborn factors and the seven factors describing the male and female infants at three months yielded two relationships of interest.

TABLE 2

Correlations Between Newborn and 3-Month Factors

| 3-Month Factors | Newborn Factors | | |
	Reactivity Irritability	Maturity	Discriminative Sucking
Males $(n = 37)$			
Tonic-active	.12	.37**	.06
Social	.07	.17	.05
Clarity	.20	—.01	.10
Females $(n = 34)$			
Active-social	.21	.17	.16
Tonic	—.09	.01	.01
Positive vocalizations	—.08	.22	.04
Clarity	.30*	—.14	.14

* $p < .10$
** $p < .02$

Two newborn factors, one for males and one for females, were correlated with factors derived from the three-month assessment. For males, newborn maturity was positively correlated with tonic-active behavior at three months. For females, newborn reactivity-irritability was positively correlated with clarity at three months. Longitudinal correlations between the newborn and three-month variables that had high loadings on the correlated factors are presented in Tables 3 and 4, respectively.

TABLE 3

Correlations Between the Defining Components of
Newborn Maturity and 3-Month Tonic-Active Behavior
for Males

Newborn Maturity	Vocali-zation	Visual Alertness	Muscle Tonus	Vocalizes	Kick & Thrash
Body size	.17	.39***	.50***	.16***	.23
Gestational age	.22	.38***	.58***	—.06	.16
Autonomic variability in quiet sleep	—.25	—.25	—.45***	—.41***	—.46***
Autonomic variability in active sleep	—.10	—.03	—.16	—.24	—.34***
Respiratory rate	—.04	.00	.00	—.01	—.02

(*n* range: 33 to 48)
** *p* < .05
*** *p* < .01

For males, four of five measures defining newborn maturity were correlated with four of five measures defining tonic-active behavior at three
months. At the newborn period, the relation was supported by body
size, gestational age, and the measures of autonomic variability during
sleep. At three months, the relation was supported by ratings of visual
alertness, vocalization, muscle tonus, and the observed behavior, kick
and thrash.

TABLE 4

Correlations Between the Defining Components of
Newborn Reactivity-Irritability and 3-Month Clarity
for Females

Newborn Reactivity-Irritability	3-Month Clarity
Reaction to aversive stimulation	.26
Reaction to aversive stimulation with intervention	—.17
Cries	—.10
Latency to cry	—.19
Latency to movement	—.06

(*n* range: 21 to 43)

For females, none of the five newborn variables defining reactivity-irritability was significantly correlated with the single measure defining three-month clarity; the relation between the factors was not supported by correlations between the defining components.

For males, the general tenor of the relations between these newborn characteristics and infant behavior might be viewed as characterizing optimal functioning. To the extent that the cluster of visual alertness, strength, and activity characterize optimal functioning at three months, the newborn measures that precede it are cast in a positive light: Within clinically normal boundaries, long gestational age, large body size, and low autonomic variability during sleep may reflect optimal birth status and homeostatic efficiency. If such an optimal functioning interpretation can be applied to these relations, it suggests that there is some *direct* continuity in functioning between these two periods.

Perhaps more important, there appears to be a substantive reorganization of behaviors between both periods. The newborn factor seems to reflect homeostatic efficiency. The three-month factor seems to reflect active physical involvement with the environment. The relation between the factors suggests that some common underlying dimension (i.e. maturity) is undergoing a major behavioral transformation between both periods.

Nonetheless, to emphasize the continuity in the underlying dimension at the expense of recognizing the substantive reorganization in behavior (or vice versa) may be inappropriate. Superimposing a common, socially valuative "template" to both periods, be it intensity or optimal functioning, only further clouds the picture (Bell, 1975). Bell's (1978) recent call for more fine-grained longitudinal analyses at more frequent intervals is one effective (if costly) way to avoid this pitfall. Repetitive measurements lessen the likelihood that transformations will go undetected and concomitantly, that speculation about underlying dimensions (intensity, optimal functioning) will become misleading.

Although Bell's call for more fine-grained analyses could not be met by the Bethesda Longitudinal Study, the analyses reported in this chapter can be recast in the direction of Bell's suggestion. Halverson, Moss, and Jones-Kearns (1977) reported that the three-month correlate of newborn maturity for males was also predictive of general activity in nursery school at three years: The *tonic-active* factor for male infants was negatively correlated [$r(44) = -.33$, $p < .02$] with a composite measure representing general activity in nursery school. Furthermore, the social factor for male infants was positively correlated with the same measure of general activity in nursery school [r (44) = .47, $p < .001$].

In light of Bell's call for fine-grained analyses, the naturally emerging question was whether the newborn measures, when combined with the measures obtained at three months, had any predictive power greater than when considered individually. If nothing else, this represented a temporally more fine-grained analysis by three months. A multiple regression analysis using newborn maturity, three-month tonic-active behavior and social behavior to predict general activity at nursery school produced a multiple correlation of 0.63.* Although sizeable, this multiple correlation was only slightly larger than that reported by Halverson, Moss, and Jones-Kearns (1977) in predicting nursery school activity from three-month behavior, excluding newborn measures [R = .58]. Apparently, little additional predictive ability was gained by including the newborn data.

Although this was only an "approximation" of a more fine-grained analysis, it seems doubtful that the lack of increase in predictive power occurred because of the poor approximation. It may be that while detailed analyses are necessary, they are not sufficient to improve our predictions. What is needed is a conceptual framework, be it Wolhwill's (1970) "developmental function" or a stage approach containing hypotheses about emergent functions. Such a framework would provide focal clarity to a plethora of measures and chronologically locate points of data collection. Essentially, Bell's call for more fine-grained analyses contains, on an implicit and minimal level, a conceptual framework: Early developmental changes are rapid and involve major reorganizations. Notwithstanding, more is needed in the form of substantive guidance regarding measures and time of data collection.

CONCLUSION

The Bethesda Longitudinal Study was a major attempt to improve on the shortcomings of other longitudinal studies. It was confined to a relatively brief period of data collection, thus preventing the continuous commitment of effort to data collection and (what would have been) the resultant lack of data analysis. The study also used independent teams of researchers to collect data at each stage, thereby avoiding the development of subtle biases on the part of the researchers. Clinical-descriptive as well as experimental procedures were used to generate

---

* This analysis was conducted in collaboration with Charles F. Halverson. Appreciation is expressed to Carol Lynn Martin for computational assistance.

data which was comprised of both behavioral observations and impressionistic ratings.

Thus, the administrative strategy and, to an extent, the methodology were well planned. What was missing was the conceptual framework, the theoretical (or proto-theoretical) substance that would have provided some degree of overall focus to the project. Such a framework, while not precluding empirical exploration of the data, would have provided direction for the selection of variables as well as initial approaches to the data. While enough of a conceptual structure was available to help determine the times at which data collection would occur, there was not enough to influence the substantive areas in which data was to be collected. Thus, while considerable energy was expended within each stage of data collection, coordinating and organizing measures, little effort was directed at coordination *between* stages.

These between stage considerations were particularly important for the Bethesda Longitudinal Study. Spanning early marriage, infancy, and early childhood, the study crossed several traditional and disciplinary boundaries. Psychological measures of adult personality in the marriage assessment, physiological measures of neonatal autonomic functioning, time-sampled observations of mother-infant interaction, and measures of early social behavior in young children were all available, presumably because they were related in some way to one another. That presumption, implicit in the design of the study, was necessary but insufficient to provide conceptual guidance in relating the stages. As indicated earlier, in the area of infancy where the traditional boundaries (physiological-psychological, beginning-end point) are blurred, this deficiency is particularly damaging.

In conclusion, it appears that Baldwin's (1960) warning that the longitudinal study was a concluding and confirmatory step in a research program and not an exploratory one is well taken, at least in the areas covered by the Bethesda Longitudinal Study. While theoretical development may have occurred within each of these areas, the unique considerations in infant research (if nothing else) made theoretical hypotheses about the interrelationships between these areas risky. Although dated, Baldwin's chariness may be as appropriate now as it was then.

13

Analyzing Behavioral Sequences: Differences Between Preterm and Full-term Infant-Mother Dyads During the First Months of Life

ROGER BAKEMAN and
JOSEPHINE V. BROWN
Georgia State University

As part of an ongoing research program concerned with the development of early mother-infant interaction, mothers with full-term and mothers with preterm infants were observed with their infants during a feeding situation just before hospital release, one month later, and three months later. Because preterm infants are at greater risk of being abused than full-term infants, we hoped that a comparison of the early interactions of mothers with preterm and full-term infants could reveal disturbed or deviant interaction patterns, patterns that might be implicated in the breakdown of interaction represented by child abuse. One purpose of this chapter is to describe the observed interactions, paying particular attention to elements that distinguish the two groups of mother-infant dyads. Such normative data should provide a reasonable basis for expectations concerning the behavior of preterm infants and should,

The work reported here was supported by Grant No. MH26131 awarded by the National Institutes of Mental Health. The authors would like to thank Mark Evans, Sandra Gentry, May Kennedy, Marion Latham, Sharon Ptacek, Polly Trnavsky, Beverly Wilkerson, Joan Wolkin, and Rick Zapf for work as behavioral observers and the mothers and infants for their participation in this study. The material presented in this chapter first appeared as a longer and more detailed technical report (Bakeman & Brown, 1977).

furthermore, document preterm/full-term interactive differences, differences that might be implicated in the etiology of child abuse.

Some behavioral differences between preterm and full-term interaction may represent reasonable adaptations of, and to, an immature organism. However, careful study is needed to reveal those differences which are adaptive and those which are maladaptive. This can best be done by relating measures of early interaction to measures of infant outcome and to later measures of infant-mother and infant-peer interaction. Subsequent reports will, in fact, examine such relationships, but the purpose of this chapter is more limited. First, it is descriptive, detailing differences in early interaction between preterm and full-term infant-mother dyads. Second, it is methodological, demonstrating how three different "levels" of analysis yield different information about preterm and full-term differences during the first few months of life.

The three levels correspond to data reduction steps. Just as the second level data are reduced or abstracted from the first level data, so the third level data are abstracted from the second. The first level is probably the most familiar. We simply describe the frequency and duration of particular discrete behaviors. The bulk of this chapter is devoted to the second level. Viewing the interaction more abstractly—as a behavioral dialogue —we focus on the frequency, flow, and patterning, not of particular behaviors but of "dialogic states." The third level is more abstract still. We are concerned not with what the particular patterns of the behavioral dialogue are, but with just how patterned or predictable a given dialogue is overall. It is our hope that clearing out the "underbrush" of specific behaviors may let us "see" aspects of interaction that might not be readily apparent to observers. The purpose of this chapter is to demonstrate some techniques for reducing interaction data and to explore their usefulness in describing preterm—full-term differences with respect to early mother-infant interaction.

METHOD

Subjects

Because subject characteristics, including demographic and sociological background information, are described extensively elsewhere (Trnavsky, Brown, & Bakeman, 1978), they will be dealt with only briefly here. All mothers were black, the majority were on welfare, and all had given birth at Grady Memorial Hospital in Atlanta, Georgia. The hospital is an urban hospital serviced by Emory University School of Medicine.

Subject Selection

To be considered for the study, mothers and infants had to meet the following criteria: no complications during pregnancy and delivery; mother and infant in reasonably good health; mother bottle-feeding the baby; mother over 18 years of age; and mother planning to remain in this geographic area. Ninety-four mothers who met these criteria were approached about participation in this study. Of those 94, 44 had just given birth to preterm infants while 50 had just delivered full-term infants. Thirty-two (72.7%) of the preterm mothers and 24 (48.0%) of the full-term mothers agreed to participate. Thus a decision to participate was significantly associated with whether the mother delivered a preterm or full-term infant (corrected chi-square $= 4.96$, $p < .05$).

In most other ways, mothers who declined were not different from mothers who decided to participate. There were no significant differences with respect to the infants' sex, birth weight, one- and five-minute Apgar scores, and gestational age (based on the mother's last menses). Furthermore, participating mothers did not differ from decliners with respect to age, parity, previous preterm infant(s), or previous abortion(s), spontaneous or otherwise. Only one bias was detected: Subjects were more likely than decliners to be living alone (29% vs. 18%) or with parents or other relatives (42% vs. 27%), while decliners were more likely to be living with a husband (52% vs. 29%). Indeed, a common reason for declining was that the husband did not approve.

Subject Loss

Over the course of the first year, only seven of the original 56 subjects left the project. One full-term mother moved away, three premature infants died, and three premature mothers did not want to continue for various reasons. All data reported here are based on the 49 mother-infant dyads who remained with the project for the full year (11 preterm and 11 full-term infants were male, 15 preterm and 12 full-term infants were female).

Observations

The observational method used here is essentially the same as that employed in an earlier study (Brown, Bakeman, Snyder, Fredrickson, Morgan, & Hepler, 1975). The recording apparatus is the same but the earlier experience suggested many changes and additions to the behavior code catalog.

Apparatus

The behaviors of the mothers and the infants were recorded with the aid of an electronic digital recording system, the Datamyte (Electro-General Corporation, model DAK-8C; this recording device is similar to the one described by Sackett, Stephenson, & Ruppenthal, 1973). This model of the Datamyte consists of a 12-button keyboard and a tape recorder for data storage.

The behaviors of the infant and those of the mother were recorded separately by two observers. In order to insure that the times entered by the two observers were synchronized, the keyboards had been modified so that both used the same clock. Mother and infant behaviors recorded during a particular session were subsequently merged on the basis of time of entry.

Behavior Codes

Approximately 82 different mother and 75 infant behavior units were encoded (these codes are listed and defined in Brown & Bakeman, 1975). Several considerations influenced the choice of these behavior units. First, they had to be appropriate to the situation, that is, represent behaviors that could occur in a half-hour session during which the infant was being bottle-fed. Second, they had to be quite concrete and require little judgment of intentionality (e.g., mother touches infant's lips or gums with nipple, and infant roots when mouth is touched by nipple). Finally, they could not present undue reliability problems. The behavior codes were actually developed by first examining the work of others (e.g., Richards & Bernal, 1971) and then successively refining the code catalog both before and after an earlier study of ours (Brown et al., 1975).

Codes were organized in a hierarchical fashion for ease of learning and so that later analyses could proceed easily on different levels of behavioral specificity. All behaviors recorded by the observers were coded in three digits. The first digit indicated a general class of mother or infant behaviors (e.g., *1xx* indicated an infant feeding response), the second digit indicated a subcategory of the first (e.g., *12x* referred to an infant feeding behavior while the bottle was in his mouth), and the third digit indicated a specific behavior within the subcategory (e.g., *126* was infant rejects nipple). Behaviors were partitioned as much as possible into mutually exclusive and exhaustive sets so that the offset of one behavior could be determined from the onset of another incompatible (i.e., mutually exclusive) behavior.

Observer Training and Interobserver Agreement

An agreement was tallied whenever both observers recorded the same behavior within five seconds of each other, a disagreement was tallied whenever the observers recorded a different behavior within a five second frame, and an omission was tallied whenever one observer recorded a behavior and the other did not. Because behaviors were recorded quite rapidly, about every eight seconds on the average, disagreements were regarded as rather more serious than omissions.

Interobserver agreement was computed by dividing the number of agreements by the sum of the number of agreements and the number of disagreements (loose definition) and also by dividing the number of agreements by the sum of the number of agreements, the number of disagreements, and the number of omissions (strict definition). Observers were trained with a combination of videotapes and live practice. Only after they reached 70% and 90% agreement (strict and loose definitions, respectively) for three "criterion" sessions in a row, were they allowed to record data. Additionally, criterion sessions were interspersed throughout the data collection period, occurring about every two weeks on the average. Interobserver agreement did not differ for preterms and full-terms or for mother and infant observers; overall it averaged 70.6% and 91.6% (strict and loose definitions, respectively).

Observation Procedure

The ongoing behaviors of the mother and infant were observed during three 1/2-hour sessions during which the mother bottle-fed her infant. The first observation took place just before release from the hospital, the second one month later, and the third three months later. All observations took place in the hospital.

Observers were instructed to interact with the mothers as little as possible, and the mothers were told that the observers would not be able to talk to them. The mothers were asked to feed and handle their babies as they normally would, and they were told that the observers were instructed to remain in the room for 30 minutes whether the mothers were finished with the feeding or not.

Age of Infants at Time of Observation

Because the focus of this study is on mother-infant interaction, we chose to equate dyads for the length of time the mothers were responsible for the care of their infants (instead of for chronological or for conceptional age). This means that we first observed mother-infant dyads just before the infant was released from the hospital. But it also means that we observed preterms and full-terms at different chronological and conceptional ages. On the average, preterms were four weeks older chronologically and four weeks younger conceptionally than the full-terms. Further, all full-terms left the hospital on the third postpartum day while preterms left seven to 59 days after birth. As a result, the standard deviations for preterms ages at time of observation are much greater than those for full-terms. Ages and standard errors are given in Table 1. These preterm/full-term differences should be kept in mind when interpreting group differences presented later in this report.

TABLE 1

Infants' Mean Chronological and Conceptional Age
by Type of Infant and Time of Observation

Age*	Hospital		1-month		3-month	
	prem	full	prem	full	prem	full
Chronological	3.6	0.4	9.0	5.4	18.1	14.0
	(0.7)	(0)	(0.8)	(0.2)	(0.7)	(0.1)
Conceptional	37.0	39.9	42.4	45.3	51.5	53.7
	(0.9)	(0.3)	(1.0)	(0.4)	(0.9)	(0.4)

* Age is given in weeks. Means are based on 26 preterm and 23 full-term infants (standard errors for the means are given in parentheses). Conceptional age is based on mother's last menses.

RESULTS

FREQUENCIES AND DURATIONS
OF SPECIFIC BEHAHIORS

The purpose of this section is to describe the feeding observations in terms of specific behaviors; that is, to describe how preterm and full-term mothers and infants spent their time and how often particular behaviors occurred during the three half-hour observation sessions. This is the first level of analysis, the level of specific, discrete behaviors.

Summary statistics for various behaviors are given in Tables 2, 3, and 4. Some selection and condensing has occurred; that is, not all summary scores for all behaviors recorded are given in these three tables. To be included, a behavior had to have been coded for at least half of the subjects during at least one of the three observations. For many behaviors,

TABLE 2

Summary Scores[1] for Infant Behaviors by
Type of Infant and Time of Observation

Infant Behavior[a]	Hospital		1-month		3-month	
	prem	full	prem	full	prem	full
a. MOTOR						
% gross motor (811)	6.7	6.6	17.4	26.4*	25.0	25.1
% fine motor (822)	15.2	18.1	17.1	16.6	16.3	13.5
% touching/grasping (823)	9.7	12.7	6.8	4.7	6.1	7.7
b. VISUAL						
# looks at mother (621)	(4)	(14)**	6.5	11.3*	8.4	8.7
# looks at surround (622)	(2)	(2)	3.9	9.6*	10.7	12.3
% eyes open (611)	28.8	40.5	60.7	72.8	80.3	71.6
% looking at mother (621)	—	2.5	12.3	15.2	12.4	10.3
% looking at surround (622)	—	—	7.7	29.6***	56.5	50.7
c. VOCAL						
# whimpers (711)	(7)	(4)	8.9	11.2	13.0	11.9
# cries (712)	(3)	(5)	(9)	(10)	(11)	(12)
# babbles/coos (721)	(0)	(1)	3.5	7.2	14.1	26.3*
# sucking noises (716)	5.8	8.1	8.8	17.5*	12.7	13.6
# other vocalizations (717)	15.0	4.9**	30.1	24.0	26.1	17.5*
% vocalizing (711, 712, 715-717, 721)	1.9	1.2	9.3	10.3	13.7	15.5
d. EXPRESSIVE						
# grimaces (635)	3.8	4.9	3.5	4.3	1.5	1.7
# yawns (636)	2.8	2.3	2.6	2.4	(15)	(9)
# opens mouth/roots (637)	2.2	6.5*	(12)	(14)	(7)	(11)
# smiles (638)	(12)	(1)**	(12)	(9)	4.2	4.8

[1] Summary scores are mean frequencies (#) and mean durations (%) based on 26 preterm and 23 full-term dyads. Mean durations are expressed as percentages of the half-hour observation sessions. If at a given observation time less than half of either premature or full-term dyads engaged in a particular behavior then the number of such dyads is noted in parenthesis, no mean frequency or duration is given, and significance was determined by corrected chi-square; otherwise two-tailed t-tests were used to determine significance.

[a] Numbers refer to specific codes; see Brown & Bakeman, 1975.

+ $p < .10$ ** $p < .01$

* $p < .05$ *** $p < .001$

TABLE 3

Summary Scores[1] for Mother Behaviors by
Type of Infant and Time of Observation

Mother Behaviors[a]	Hospital prem	Hospital full	1-month prem	1-month full	3-month prem	3-month full
a. VISUAL/VOCAL/EXPRESSIVE						
# looks at infant (1611)	29.0	30.6	13.4	12.3	15.4	13.7
# smiles (1626)	14.3	11.7	10.6	13.5	17.0	17.9
# directive commands (1711)	9.6	3.4*	8.6	5.5	9.6	5.2+
# expressive vocalizations (1712)	19.5	17.3	28.7	24.2	34.1	26.4
# other vocalizations (1713-16)	2.1	2.3	4.8	3.9	7.4	4.9
% looking at I (1611)	92.3	91.7	94.3	94.4	95.8	84.0*
% vocalizing to I (1711-16)	13.6	8.1	17.8	15.1	25.7	15.8
b. TACTILE STIMULATION						
# pats (1411)	6.5	7.9	8.0	8.8	8.0	6.0
# rubs (1412)	4.1	3.8	2.4	2.5	1.9	0.9
# inspects (1413)	4.9	3.1	2.9	3.2	3.8	1.7
# thumps/pokes/pinches (1414)	12.8	2.9***	5.4	2.7	(19)	(11)
# grooms (1415)	1.0	2.3*	1.3	1.8	3.0	3.1
# kisses (1417)	(7)	(10)	(15)	(9)	6.2	4.5
# elicits grasp (1418)	5.7	5.3	1.8	1.8	2.0	1.9
% tactile stimulation	26.7	20.0*	16.2	15.3	13.4	10.7
c. VESTIBULAR STIMULATION						
# rocks (1421)	13.3	9.1	12.8	10.6	10.3	8.7
# bounces/jiggles (1423)	(9)	(11)	5.7	4.4	4.2	6.0
% vestibular stimulation (1421-23)	19.3	9.8*	17.9	11.5	13.4	7.9

[1] Summary scores are mean frequencies (#) and mean durations (%) based on 26 preterm and 23 full-term dyads. Mean durations are expressed as percentages of the half-hour observation sessions. If at a given observation time less than half of either premature or full-term dyads engaged in a particular behavior then the number of such dyads is noted in parenthesis, no mean frequency or duration is given, and significance was determined by corrected chi-square; otherwise two-tailed t-tests were used to determine significance.

[a] Numbers refer to specific codes; see Brown & Bakeman, 1975.

+ $p < .10$ * $p < .01$
* $p < .05$ *** $p < .001$

both frequency of occurrence and duration were computed. Rather than report both frequencies and durations for all such behaviors, we have reported frequencies for specific behaviors within a class and durations for the class of behaviors (durations are expressed as percentages of the half-hour observation sessions). The purpose of these selections and condensations is to reduce the information presented to a manageable size.

Developmental Trends

The increasing behavioral repertoire of the infants, more than any other factor, accounted for how the mother-infant dyads spent their time during the three feeding observations. Infant (preterm/full-term) by sex (male/female) by time of observation (hospital, one month, three months) analyses of variance for the duration of summary behaviors (indicated with a "%" in Tables 2-4) revealed very strong effects for time, but few infant by time interactions (see Table 5). With time, the infants simply did more: They kept their eyes open more and looked at their mothers and the surrounding environment more, they vocalized more, and were more physically active. Mothers, too, became more vocal, but engaged in less tactile stimulation.

Differences Between Full-term and Preterm Infants

Activity level. Contrary to our expectations, full-terms were in general *not* more active than preterms during a feeding. Although at one month full-terms were more active than preterms (as indexed by differences in gross motor activity), this difference was not a lasting one and had disappeared by three months.

Visual behaviors. Full-terms were more visually alert in the hospital and at one month. They looked more at their mothers (in the hospital and at one month) and more at the environment around them (at one month). Three months after hospital discharge, however, full-terms and preterms no longer differed with respect to their visual behaviors.

Vocal behaviors. In the hospital, full-terms were less vocal than preterms. The vocalizations of the preterms, however, consisted primarily of gasping inhalation sounds characteristic of preterm infants (coded as "other vocalizations"). By three months, full-terms babbled and cooed more than preterms while the preterms continued their earlier gasps and sighs.

TABLE 4

Summary Scores[1] for Feeding Behaviors by
Type of Infant and Time of Observation

Feeding Behaviors[a]	Hospital prem	full	1-month prem	full	3-month prem	full
a. MOTHER						
# stimulates I to suck (1112)	5.3	4.0	(18)	(9)	(10)	(6)
# inserts nipple (1122)	5.3	7.8*	6.5	9.5+	5.6	8.9+
# nipple out slightly (1125)	3.7	3.1	6.3	5.6	2.3	3.0
# jiggles nipple (1191)	7.7	6.2	8.4	3.1	(12)	(12)
# checks amount (1192)	1.4	2.3	1.1	1.4	(10)	(8)
# starts spoon feeding (1211)	(0)	(0)	3.0	3.7	3.0	4.1
# wipes I's mouth (1467)	4.6	8.5***	7.5	7.1	7.5	7.5
# moves I to shoulder (1324)	2.5	4.7**	2.8	4.7**	3.1	3.1
b. INFANT						
# refuses nipple (116)	6.5	4.7	(18)	(9)	(4)	(5)
# milk dribbles from mouth (191)	3.3	4.8	4.4	3.3	1.7	1.9
# chokes/spits up (192)	0.8	1.3	2.4	1.5	2.5	3.3
# burps (193)	1.1	1.9*	2.0	2.4	1.5	1.5
# bottle feeding episodes (121)	5.0	7.6*	6.4	8.6	5.5	7.8
# spoon feeding episodes (221)	(0)	(0)	2.5	3.8	2.4	3.5
% bottle feeding episodes (121)	20.4	33.1***	27.7	28.4	16.3	20.3
% spoon feeding episodes (221)	—	—	10.9	11.3	14.9	14.0

[1] Summary scores are mean frequencies (#) and mean durations (%) based on 26 preterm and 23 full-term dyads. Mean durations are expressed as percentages of the half-hour observation sessions. If at a given observation time less than half of either premature or full-term dyads engaged in a particular behavior then the number of such dyads is noted in parenthesis, no mean frequency or duration is given, and significance was determined by corrected chi-square; otherwise two-tailed t-tests were used to determine significance.

[a] Numbers refer to specific codes; see Brown & Bakeman, Note 2.

+ $p < .10$
* $p < .05$
** $p < .01$
*** $p < .001$

TABLE 5

Analysis of Variance *F*-ratios[1]
for Duration Behaviors

Behavior	Infant[a]	Sex[a]	IxS[a]	Time[b]	TxI[b]	TxS[b]	TxIxS[b]
				Source			
GROSM				40.9***	2.9		
FINEM						2.6	
GRASP				7.3***			2.5
IOPEN				27.1***			
LOOKM				14.0***		3.3*	
LOOKS	3.0			99.6***	7.6***		
IVOC		3.6		31.9***		2.9	
MLOOK	3.1		4.3*		3.0		
MVOC				7.2***			
TSTIM	3.8			21.7***			
VSTIM	4.9*						
BFEED	3.7	3.2		6.5**			
SFEED				33.4***			

[1] Only *F*-ratios whose probabilities were less than .10 are given here. Descriptions of the behaviors, represented here by mnemonics, are given in Tables 2-4.
   a df = 1/45
   b df = 2/90
   * p < .05
   ** p < .01
   *** p < .001

Expressive behaviors. In the hospital, 12 preterm infants smiled while only one full-term infant did so. However, according to our observers, the smiles of the preterms were nondirective and did not seem to be elicited by any external stimulus.

Differences Between Mothers of Full-term and Preterm Infants

Tactile and vestibular stimulation. Mothers of preterms gave more tactile and vestibular stimulation to their infants than mothers of full-terms. However, these differences in stimulation were only significant in the hospital.

Differences in Feeding Behaviors of Full-term and Preterm Dyads

Infants. During the first observation, full-term were more lusty feeders than preterms. They signaled their readiness to feed by opening their mouths and by rooting in the absence of any nipple stimulation more so than preterms. Full-terms spent about a third of the session actively feeding while preterms did so during only about one-fifth of the session.

Mothers. Again, during the first observation, mothers of full-terms experienced more successful feedings than mothers of preterms. Mothers of full-terms engaged in more bottle feeding episodes with their infants, they wiped their infants' mouths more, and burped their infants more. Mothers of preterms, on the other hand, spent more time trying to get their infants to feed. They issued more directive commands, and thumped, poked, pinched, and rocked their infants more, presumably in order to get them to feed. But few differences were detected for the last two observations.

Summary

Although there were many differences in the behaviors of full-term and preterm infants and their mothers in the hospital, most of these differences in the specific behaviors described here had disappeared by one and three months after hospital discharge. The general sense of these data, then, is that the full-term infants appeared to be more fun to interact with and more satisfying to feed, but that most specific behavioral differences disappeared during the first three months after hospital discharge.

BEHAVIORAL DIALOGUES: RATES OF DIALOGIC STATES

The purpose of this section is to describe the feeding observations, not in terms of specific behaviors as in the previous section, but in terms of the amount of interactive behaviors in general. This is the first of three sections representing what we have termed the second level of analysis.

Mother-infant interaction is viewed in this and the following two sections as a "dialogue" or "conversation," the elements of which are not just vocalizations but a broader class of communicative behaviors. (This approach is discussed in more detail in Bakeman & Brown, 1977). In a sense, a class of interactive behaviors or "communicative acts" is equated to the phrases and sentences of adult conversation, and the entire interaction is reduced to sequences of mother "talks" (M, mother acting), infant "talks" (I, infant acting), both "talk" (C, mother and infant co-acting), or neither "talks" (Q, both quiescent). An advantage of viewing mother-infant interaction as a sequence of these four "dyadic states" is that certain characteristics of the interaction can easily be quantified (e.g., the proportion of time spent in the various dyadic states and the probability with which various states follow each other). Because these characteristics are not tied to specific behaviors we regard them as relatively "content-free" indices of interaction.

Specifically, 42 behaviors from the code catalog were designated "mother communicative acts" and 30 were designated "infant communicative acts." These included such behaviors as the mother rocks, rubs, pats, pokes, vocalizes, shifts position, offers bottle, etc., and the infant cries, whines, babbles, burps, looks to mother, smiles, wiggles, waves arms, rejects nipple, etc. (a complete list is given in Table 6). Because our code catalog is quite exhaustive, and because we wanted to include all communicative behaviors—that is, those infant behaviors and mother behaviors to which the other might respond—the list is quite long.

Then each ½-hour session was segmented into 360 five-second intervals, and each interval was categorized as quiescent (Q) if none of the mother and none of the infant communicative acts occurred within it, as infant-alone (I) if one or more infant communicative acts occurred but no mother communicative acts, as mother-alone (M) if one or more mother but no infant communicative acts occurred, and as co-acting (C) if one or more infant and one or more mother communicative acts occurred. Although the resolution of the Datamyte clock is one second, we believe that a five-second interval more accurately reflects the precision of the total observation system including the human observers (which is why, when computing interobserver agreement, we defined agreement as both observers entering the same code within five seconds of each other). Thus the behavioral dialogues described here have a certain resilience; co-action, for example, means not split second reactions but behaviors in the near neighborhood of each other.

In summary, observation sessions were reduced to sequences of the four dyadic states defined here. A segment of an interaction then might "look" like this: QQQQMMMCIICMMMCMMQQQIIIQQ . . . etc. Once an interaction is viewed and encoded in this way, a variety of interaction indices can be defined and computed. The simplest would be unconditional (as opposed to conditional) probabilities for the various dyadic states. For example, if the sequence of 25 states given earlier in this paragraph constituted the entire interaction, then the $p(M) = 8/25 = .32$, $p(C) = 3/25 = .12$, and the $p(M + C) = 11/25 = .44$.

Developmental Trends

The rate of most specific infant behaviors increased with time and so it is not surprising that the overall rate of infant activity [$p(I + C)$, the probability of the infant acting alone plus the probability of co-action],

TABLE 6

Mother and Infant Communicative Behaviors*

a. Infant communicative behaviors   b. Mother communicative behaviors

115	roots, opens mouth
116	refuses nipple
126	rejects nipple
191	milk dribbles
192	regurgitates
193	burps
619	opens eyes
629	looks to mother
635	grimaces
636	yawns
637	roots, opens mouth
638	smiles
711	whimpers
712	cries
715	sneezes
716	makes sucking noises
717	other vocalizations
721	babbles, coos
832	hand, finger in mouth
835	touches mouth
836	rejects pacifier
839	accepts pacifier
815	startles
819	begins gross movements
821	trembles
825	swipes, hits
826	turns head
829	begins fine movements
842	grasps, touches

1112	stimulates I to suck
1125	pulls nipple out slightly
1129	inserts nipple
1139	removes nipple
1191	jiggles, rotates bottle
1125	fetches spoonful of food
1329	shifts position
1352	restrains I's hand
1355	pushes I's hand from mouth
1411	pats, rubs
1412	rubs, nuzzles
1413	inspects, grooms with hand
1414	tactually stimulates body parts
1415	grooms with object
1416	tactile play
1417	kisses
1418	elicits grasp reflex
1421	rocks, close contact
1422	rocks, no close contact
1423	bounces, jiggles
1431	presents face
1432	presents object
1433	visual play
1441	makes noise
1455	places I's hand on object
1456	places object in I's hands
1457	removes I's hands from object
1461	changes diaper
1462	changes clothes
1465	checks diaper
1466	arranges blanket, bib
1467	wipes I's mouth
1475	offers pacifier
1476	removes pacifier
1625	makes faces
1626	smiles
1711	directive command
1712	social expressive vocalization
1713	imitates I's vocalizations
1714	praises
1715	reprimands
1716	referential speech

* More complete definitions are given in Brown & Bakeman, Note 2. All behaviors which we defined as communicative are given here, including some that never or rarely occurred. For a sense of the frequency with which behaviors occurred see Tables 2-4.

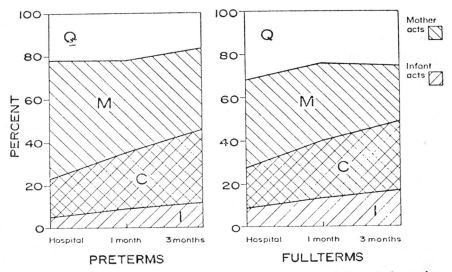

FIGURE 1. Mean dyadic state probabilities by type of infant and time of observation.

also increased with time (see Tables 7-8 and Figure 1). The mother's rate of activity [p (M + C)], however, was quite stable. As a result of increased infant activity and stable mother activity, the probability of co-action [p (C)] increased and the probability that the mother would be acting alone [p (M)] decreased. And so with time, as the infant engaged in more communicative acts, the interactions became characterized by more concurrent activity and less mother acting alone time. This was generally so both for preterm and full-term dyads.

Differences Between Preterm and Full-term Dyads

While the frequencies and durations of specific behaviors distinguished preterm and full-term dyads only slightly, the values of the dyadic state probabilities distinguished preterm and full-term dyads quite sharply. Mainly, mothers of preterms were considerably more active [p (M + C)] than mothers of full-terms, while the preterm infants were somewhat less active [p (I + C)] than full-terms ($p < .06$). Since the rate of concurrent activity [p (C)] was about the same for both groups of dyads, this means that mothers of preterms acted alone more often than mothers of full-terms, while preterm infants acted alone less often than full-terms infants. It almost seems as though the mothers had a notion of an "appropriate" amount of concurrent activity and strove to meet that "quota." Because preterm infants were less active, their mothers exerted considerably more effort in reaching the quota, while mothers of full-terms, who reached their quota with considerably less effort, were then free to let their infants act alone more.

BEHAVIORAL DIALOGUES: FLOW ANALYSIS

The above analyses examined simple or unconditional probabilities for three of the four dyadic states [p (C), p (I), and p (M); p (Q) was not

TABLE 7

Mean Dyadic State Probabilities by Type
of Infant and Time of Observation*

Dyadic State	Hospital prem	full	1-month prem	full	3-month prem	full
p (I + C)	.23	.27	.35	.40	.45	.49
	(.01)	(.02)	(.02)	(.03)	(.03)	(.04)
p (M + C)	.72	.59	.70	.63	.73	.57
	(.03)	(.03)	(.04)	(.03)	(.03)	(.04)
p (C)	.18	.18	.26	.27	.34	.32
	(.01)	(.02)	(.02)	(.02)	(.03)	(.04)
p (I)	.05	.09	.09	.13	.11	.17
	(.01)	(.01)	(.01)	(.01)	(.02)	(.02)
p (M)	.55	.41	.43	.36	.38	.25
	(.03)	(.02)	(.03)	(.03)	(.02)	(.03)

* Means are based on 26 preterm and 23 full-term dyads (standard errors for the means are given in parentheses). "1" indicates infant active alone, "M" mother active alone, and "C" both co-active, so "I + C" indicates infant active total and "M + C" mother active total.

TABLE 8

Analysis of Variance F-ratios[1] for
Dyadic State Probabilities

Dyadic State	Source						
	Infant[a]	Sex[a]	IxS[a]	Time[b]	TxI[b]	TxS[b]	TxIxS[b]
p (I + C)	3.9			43.9***			
p (M + C)	8.8**						
p (C)			3.4	27.8***			
p (I)	11.6***			20.8***			
p (M)	18.7***			25.2***			

[1] Only F-ratios whose probabilities were less than .10 are given here.
[a] df = 1/45
[b] df = 2/90
* $p < .05$
** $p < .01$
*** $p < .001$

analyzed because it is determined by the other three] and for two compound dyadic states [p (I + C) and p (M + C)]. But these dyadic states are imbedded in sequences of dyadic states. Descriptions of the analyses of these sequences—both how they "flow" (this section) and how they are "patterned" (next section) continue the second level of analysis begun in the last section.

Sequential analysis is not yet a simple and codified matter with commonly agreed upon procedures (for a discussion of various techniques see Bakeman, 1978; Bakeman & Brown, 1977; Bakeman & Dabbs, 1976; Gottman & Bakeman, 1979). The procedures one chooses depend in part on the sorts of questions asked. An important distinction in this regard is between asking how an interaction *flows* (taking into account how long each dyadic state lasts) and how it is *patterned* (ignoring how long each dyadic state lasts). This distinction is adhered to in the following discussion. First, the "flow-analysis" is concerned with how the interaction proceeds in time; the data analyzed look like the example given earlier (QQQQMMMCIICMMMCMMQQQIIQQ . . . etc.) in which each symbol represents a unit of time. Second, the "pattern-analysis" is concerned simply with the patterns in the sequence, ignoring how long a dyadic state lasts, and so the sample of data above would be condensed to this: QMCICMCMQIQ. The former we term "timed-event sequence" data and the latter "event sequence" data (see Gottman & Bakeman, 1979).

Transitional probabilities are commonly used to describe the flow of interaction (e.g., Stern, 1974b). (Note: A conditional probability is the probability of one event given another; a transitional probability is the probability of one event given another previous in time.) For example, if four out of 10 times a quiescent interval followed an infant-alone interval, then the transitional probability for a quiescent state, given an immediately preceding infant-alone state [p (Q/I)], would be .4. Transitional probabilities, arranged in matrix form, are given in Table 9. (Note that because of the way transitional probabilities are defined, rows in a transitional probability matrix sum to 1.)

Before proceeding we would like to make a minor technical point. It may seem to the statistically concerned reader that we are rather cavalier with statistical tests. Indeed, a problem of observational research in general and of sequential analyses in particular is that a great many numbers are generated. By subjecting all those numbers to statistical tests, we clearly run the risk of capitalizing on chance. Our solution to this dilemma is to regard test results as helpful descriptive devices, but to base interpretation only on coherent patterns of results. Ultimately, of course, only replication can provide confirmation for the patterns of preterm/full-term differences described here.

Developmental Trends

Mothers tended to be persistent; that is, if a mother was acting alone in one interval, she was probably acting alone in the following interval as well [overall, p (M/M) = .57]. With time (i.e., over the three observations), however, this tendency decreased [F (2/90) = 15.7, $p < .001$]. Complementing the decrease in maternal persistence, and like it, no doubt, affected by the general increase in infant activity over time, was an in-

TABLE 9

Mean Transitional Probabilities[1] by Type
of Infant and Time of Observation

A. Hospital

t	preterm Q	preterm I	preterm M	preterm C	full-term Q	full-term I	full-term M	full-term C
Q	.51	.10	.30	.08	.59	.12	.20	.08
I	.46	.11	.26	.17	.42	.18	.24	.16
M	.11	.03	.68	.18	.17	.05	.59	.19
C	.10	.04	.57	.28	.15	.08	.44	.33

B. 1-month

t	preterm Q	preterm I	preterm M	preterm C	full-term Q	full-term I	full-term M	full-term C
Q	.49	.13	.26	.11	.49	.21	.19	.11
I	.37	.21	.17	.24	.34	.26	.19	.22
M	.12	.05	.60	.23	.12	.08	.53	.27
C	.10	.09	.41	.40	.11	.09	.39	.41

C. 3-month

t	preterm Q	preterm I	preterm M	preterm C	full-term Q	full-term I	full-term M	full-term C
Q	.39	.16	.30	.16	.53	.18	.16	.13
I	.27	.25	.18	.30	.26	.35	.11	.28
M	.10	.06	.56	.29	.15	.08	.46	.30
C	.08	.10	.33	.49	.08	.15	.25	.51

[1] Means are based on 26 preterm and 23 full-term dyads. Particular preterm and full-term transitional probabilities which differ significantly from each other ($p < .05$, determined by two-tailed *t*-test) are italicized. Standard errors are typically .02 or .03; none exceeds .04.

crease in the tendency for the infant-alone and the co-acting states to follow themselves [F (2/90) = 16.6 and 24.4, respectively, $p < .001$ for both].

Differences Between Preterm and Full-term Dyads

While all mothers tended to be persistent, mothers of preterms were especially so [F (1/45) = 17.1, $p < .001$]. Correspondingly, preterm infants were less likely than full-terms to persist in the infant-alone state [F (1/45) = 8.0, $p < .01$].

These findings suggest that preterm mothers bore an unequal share of the responsibility for the flow of the interaction. An examination of group differences with respect to which partner was more likely to start when no one was acting (i.e., to break the quiescent state) and which partner was more likely to quit when both were co-acting (i.e., to break off the co-acting state) gives further support to this impression. At all three observation times mothers of preterms were more likely than their infants to initiate behavior; p (M/Q) was greater than p (I/Q) for 23 of the 26 preterm dyads during the hospital observation ($p < .001$ by two-tailed sign test); and p (M/Q) was greater than p (I/Q) for 21 of the dyads at one month and 20 of the dyads at three months ($p < .01$ for both). In contrast, mothers and infants in full-term dyads split the responsibility more evenly. Although mothers of full-terms dominated initiation in the hospital [p (M/Q) was greater than p (I/Q) for 18 of the 23 full-term dyads, $p < .05$], no such domination was evident during the one month and three months observations [p (M/Q) was greater than p (I/Q) for 10 of the 26 dyads at one month and 8 of the 26 dyads at three months, both nonsignificant].

Almost invariably, infants were more likely than their mothers to break off the co-acting state [p (M/C) was greater than p (I/C) for all dyads in the hospital, and for 24 and 23 of the 26 preterm and for 21 and 21 of the 23 full-term dyads at one month and three months, respectively, $p < .001$ for all]. That is, the infants typically broke off the co-acting state, leaving the mother acting alone. Though this tendency decreased with time [F (2/90) = 42.9, $p < .001$], preterms were more likely to break off the co-acting state than full-terms [F (1/45) = 7.9, $p < .01$].

Summary and Discussion

The important differences between preterm and full-term dyads in the flow of their interactions can be summarized as follows: (1) Mothers of preterms were more persistent and were more likely to initiate and continue behavioral episodes than mothers of full-term. (2) Over time all infants were more likely to initiate and continue behavioral episodes so that the balance between mother and infant dialogues became more even; however, this tendency was evident to a lesser extent for the preterm than for the full-term infants.

In one sense, it is not surprising that those transitional probabilities which distinguished preterm from full-term dyads were transitions to the mother-alone state, and to a lesser extent to the infant-alone and quiescent states (see Table 9). Because the simple probabilities for the mother-alone state, for example, were higher for preterms, transitions to it were also more likely for preterms: It was simply a more frequent state in the stream of behavior. But it would be wrong to dismiss preterm/full-term differences with respect to transitional probabilities as simply "caused" by the simple dyadic state probability differences (noted in Tables 7 and 8). We could just as well say that transitional probability differences "explain" how the simple dyadic state probability differences came about.

The point to be emphasized here is that both simple and transitional probabilities serve our primary goal—describing mother-infant interaction and explicating preterm/full-term differences—and that the latter provides a type of sequential description that the former does not. For example, we might speculate that the reason p (M) was greater for preterms was because preterm mothers were very persistent. If that were the only explanation, then p (M/M) would be greater for preterms but p (M/Q), p (M/I), and p (M/C) would not. In fact, all transitions to the mother-alone state were typically higher for preterms, suggesting multiple causes for the increased probability of that state: Not only were preterm mothers more persistent [p (M/M)], but they were also more likely to initiate behavior [p (M/Q)] and more likely to find themselves acting alone [p (M/C)] after their infant quit.

We might further speculate that the reason p (I) was greater for full-terms was because full-terms were both more likely to initiate behavior and more likely to persist in the infant-alone state than preterms. Actually, the evidence is equivocal: p (I/Q) did distinguish the groups, but only at one month, and p (I/I) distinguished the groups only in the hospital (although $p < .07$ at three months). A better interpretation of the findings might be that full-term infants were more often in the infant-alone state because full-term mothers were more likely to inhibit their own behavior, and indeed p (I/M) and p (I/C) were greater for full-terms at two of the three observation times. This latter interpretation is supported by the fact, noted earlier, that full-term mothers and infants were about equally likely to initiate behavior (at least at one month and three months), while preterm mothers were twice as likely (three times as likely in the hospital) as their infants to break the quiescent state. But independent of the validity of the above speculations, a major point of this and the preceding paragraph is that transitional probabilities provide a level of descriptive information not available from simple probabilities alone.

BEHAVIORAL DIALOGUES: PATTERN ANALYSIS

The only difference between what we have termed here "flow" analysis and "pattern" analysis lies with the data analyzed and with the questions asked and not with the techniques employed. In the previous section we described the lag one transitional probabilities (the probability of an event at time $t + 1$ given another at time t) for "timed-event sequence" data (QQQQMMMCII . . .). We could also compute lag one transitional probabilities for "event sequence" data (QMCI . . .) as well. In that case, the lag would refer to an event position and not to a time interval, and so, e.g., the p (M/M) would be zero since by definition an event cannot follow itself. In fact, we reduced the timed-event sequence data analyzed in the previous section to event sequence data and computed lag one transitional probabilities; our conclusion was that those analyses added little to the "flow" analyses of the timed-event sequence data already presented.

But if one is concerned with patterns of interaction, it makes sense to analyze event sequence data. For example, QQMCC, QMMMC, and QMCCC (timed-event sequence data) would appear as different patterns, but if reduced to event sequence data (QMC) would be detected as instances of the same pattern. In principle, the two techniques discussed below for "pattern" analysis would work with timed-event sequence data, but in most cases we suspect that variability in the length of different dyadic states would obscure whatever patterns exist in the data and for that reason we present them as techniques appropriate for event sequence data.

The first technique has been well described by Sackett (1977) and will be mentioned only briefly here. He constructs "probability profiles" for various pairs of events—i.e., he graphs the probability of event B a time $t + 1$, $t + 2$, $t + 3$, etc., given event A at time t—and from these profiles constructs probable sequences or probable patterns of behaviors (for an example see Gottman & Bakeman, 1979).

The second technique—computing simple probabilities for all possible two-event sequences, all possible three-event sequences, and so forth—is relatively simple and straightforward but becomes unwieldy if more than four or five events or dyadic states are defined (as the number of possible events increases, the number of possible sequences becomes unmanageably large). But if the number of possible events is small, as is the case here with only four dyadic states, then these computations are practical and provide an efficient way to describe how interaction is patterned.

Consider the example given earlier: QMCICMCMQIQ. This 11-event chain consists of ten two-event chains, nine three-event chains, and so forth. With four event types (Q, I, M, and C), 12 different two-event chains are possible. In this simple example, only 8 occurred: QM, MC, CI, IC, CM, MQ, QI, and IQ. The frequencies for these were 1, 2, 1, 1, 2, 1, 1, and 1 and the probabilities were thus .09, .18, .09, .09, .18, .09, .09, and .09 respectively.

The results of a two-event chain analysis are presented in Table 10 and Figure 2. The chains were selected as follows: If the mean probability of a particular two-event chain was greater than .083 for either preterms or full-terms at any one of the three observation times, it was tabled and included in the figure. (The rationale for the .083 cutoff is that it represents a chance value; all other things being equal, the chance value for any one of 12 possible chains is .083.) By this rule, eight chains were included and four excluded; these latter four represented "abrupt" transitions (QC, CQ, IM, MI).

TABLE 10

Mean Probabilities for Selected Two-Event Chains
by Type of Infant and Time of Observation*

Chain	Hospital prem	full	1-month prem	full	3-month prem	full
MC	.235	.167	.224	.188	.236	.151
CM	.237	.167	.226	.199	.237	.154
MQ	.122	.135	.092	.082	.071	.077
QM	.125	.133	.101	.081	.072	.073
QI	.058	.084	.057	.090	.054	.093
IQ	.059	.081	.066	.089	.055	.090
CI	.016	.029	.042	.045	.061	.098
IC	.017	.029	.043	.053	.061	.102

* If a mean probability was greater than .083 (1/12) for either preterms or full-terms at any of the three observation times, it is tabled here. Values significantly different from each other ($p < .05$ by two-tailed t-test) at a given observation time are italicized.

Below we discuss specific patterns, but first we move to a third level of analysis, one that uses information theory measures to characterize the interaction as a whole.

Predictability of Patterns: Third Level Analysis

Interactions of preterms with their mothers were more patterned and stereotyped than were those of full-terms. Two chains dominated preterm interaction and the probabilities for the other chains above the cutoff point differed considerably, while the probabilities for the chains above the cutoff point in full-term interaction were more similar in value (see Figure 2). As a result, preterm interaction was less varied; some chains occurred often, some very little. No particular chain dominated full-term interaction to the same extent and so full-term interaction was more varied.

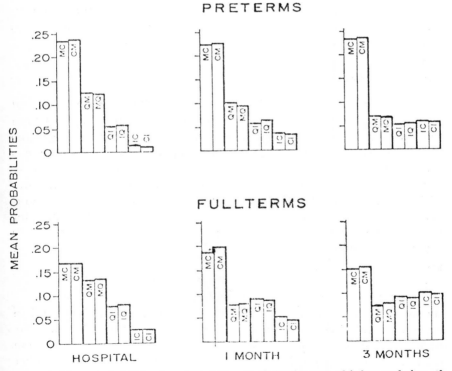

FIGURE 2. Mean probabilities for selected 2-event chains by type of infant and time of observation.

In information theory terms, the average information value of an episode in preterm sequences was lower than the average value in full-term sequences; when events are less varied (and so more predictable), their information value is less. After all, knowing relatively predictable events reduces uncertainty less than knowing less predictable events; one was more certain to begin with. The usual measure of average information value is H and in particular H_2 is the average value of an episode when the previous episode is known, that is, when the sequence is viewed from the point of view of 2-event chains (for further discussion of information analyses and appropriate references see Gottman & Bakeman, 1979). Here the mean values of H_2 (in bits) were 1.12 and 1.28 (with standard errors of .04 and .03) for preterms and full-terms, respectively. An infant by sex by observation time analysis of variance revealed only an infant effect [$F(1/45) = 9.5$, $p < .01$]. Thus, average information value did distinguish preterm and full-term interaction; preterm interaction was less varied and more predictable, and this was so at all three observation times. Unlike many of the other measures of interaction described earlier in this chapter, the information measures showed no developmental trend.

Analysis of Specific Patterns

In addition to the greater disparity of probability values for two-event chains among preterms, quite specific information can be gleaned from the two-event chain profiles presented in Figure 2. Most striking is the arrangement of these chains into pairs of the form *ab/ba*. This suggests that a common feature of the interactions we observed was the chaining of alternating episodes; the most common alternating sequence was MCMCM . . . but MQMQM . . ., QIQIQ . . ., and CICIC . . . also occurred. This notion is confirmed by examining the probabilities for three-episode chains (see Table 11); only five of these three-episode chains were not of the form *aba*, and three of those had the lowest probabilities.

While many of the QM and MQ chains occurred in an MQMQM . . . alternating sequence, others served to begin and end the MCMCM . . . chains; that is, a common pattern was QMCMC . . . CMCMQ (and in fact the probabilities for QMC and CMQ chains were usually just somewhat lower than those for MQM and QMQ). In sum, the most common pattern for both types of infants at all time periods consisted of a mother beginning and maintaining her activity and being joined from time to time by her infant. Judging from the probabilities for the MC and CM

TABLE 11

Mean Probabilities for Selected Three-Event Chains
by Type of Infant and Time of Observation[1]

Chain	Hospital prem	full	1-month prem	full	3-month prem	full
MCM	.206	.129	.186	.154	.195	.106
CMC	.174	.109	.177	.145	.189	.109
MQM	.079	.077	.057	.038	.039	.038
QMQ	.060	.074	.050	.036	.029	.036
QMC	.050	.044	.034	.027	.031	.024
CMQ	.049	.044	.033	.031	.030	.030
QIQ	.040	.057	.038	.057	.030	.057
IQI	.029	.038	.028	.046	.026	.052
CIC	.004	.012	.021	.022	.037	.069
ICI	.002	.007	.016	.021	.028	.056
MQI	.021	.031	.019	.027	.016	.025
IQM	.024	.030	.025	.026	.015	.022
ICM	.011	.015	.019	.022	.022	.031

[1] If a mean probability was greater than .028 (1/36) for either preterms or full-terms at any one of the three observation times, it is tabled here. Values significantly different from each other ($p < .05$ by two-tailed t-test) at a given observation time are italicized.

chains, the frequency of this pattern (MCMCM . . .) did not change over time, but was more characteristic of the preterm dyads (see Table 12).

TABLE 12

Analysis of Variance F-ratios for Selected Compound
Two-Event Chain Probabilities[1]

Compound	Source Infant[a]	Sex[a]	I×S[a]	Time[b]	T×I[b]	T×S[b]	T×I×S[b]
MC+CM	8.5**						
MQ+QM				20.7***			
QI+IQ	7.0*	3.2					
CI+IC	9.7**			40.1***	3.1		

[1] Only F-ratios whose probabilities were less than .10 are given here. Similar results were obtained by analyzing each 2-episode chain probability separately, but because certain pairs of those probabilities were typically similar, it seemed more economical to analyze the sum of the two probabilities in the pair.
a df = 1/45
b df = 2/90
* $p < .05$
** $p < .01$
*** $p < .001$

Other aspects of the data support the notion that the mother was typically the initiator of joint action. Alternating quiescent and infant-alone episodes rarely resulted in co-action; instead this sequence was most likely to end on a quiescent episode, which was then followed by a mother-alone episode (QIQ was always more likely than IQI; IQM was always more likely than IQC or QIC). Further, alternating co-acting and infant-alone episodes typically were preceded by a mother-alone episode (CIC was always more likely than ICI; MCI was always more likely than QCI or QIC—exception: p (MCI) = .016 but p (QIC) = .017 for full-terms at the one month observation). Now we can expand the pattern described in the previous paragraph and say that sometimes the "interactive burden" shifted from mother to infant, that is, periods of maternal activity which the infant occasionally joined were followed by periods of infant activity which the mother occasionally joined (. . . MCMCMCICI . . .). Judging from the probabilities for the IC and CI chains, this became more common over time and was always more characteristic of the full-term dyads (see Table 12).

Summary

In summary, the "pattern" analysis supports the general conclusion of the "flow" analysis: With time full-term infants took more responsibility for the interaction than preterm infants did. And the pattern analysis reveals that although mothers of preterms and full-terms were both required to do a certain amount of "interactive pump priming," full-term infants contributed to the interactive flow more than preterms while the burden of maintaining that flow fell disproportionately on the mothers of preterms. Still, most of these second level analyses reflect that all infants, preterm and full-term, became more active over these three months. What the third level of analysis reveals is this: the amount of patterning (as measured by H_2) in the behavioral dialogues did not change. From the beginning full-term interaction was more varied than preterm.

STABILITY OF LEVEL 1, 2, AND 3 VARIABLES

A major purpose of this chapter has been to develop indices of mother-infant interaction that tap structural aspects of the interaction and that are not particularly tied to specific behaviors, and indeed various measures (Level 2 and 3 variables), based on viewing that interaction as a "behavioral dialogue," have been developed above. But precisely because these indices are rather abstract and do not measure some quality immediately apparent to an observer, it is reasonable to ask just how "meaningful" they are. For that reason, their relationship to other measures—observers' ratings—was examined and found to be sensible and consistent (Bakeman & Brown, Note 3).

We can also ask how stable these measures were, that is, did high scorers at one observation also score higher later. If the measures turn out to be unstable, it could be because the characteristics they measure

TABLE 13

Stability of Selected Variables[1]

Variable	H to 1	H to 3	1 to 3
GROSM	. . .	. . .	.30*
FINEM	. . .	. . .	. . .
GRASP	. . .	. . .	. . .
IOPEN	. . .	. . .	. . .
LOOKM	—	—	. . .
LOOKS	—	—	. . .
IVOC	. . .	.21	. . .
MLOOK	. . .	. . .	. . .
MVOC	.66***	.55***	.65***
TSTIM	.22	. . .	. . .
VSTIM	.20	. . .	.66***
BFEED	. . .	. . .	.24
SFEED	—	—	.53***
p (I + C)	. . .	. . .	.27
p (M + C)	.47***	.47***	.54***
p (C)	.27	.23	.42**
p (I)	.33*	.32*	.53***
p (M)	.38**	.37**	.35*
p (Q)	.43**	.30*	.41**
MC + CM	.50***	.41**	.56***
MQ + QM	. . .	. . .	. . .
QI + IQ	.29*	.31*	.49***
CI + IC	. . .	. . .	.22
H_2	.28	.30*	.40**

[1] Correlations less than .20 are not given. If less than half of the dyads engaged in a particular behavior at an observation time then a correlation was not computed (indicated by dashes). Significance levels are two-tailed. The variables are defined in previous tables and in the text. These correlations are based on 49 mother-infant dyads.
* $p < .05$
** $p < .01$
*** $p < .001$

were unstable or because the indices really measure "noise" more than any coherent characteristic of the interaction. But if the measures were stable, then we can be reasonably confident that they measure coherent and meaningful qualities of the interaction. In fact, the indices based on viewing the interaction as a behavioral dialogue were quite stable, considerably more so than specific behavior rates (see Table 13). In general, qualities associated with the mother were more likely to be stable than ones associated with the infant (e.g., the probability that the infant was active overall, $p(I + C)$, was not stable), and all characteristics tended to be more stable from the one-month to the three-months than from the hospital to the one-month observation. In conclusion, the pattern of correlations displayed in Table 13 (together with the correlations with the observers' ratings) suggests that the various indices of mother-infant interaction developed here measure stable, coherent, and meaningful aspects of the interactions we observed.

SUMMARY

This chapter compares early interaction between mothers and preterm infants with that between mothers and full-term infants. Specifically, mother-infant dyads were observed during a feeding session just before hospital release, one month later, and three months later. The interaction between preterm infants and their mothers seemed quite different from that between full-term infants and their mothers, enough so that it makes sense to speak of a different modal interaction style for preterm dyads. This does not necessarily mean that preterm infants engaged in "worse" interaction than full-terms or that their interaction style led to deficient outcomes. Such questions are obviously important, however, and will be addressed in subsequent reports (e.g., Brown & Bakeman, in press). But the purpose of this chapter is quite narrow; it is simply to document differences with respect to early mother-infant interaction and to demonstrate the utility of various data reduction techniques. The major findings are summarized below.

(1) When the frequencies and durations of specific behaviors were analyzed (first level analyses), preterm dyads differed from full-term dyads in several ways just before being released from the hospital, in a few ways a month later, and in very few ways three months later. During the hospital observation, full-term infants were more visually active and were more active feeders while mothers of preterm infants were more likely to say something in a directive way to their infants and spent more

time stimulating their infants. We infer that full-term infants were more rewarding and satisfying to their mothers initially. But three months later, preterm and full-term dyads differed hardly at all, at least with respect to frequencies and durations of specific behaviors.

(2) When mother-infant interaction was viewed more abstractly—as a "behavioral dialogue" between mother and infant (second level analyses)—differences between preterm and full-term dyads remained stable across the three observation sessions. Mothers of preterms were more active generally and in particular were more persistent and were more likely to initiate and continue behavioral episodes than the mothers of full-terms. While all infants contributed more to the interactive flow as they became older, the burden of maintaining that flow still fell disproportionately on the mothers of preterms.

(3) Even though the various behavioral dialogic indices revealed consistent differences between preterm and full-term dyads, they still changed over time, reflecting, perhaps, the development of the infants. What remained unchanged was the variability of the behavioral dialogues (third level analyses). Preterm interaction was more patterned and stereotyped while full-term interaction was more varied, and this was so at all three observation periods. For the first three months at least, this particular attribute of mother-infant interaction distinguished preterm and full-term dyads and was apparently unaffected by development.

(4) We conclude that viewing early mother-infant interaction as a behavioral dialogue is useful. Various measures derived from this approach correlated in sensible ways with observers' ratings and the measures demonstrated stability over the three observation sessions. Moreover, the pattern of differences between preterm and full-term dyads changed little during the three months and so we think it makes sense to speak of different modal preterm and full-term interaction styles. What consequences, if any, such early differences have for later development will be discussed in subsequent reports.

14

Lag Sequential Analysis as a Data Reduction Technique in Social Interaction Research

GENE P. SACKETT

University of Washington

Research using human observers to encode social behavior is becoming increasingly popular. These studies, conducted in laboratory, natural, and seminatural settings, have achieved their popularity for at least three reasons.

Biological approaches to behavior including ethology, ecology, and sociobiology are influencing most experimental behavior sciences (e.g., Wilson, 1975; Bateson & Hinde, 1978; Crook, 1970). These theories propose that environmental factors, including social organization, are major determinants of both behavioral evolution and current behavioral phenotypes in all animal species. Understanding behavior, according to these views, best proceeds by first describing typical behavioral repertoires of a species and the physical and social environments in which these repertoires occur (e.g., Miller, 1977). This description provides a baseline from which specific hypotheses are tested. Observational data often yield the major baseline information. Many behavioral scientists, including even psychologists, recognize the importance of such information and are gathering large amounts of descriptive baseline data in many human settings.

Direct observation is also on the rise in behavior development research

Preparation of this paper was supported by grant RR-00166 from NIH Animal Resources Branch to the Regional Primate Research Center, University of Washington. I wish to thank my colleague Dr. Jonathan Lewis for his mostly helpful comments on the methods presented here and for his encouragement in developing the Angles of Sequential Significance.

300

(e.g., Bronfenbrenner, 1977; Parke, 1978). Examples include describing interactions of parents with young, relating early life social interactions to later behavior, assessing effects of infants upon caregivers, and evaluating the role of socialization in producing sex differences. Such research is generating social behavior data in both laboratory and real-world situations. Much of this work is not only of theoretical value, but may have application to important human problems such as prematurity and postmaturity, child abuse, learning failures, and social-emotional abnormalities (e.g., Sameroff, 1975a).

A third factor influencing the proliferation of direct observation is technological. Electronic gadgets for coding behavior occurrences, durations, and sequences (e.g., Sackett, Stephenson, & Ruppenthal, 1973; Stephenson, Smith, & Roberts, 1975) can generate astronomical amounts of data in even a single study. There is also ready access to computers by investigators. In principle, computers can reduce the almost limitless original observations to a smaller set of comprehensible numbers. These numbers may summarize anywhere from a few observed behaviors to dozens or even hundreds of different acts. Studies of social interaction often measure sequential dependencies among the behaviors of two or more individuals to identify patterns of simultaneous or successive responses occurring in a given time period. Unfortunately, computer summaries can yield more dependency measures than the original number of raw observations. Although computers permit complex analyses of complex phenomena, potential information gains may be offset by inability of even intelligent investigators to comprehend the typically huge amounts of output (e.g., Altmann, 1965).

Scientifically valuable data must be comprehensible to at least some investigators or theoreticians, and must be transportable via publication. Unfortunately, many observational studies yield reports concerning only a small fraction of the data collected. The rest lies unanalyzed or indigestible in cabinets and on computer tapes. Most sequential dependency studies analyze only pairs of behaviors occurring simultaneously or in one-step sequences. This barely scratches the surface of potentially important sequential relationships, and may waste much of our computing power. Two reasons for difficulty in handling sequential data and wasting technological power are probably (1) lack of appropriate yet relatively simple data analysis models, and (2) lack of comprehensible methods for summarizing and representing complex sequential relationships among behaviors.

Accordingly, this paper has three main purposes. The first is to present one model for extracting sequential information from observational data. The second is to illustrate how large quantities of sequential information can be summarized for individual subjects or behaviors in a small number of statistics. The third is to describe a method for quantifying sequential relationships from a whole experiment in just a few numbers.

THE LAG MODEL FOR SEQUENTIAL ANALYSIS

Computing Lag Probabilities

Sequential analysis involves prediction of future behavior from knowledge of current behavior. This is a problem of temporal correlation. A relatively simple example is measuring diurnal cyclicity. Table 1 presents hypothetical sleep-wakefulness data for an adult human observed once per hour on seven consecutive days. Each observation rates whether the person is behaviorally asleep (*S*), awake but inactive (*I*), or actively engaged in motor or intellectual activity (*A*). Simply scanning the table rows reveals that one typical state occurs on most hours across days. We can measure the extent of this temporal dependency, within and between states, by calculating lag probabilities as follows:

(1) Choose any one of the states as a *criterion* behavior.
(2) Count the number of times that each behavior—including the criterion itself—*matches* each occurrence of the criterion as (1) the very next behavior (Lag 1), (2) the second behavior after each criterion occurrence (Lag 2), (3) the third behavior after the criterion (Lag 3), . . ., (4) the *Maximum Lag* behavior after the criterion. The Maximum Lag is the largest sequential step of interest.

A complete analysis uses every behavior as criterion, matched against all other behaviors up to the *Maximum Lag*. The procedure yields a frequency count of the number of times each criterion behavior is followed by each matching behavior at each lag.

To illustrate, let us use the inactive state as criterion matched against itself. Self-matching is termed autolags, analogous to the idea of autocorrelation in a time series analysis (e.g., Jenkins & Watts, 1969). Matching of other behavior to the criterion is termed crosslags, analogous to the idea of crosscorrelation.

Inactive occurred 33 times out of the total 168 events. Thus, the unconditional probability of *I* is $33/168 = .20$. Among these 33 instances,

Table I. Sleep-wakefulness data used to illustrate calculation of lag conditional probabilities (S=Sleep, I=Inactive, A=Active).

Time (Hours)	Day 1	Day 2	Day 3	Day 4	Day 5	Day 6	Day 7
1	S	S	S	S	S	S	S
2	S	S	S	S	S	S	S
3	S	S	S	S	S	S	S
4	S	S	I	S	S	S	S
5	S	I	S	S	S	S	S
6	I	S	S	I	I	S	I
7	A	A	I	A	I	I	A
8	A	A	A	A	A	I	A
9	A	A	A	A	A	A	A
10	I	I	A	I	A	A	I
11	A	A	I	A	A	I	A
12	A	A	A	A	A	A	A
13	A	A	A	A	A	A	A
14	A	I	A	I	A	A	I
15	I	A	I	A	A	I	A
16	A	A	A	A	S	A	A
17	A	A	A	A	A	A	A
18	A	I	A	A	A	A	A
19	I	A	I	I	A	A	I
20	A	A	A	A	A	A	A
21	A	I	A	A	I	I	A
22	I	S	A	A	S	I	I
23	S	S	S	A	S	S	S
24	S	S	S	S	S	S	S

I followed itself as the very next behavior three times (Day 5 at hours 6-7, Day 6 at hours 7-8 and 21-22). So, the autolag 1 probability for *I* following itself is $3/33 = .09$. *I* never followed itself two hours after its occurrences, so the autolag 2 probability is $0/33 = .00$. At lag 3 *I* could only be followed 32 times. This decrease in the sample size available for lagging happened because the final *I* occurrence at hour 22 on Day 7 left only two events remaining. Thus, lags greater than 2 were impossible after this *I* occurrence due to "falling off at the sample end." At autolag 3 *I* followed itself five times (Day 1 at hours 19-22, Day 2 at hours 18-21, Day 3 at hours 4-7, Day 6 at hours 8-11, Day 7 at hours 19-22), yielding a probability of $5/32 = .16$.

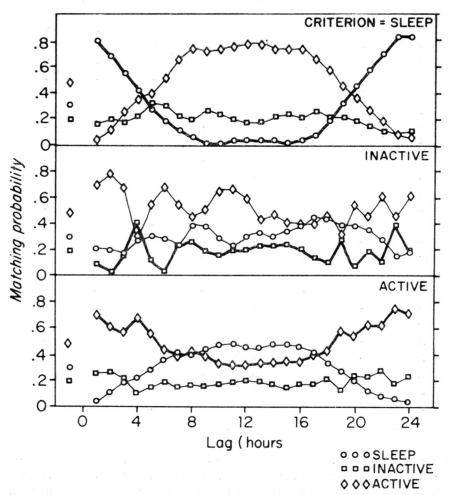

FIGURE 1. Auto and cross lag probabilities showing diurnal cyclicity and phasic relationships between sleep, inactive, and active states of one person measured hourly over seven days.

Table 2 presents the complete analysis of *I* as criterion and all three states as matches for 24 one-hour lags. The 24-hour period represents one complete diurnal cycle. The first row gives the overall frequency and unconditional probability for each state in the total sample. The next 24 rows show the total *I* instances available for matching (Total Freq), and the frequencies and probabilities with which each state actually matched *I*. The middle panel of Figure 1 plots each of these probabilities against lag. This display shows the degree to which *I* predicts its own recurrences and predictability of the other two states given that *I* has occurred up to 24 hours previously. A rough estimate of prediction "goodness" is obtained by comparing the unconditional probability (U) of the matching behavior with lag probability. If chance alone were operating, a behavior should match any other including itself in proportion to its overall probability in the sample. This unconditional probability is used in all current sequential analysis models as an expected value for random matching.

Relative to the .20 expected value for *I* following itself (1) *I* was *inhibited*—below its expected value—at lags, 1, 2, 5, 6, 17, 18, 20 and 22; (2) *I* was *excited*—above its expected value—at lags 4, 19 and 23; and (3) *I* was at or near the expected value at all other lags. In other words, the occurrence of *I* led immediately to its own inhibition, followed by one hour of excitation and two hours of inhibition, with this pattern repeating 12 hours later. The two crossing functions reveal some degree of predictability for both sleep and awake following inactivity. (4) Starting with weak inhibition, the probability of sleep gradually rises to a peak at 17 hours after inactivity, then falls to an inhibited level. (5) Active has strong excitation for three hours after inactivity, is sharply inhibited for one hour, has a repeating cycle of excitation-inhibition for the next nine hours, then gradually rises to a peak at 24 hours.

Figure 1 also displays sleep and active as criteria. (1) Sleep (upper panel) shows very strong diurnal cyclicity. High lag probabilities occur for four hours after sleep, inhibition for about 13 hours, then strong excitation at 20-24 hours. As we would expect, the active state is strongly and inversely related to sleep occurrence. Inactivity shows weak excitation five-six hours after sleep and weak inhibition 22-24 hours after sleep. (2) Active (lower panel) is diurnally cyclic with itself, is inversely related to sleep, and has only very weak relationships with inactivity.

This section presented the basics of the lag technique, illustrating the relative simplicity of calculating lag probabilities and visualizing auto and cross lag functions. These functions display one-step dependencies, more complex multi-step contingencies, repetition, and cyclicity. How-

Table 2. Matching frequencies and probabilities for lags 1-24 with <u>Inactive</u> as the criterion behavior matched against itself, Sleep, and Active (from the Table 1 data).

Lag	Sleep Freq.	Sleep Prob.	Inactive Freq.	Inactive Prob.	Awake Freq.	Awake Prob.	Total Freq.
Overall	52	.31	33	.20	83	.49	168
1	7	.21	3	.09	23	.70	33
2	7	.21	0	.00	26	.79	33
3	5	.16	5	.16	22	.69	32
4	9	.28	13	.41	10	.31	32
5	10	.31	4	.12	18	.56	32
6	9	.29	1	.03	21	.68	31
7	7	.23	7	.23	17	.55	31
8	12	.39	8	.26	11	.36	31
9	12	.39	6	.19	13	.42	31
10	9	.29	5	.16	17	.55	31
11	7	.23	6	.20	17	.57	30
12	9	.30	6	.20	15	.50	30
13	10	.33	7	.23	13	.43	30
14	9	.30	7	.23	14	.47	30
15	10	.37	7	.24	12	.41	29
16	11	.38	6	.21	12	.41	29
17	13	.45	4	.14	12	.41	29
18	13	.45	3	.10	13	.45	29
19	11	.39	8	.29	9	.32	28
20	11	.39	2	.07	15	.54	28
21	10	.36	5	.18	13	.46	28
22	8	.29	3	.11	17	.61	28
23	4	.14	11	.39	13	.46	28
24	5	.18	6	.21	17	.61	28

ever, the presentation was overly simple. Lag analysis and all other sequence or pattern detection methods are fraught with measurement and research design problems. These issues have been described in great detail (Bakeman, 1978; Sackett, 1978), and most will not be treated here. Interested researchers are urged to consult these references before applying the techniques described below. Especially important are sampling and measurement problems resulting in lack of independence among behavioral categories, simultaneous occurrence of more than one behavior, analysis of event sequences regardless of duration as opposed to actual time-based dependency, and identification of exact simultaneous or successive behavior patterns.

LAG SEQUENTIAL ANALYSIS OF A COMPLETE OBSERVATIONAL STUDY

Research designs for collecting sequential data employ three basic types of behavior-subject sampling strategies. These are (1) a single behavior emitted successively by a number of potential interactors, (2) many behaviors emitted by a single individual, and (3) a target behavior emitted by a single individual followed by many behaviors of one or more other subjects. Each of these strategies yields data appropriate for the same methods of lag analysis. The remainder of this paper deals with a study concerning a single behavior emitted by a number of interacting people. The similarity of these data to the other two behavior-subject strategies will be described as appropriate. The analysis illustrates display and significance tests of lag probabilities, autocontingency effects on social interaction data, and reducing large quantities of sequential dependencies to a small set of psychologically meaningful numbers.

Subjects and Setting

Sixteen eminent observational researchers, plus myself, gathered to confer on analysis of social interactions. These 16 people were the subjects. To effect privacy and avoid embarrassment and civil suits these people will remain anonymous.

The Sampled Behavior: Definition and Procedure

The conference lasted for 2.5 days. It occurred in 17 20-40 minute sessions during which each participant led a discussion of his or her favorite analysis problem. During 16 of these sessions the experimenter

Table 3. Complete lag sequential analysis with Speaker D as Criterion and the remaining 15 speakers as matches. The experimenter's data are included only to calculate total Ns. (Decimals have been omitted for all probabilities and negative z values are underlined).

		A	B	C	D	E	F	G	H	I	J	K	L	M	N	O	P	(me)	TOTAL FREQ
OVERALL	N	63	89	170	101	46	151	72	113	87	40	48	113	139	35	100	61	(78)	1506
	Pun	042	059	113	068	030	103	048	074	056	027	032	074	092	023	066	040	(052)	
								SPEAKER D AS CRITERION												
LAG 1	Nmatch	0	4	17	—	6	8	3	7	12	3	3	2	6	1	13	7	(111)	103
	Pbos	000	039	165	—	058	078	029	068	117	029	029	019	058	010	126	068		
	Nposs	63	89	170	—	46	151	72	113	87	40	48	113	139	35	100	61	(78)	1405
	Pexp	045	063	121	—	033	108	051	081	062	034	034	081	099	025	071	043		
	SD	020	024	032	—	018	031	022	027	024	016	018	027	029	015	025	020		
	Z	2.20	1.02	1.36	—	1.45	.98	1.02	.47	2.29	.04	.28	2.28	1.39	.99	2.17	1.22		
	Pz	014	154	087	—	074	164	154	319	011	484	390	011	082	161	015	111		
	Pbinomial	009	216	114	—	126	206	224	398	026	577	534	008	106	268	031	156		
LAG 2	Nmatch	4	3	5	43	3	5	1	4	4	1	3	5	5	0	6	3	(8)	103
	Pobs	039	029	049	417	029	049	010	039	039	010	029	049	049	000	058	029		
	Nposs	63	85	153	101	40	143	69	106	75	37	45	111	133	34	87	54	(67)	1403
	Pexp	045	061	109	072	029	102	049	076	053	026	032	079	095	024	062	038		
	SD	020	024	031	025	016	030	021	026	022	016	017	027	029	015	024	019		
	Z	.30	1.34	1.97	13.6	.04	1.79	1.85	1.41	.66	1.06	.17	1.15	1.60	1.60	.16	.49		
	Pz	382	090	024	0001	484	037	032	079	255	145	432	125	055	055	436	312		
	Pbinomial	504	120	026	0001	577	042	036	101	358	249	580	168	066	082	543	447		
	Nmatch	1	3	14	7	6	8	4	8	13	2	2	1	4	1	13	7	(9)	103
	Pobs	010	029	136	068	058	078	039	078	126	019	019	010	039	010	126	068		

Table 3 continued

		A	B	C	D	E	F	G	H	I	J	K	L	M	N	O	P	(me)
																		(70) 1403
LAG 3	Nposs	59	86	165	58	43	146	71	109	83	39	45	108	134	35	94	58	
	Pexp	042	061	118	041	031	104	051	078	059	028	032	077	096	025	067	041	
	SD	020	024	032	020	017	030	022	026	023	016	017	026	029	015	025	020	
	Z	1.64	1.36	.58	1.36	1.63	.88	.55	.01	2.88	.52	.73	2.56	1.96	.99	2.40	1.36	
LAG 4	Pobs	020	040	059	406	050	099	030	050	030	010	000	030	020	010	020	040	
	Z	1.19	.91	1.66	13.6	1.27	.10	.88	.97	1.04	1.06	1.85	1.86	2.60	.94	1.76	.06	
LAG 5	Pobs	000	029	165	097	039	068	019	058	107	058	019	019	068	010	117	029	
	Z	2.16	1.34	1.53	2.73	.58	1.09	1.39	.71	2.01	1.88	.82	2.22	1.01	.96	1.86	.59	
LAG 6	Pobs	039	029	059	343	078	108	029	020	029	000	000	059	049	000	078	039	
	Z	.28	1.34	1.63	11.4	2.87	.17	.95	2.16	1.10	1.59	1.86	.76	1.56	1.59	.65	.11	
LAG 7	Pobs	010	038	154	096	019	058	058	058	115	038	000	038	029	000	125	048	
	Z	1.65	.97	1.18	2.37	.49	1.43	.40	.81	2.39	.61	1.92	1.45	2.31	1.63	2.45	.39	
LAG 8	Pobs	029	029	127	363	059	088	039	039	029	020	010	039	029	010	029	010	
	Z	.73	1.32	.57	12.2	1.59	.58	.37	1.41	1.08	.39	1.36	1.45	2.31	.98	1.37	1.55	
LAG 9	Pobs	029	019	096	115	048	048	029	058	135	048	038	048	067	000	087	029	
	Z	.70	1.79	.51	3.41	1.20	1.79	.93	.76	3.22	1.32	.28	1.13	1.02	1.61	.70	.70	
LAG 10	Pobs	000	019	146	320	087	049	029	078	019	000	010	058	049	010	039	029	
	Z	2.15	1.79	1.01	10.7	3.50	1.85	.94	.05	1.49	1.62	1.26	.71	1.58	.99	1.07	.62	
								$\Sigma Z / \sqrt{N}$											
Overall		4.11	4.17	.14	23.8	4.31	3.24	2.68	2.74	2.35	.76	3.15	4.92	5.48	3.88	1.41	.33	
Odd Lags		3.73	2.90	1.85	4.94	4.15	2.76	1.56	1.23	5.72	1.49	1.55	4.31	3.44	2.76	3.66	.75	
Even Lags		2.08	3.00	1.65	27.5	1.95	1.82	2.23	2.64	2.40	2.56	2.91	2.65	4.32	2.73	1.66	1.21	

(me) recorded *the order in which participants held the floor.* I call this "speakership" data. Recording was not done during my turn as discussion leader because I could not record, attempt to think, talk and answer questions at the same time.

Of the 1506 speakership changes, 95% were initiated by one, and only one, person. The others appeared to be either listening, thinking, chatting, or sleeping. The remaining 5% of speakership changes found two, and only two, people trying to talk at once. On all but 10 of these 75 occasions it was obvious to me that the group was attending to only one of these buttinskies, who therefore was credited with that speakership. This left only 10 speakership changes (.6%) on which two people obtained the floor simultaneously. These speakerships were given to each buttinsky, which produces 10 more events in the data as a whole than actually occurred.

Reliability

Between-observer agreement was checked for two 15-minute periods; once by me and my right-hand neighbor and once by me and the person on my left. Only one mismatch occurred out of the 44 speakership changes during the reliability period. This yielded an overall agreement of 98%, uncorrected for chance (Hollenbeck, 1978). So, I figured that real behavior was being scored—whatever its importance—and the scoring was reasonably consistent. Next, a lag analysis was performed with little regard for the Pandora's boxes that might be opened.

Lag Analysis with Speaker D as Criterion

Table 3 presents a complete computer-generated lag analysis of a single criterion event (speakerships by Subject D). Compared to other behavior-subject data types, this could be an analysis of one among 17 behaviors by a single individual. It could also be an analysis of a target behavior by one individual, perhaps a mother looking at her infant. The remaining events might be 16 behaviors by the infant, or eight infant behaviors and eight behaviors emitted by the father.

Rows one and two present overall speakership frequency and unconditional probability for each of the 17 people. My own speakerships were included for calculating unconditional probabilities, but were excluded in the detailed analysis due to the "unnatural" nature of my participation as both speaker and data taker. *N,* the total number of speakerships per person, varied from 35 to 170 (Mean = 88.6, SD = 39.6), revealing a wide range in active participation among the 17 conference members.

The remainder of Table 3 deals specifically with Speaker D as criterion and the 15 people other than myself as matches. The analysis concerns prediction of who will talk following D speakerships. Ten lags were studied. Lags 1-3 are presented in complete detail to illustrate a number of computational fine points.

Lag 1

The first row for lag 1 gives the number of times each person followed D as the very next speaker (N_{match}). There were 103 instances (Total Freq) of D being followed immediately after he held the floor. This is an apparent anomaly, as D actually held the floor only 101 times. However, two of these were buttinskies, two people speaking at once and neither dominating. This produced an excess of two over the actual total.

Row 2 presents the lag 1 observed probabilities (P_{obs}). These are obtained dividing each N_{match} by the total number of 103. Note that person D (autolag) does not appear in the lag 1 data. Given the data collection method, D cannot lose the floor and immediately get it back again. So, an autocontingency at lag 1 does not exist.

Row 3 presents the number of times each person could possibly follow D at lag 1 (N_{poss}). These values are identical to N in the overall data. However, the total of possible lag 1 following events is not 1506 as in the overall data. Because the 101 D speakerships cannot be followed by D at lag 1, the total N_{poss} is 1506-101 = 1405. Chance expected values, the unconditional probabilities shown in row 4 (P_{exp}), are obtained by dividing each N_{poss} by 1405.

Next, we test each lag probability for departure from chance. The standard deviation (SD) of each expected probability is the square root of $[P_{exp} - (1-P_{exp})]/$Total N_{match}. Then $Z = (P_{obs} - P_{exp})/SD$ is calculated. The normal curve probability of this Z is an approximation to the exact binomial probability for each N_{match}, given its corresponding expected probability (see any introductory statistics text for reference). SD, Z, and P_z are shown in rows 5-7. For comparison purposes, exact binomial probabilities are given in the final row. One-tailed values are given as it is easier to calculate their binomial probabilities with differential N and skewed expected values. However, 2-tailed tests would ordinarily be made, unless specific predictions were available for the direction of

$P_{obs} - P_{exp}$ differences. These comparative probabilities will be discussed below.

Nine of the 15 Z values were negative, two with significance beyond the .05 level (using the appropriate 2-tailed test). Six Z values were positive, with two again significant. Thus, at lag 1, speakers I and 0 were excited (above chance) immediately following D, speakers A and L were inhibited (below chance), and the remainder did not differ markedly from chance.

Lags Greater Than 1

Lag 1 data constitute the vast bulk of sequential analyses in observational literature. A few studies deal with complex pattern dependencies (see Gottman and Notarius, 1976, for examples), in which the exact order of several behaviors following each other is studied. Such Markovian analyses search for all patterns of events occurring out to some maximum pattern size. When this size exceeds four or five consecutive events the number of conditional probabilities, intellectual load, and difficulty in generating expected values become rapidly prohibitive (e.g., Altmann, 1965). However, in lag analysis the study of dependencies more than one step from criterion events is no different than at lag 1. The third section of Table 3 illustrates computations for lag 2. The number of times people matched Speaker D, including D himself, two steps from each D speakership is in row 1. Lag 2 observed probability is in row 2.

Now we come to a fine point. The number of times each person can possibly follow Speaker D at lag 2 (N_{poss}) is not N from the overall data. A person cannot immediately follow him or herself. Therefore, the number of events that can theoretically occur after the criterion is the total N of events in the data as a whole minus the number of matches at the *immediately preceding* lag. For example, person B had 89 speakerships. Four occurred following D at lag 1. These four cannot occur at lag 2 due to restrictions of the sampling method. Thus, the number of lag 2 B speakerships that can possibly follow D is $89-4 = 85$. N_{poss} was calculated in this manner for each person, and the sum across all 17 people yields a Total Freq of 1403. This total can also be obtained by subtracting the number of times D was matched by anyone at lag 1 (Total $N_{match} = 103$) from the total N of 1506 speakerships in the data as a whole.

Expected probabilities (N_{poss}/Total Freq N_{poss}), standard deviations, Z values, and Z and binomial probabilities are calculated in the same way as for lag 1. The results produced 14 of 15 negative crosslags, with only Speaker C reaching the .05 significance level. The autolag probability of

.417 exceeded its expected value by .320, and was highly significant ($p < .00001$). Thus, at lag 2 we find that D had a good chance of following himself, with most of the others moderately inhibited.

Lag 3 calculations are identical. The number of matches three steps from each D speakership are counted and observed probabilities are computed. The N_{poss} at lag 3 for each person is found by subtracting that person's N_{match} at lag 2 from his N in the data as a whole. The results produced 10 negative and five positive crosslags, and a nonsignificant positive autolag. As occurred at lag 1, speakers I and O were significantly inhibited at lag 3, but not at lag 1. Next, Table 3 presents the *observed probabilities* and corresponding Z values for lags 4-10.

From 101 D speakerships we have generated nine autolag and 150 conditional probabilities with Speaker D as criterion. This gives us a picture of D as a "leader" and the rest of the group as "followers." We can do exactly the same analysis with D *as follower* by computing all dependencies out to lag 10 with the 15 others as criteria and D as match. This was done, and the resulting 150 crosslag Z values are presented in Table 4. We now possess 309 lag probabilities: 150 relate D to 15 other people as a discussion leader, 150 relate D to the others as a discussion follower, and nine autocontingencies measure the extent to which D follows himself.

Statistical Significance of Lag Probabilities

Bakeman (1978) uses Z scores calculated in the manner described above as relative indices of sequential dependency. He does not, however, seriously consider the Z probabilities in their usual hypothesis testing sense. Their approximation to exact binomial probabilities is poor unless sample sizes are over 30 and expected values are not skewed beyond .1-.9 (McNemar, 1955). Bakeman is certainly justified in using these relative Z. The mean difference between binomial and Z probabilities was .059

Table 3 presented Z and exact binomial probabilities for crosslags 1 and 2. The Total N_{match} of 103 was well beyond the magic sample size of 30, but expected values were markedly skewed from .024-.121. For 28 of the 30 pairs the binomial probability exceeded that of its corresponding Z. The mean difference between binomial and Z probabilities was .059 ($SD = .046$). The product moment correlation between the 30 expected values and their corresponding binomial probability minus Z probability differences was $-.615$ ($p < .001$). This all suggests that McNemar was

Table 4. $\underline{Z}$ values for lag probabilities with Speaker $\underline{D}$ as match and the 15 other people as criteria (negative values are underlined).

LAG	A	B	C	E	F	G	H	I	J	K	L	M	N	O	P
														SPEAKER	
1	-1.19	2.20	.86	1.64	2.08	-.52	-.10	1.96	1.96	-.85	2.67	-1.10	-.31	2.25	1.77
2	-1.16	.56	-1.24	.04	1.58	.49	-1.77	.18	-1.67	-1.87	-1.56	2.26	-1.59	-.16	-.60
3	.34	1.70	.54	2.97	1.89	.88	.72	2.10	-.47	-.75	-1.51	-1.71	-.31	1.65	.86
4	1.61	.95	-.67	.12	-1.35	-1.05	-1.72	-1.13	-.44	-1.87	2.17	2.33	.92	-1.00	2.52
5	-1.71	.51	-.22	5.46	-1.50	.98	.33	2.40	-1.70	-.18	-1.88	-.42	-.96	1.86	.06
6	.71	.86	.39	-1.03	1.87	0.00	-1.45	.21	-1.10	-1.28	-1.82	3.19	-.30	-.96	.32
7	-1.14	2.15	-1.27	5.58	-1.28	.96	.06	1.75	-.46	-.77	-1.87	.45	-.95	2.64	.44
8	.27	-1.77	.53	.29	2.11	-.03	-.65	-.76	-1.70	.69	-1.13	2.48	-.93	-1.35	.45
9	1.62	-1.38	-.65	-5.78	-1.94	-1.35	.13	2.48	-1.10	-1.30	-1.85	-1.39	-.30	1.90	.45
10	.76	1.32	-.23	.97	1.54	.51	.32	1.45	.17	.77	-1.84	2.26	.92	.57	.41
							$\Sigma\, \underline{z}\,/\,\sqrt{N}$									
All	2.94	4.24	-.62	6.29	5.42	2.14	-1.72	3.36	2.06	3.27	5.79	5.28	2.37	1.98	2.11
Odd	2.38	3.55	-.33	9.58	3.89	2.10	.22	4.78	-.79	-1.72	-4.37	-1.86	-1.27	4.61	1.60
Even	-1.78	2.44	-.55	.69	3.78	.93	2.64	-.02	2.12	2.90	-3.81	5.60	-2.08	-1.81	1.39

correct. Smaller (more skewed) expected values produced increasingly poorer fit between exact and estimated probabilities.

However, among the 7 significant (2-tailed .05 level) Z values all corresponding binomial probabilities except for person C at lag 2 were also significant. Even though the expected values for these seven tests ranged from .025-.103, the mean binomial-Z difference for these seven pairs was only .005 ($SD = .008$). Thus, from this limited sample size we can conclude that (1) in general with skewed expected values binomial probabilities are larger than their Z estimates; but (2) even with marked skew, statistically reliable binomial tests have remarkably good fit with their Z estimates. Obviously, a Monte Carlo computer simulation varying degree of expected value skew, sample size, and size of observed probabilities would provide a better answer. Nevertheless, it appears that Z probabilities can be used for lag data to infer statistical significance as long as conservative alpha levels and interpretations are employed.

Two other problems with lag probability significance involve potential lack of independence due to the highly correlated nature of most, if not all, observational data and type I error. The independence problem is too intricate to treat here, although some aspects will be discussed below. Type I error can be controlled to some extent by showing that more significant conditional probabilities occur than would be expected by chance. For lags 1 and 2 we would expect 1.5 of the 30 tests to be significant by chance, yet we obtained seven that reached or exceeded the .05 level ($p = .0012$).

Display of Autolags

Having generated 309 lag probabilities and associated statistics for Speaker D, we now face the problem of figuring out what, if anything, these numbers mean. One aspect deals with autolags—the degree to which Speaker D follows himself (Table 3, D column). These are displayed in the upper right hand corner of Figure 2, which presents the unconditional probability, autolag 2-10 observed probabilities, and 95% confidence bands. The confidence points were calculated from $P_{exp} \pm$ (1.96 * SD) at each autolag. The function exhibits strong repetition, with excited probabilities on even lags and probabilities near the upper confidence band on odd lags. The picture is one of a basic conversation. Given that D just talked, (1) he cannot talk one step away, thus no autolag 1; (2) he is well above chance two steps away; (3) he decreases to chance three steps away; and (4) he repeats this "I talk-You talk" conversational pattern over the remaining seven lags.

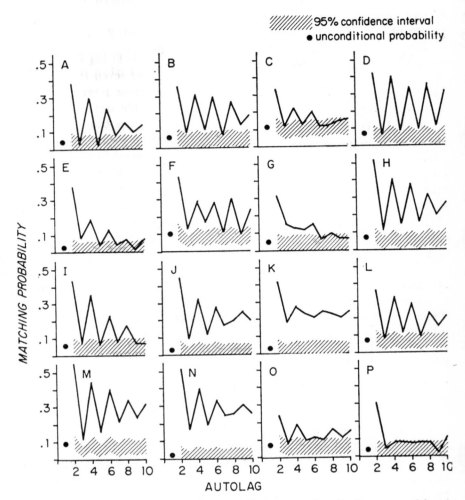

FIGURE 2. Autolag functions for the 16 Madison Interaction Conference participants showing the probability that each person will follow himself as speaker on lags 2-10.

Figure 2 also displays autolag functions for the 15 other speakers. All exhibit two basic properties: (1) *Magnitude,* the degree to which the function exceeds chance in either direction; and (2) *Cyclicity,* the degree to which a repetitive pattern occurs over the whole function.

Magnitude can be measured by the mean of the absolute Z values at each autolag. The larger these values, in either excited or inhibited direction, the greater is the predictability of the autocontingent event. Measuring cyclicity, a bit more complicated, can be done by subtracting successive Z scores that are one autolag apart. The mean absolute value of these differences will index the relative degree of "ups and downs" in the function. For example, the 9 autolag Z values for Speaker D were 13.57, 1.35, 13.62, 2.73, 11.41, 2.37, 12.21, 3.41, and 10.69. Their mean of 7.93 indexes relative autolag magnitude. The absolute values of one step

Table 5. Zsums, means, and analysis of variance for dependency relationships of Speaker D in leader and follower roles to conference participants having the greatest and least frequent overall number of speakerships (N).

Group	Speaker	N	Speaker D Role Criterion	Match	Mean
TALKERS	C	170	0.14	-0.62	-0.24
	F	151	-3.24	-5.42	-4.33
	M	139	-5.48	-5.28	-5.38
	H	113	-2.74	-1.72	-2.23
	L	113	-4.92	-5.79	-5.36
	Mean	137	-3.25	-3.77	-3.51
THINKERS	N	35	-3.88	-2.37	-3.13
	J	40	-0.76	-2.06	-1.41
	E	46	-3.24	6.29	1.53
	K	48	-3.15	-3.27	-3.21
	A	63	-4.11	-2.94	-3.53
	Mean	46	-3.03	-0.87	-1.95

Source	DF	Mean Square	F	p
Group	1	12.14	1.29	.29
Error	8	9.43		
Role	1	3.36	0.68	.43
Group x Role	1	8.95	1.82	.21
Error	8	4.92		

successive autolag differences are $(1.36\text{-}13.57=)12.21$, $(13.62\text{-}1.36=)$ 12.26, $(2.73\text{-}13.62=)10.89$, 8.68, 9.04, 9.84, 8.80, and 7.28. The mean of 9.88 indexes relative autolag cyclicity.

Table 5 presents these magnitude and cyclicity indices measuring the relative extent of autocorrelation in the 16 functions of Figure 2. Mean magnitude was based on nine Z values per speaker, mean cyclicity on eight one-lag step differences. One-way analysis of variance, with speakers considered as "independent groups" and Z values or differences as replicated scores, yielded an individual difference main effect reliable beyond the .0001 level (bottom of Table 5). The Pearson correlation between magnitude and cyclicity means was $+.44$ $(p=.09)$, suggesting that these measures are largely independent. An extreme example of this independence is Speaker K, who achieved rank 3 in magnitude but was 15th in cyclicity.

Speakers were grouped by dividing the ranked means at each point where two consecutive means differed by more than one standard error. A statistically more precise division could, of course, be made using Duncan's or Newman-Keuls' tests (Winer, 1971). Nevertheless, with little overlap, these groupings have interesting psychological interpretations when compared with the autolag functions of Figure 2.

Magnitude. There were five magnitude groupings. Speaker N formed grouping 1. He excited himself over all lags, with each probability well above chance. Group 2 (M, K) and Speakers H and J of group 3 showed this same pattern. Once they began talking they did not give up the floor, relative to their overall conference participation (i.e., unconditional probability) for at least 10 future speakerships. This "I talk-I talk- . . . I talk" pattern might be called *floor hog*. In group 3, Speaker D also had a high magnitude. However, he was much more lax than other magnitude speakers, ceding the floor on odd lags. Group 4 speakers (F, B, L, A, I) had intermediate magnitudes, and like Speaker D allowed others to talk between their even-lag speakerships. This "I talk-You talk" pattern might be called *floor sharer*. Group 5 speakers (G, E, O, P, C) had the lowest magnitudes, being above chance at early lags but quickly dropping near or into the confidence band. They appear to get their two cents worth in, then stop. This "I talk-You talk-I quit" pattern might be called *floor yielder*.

Cyclicity. There were three cyclicity groupings. Speaker D, who formed group 1, was an almost perfect floor sharer. (In fact, he was chosen to illustrate lag computations as a reward for this behavioral style.) Group 2 contained nine speakers who had generally higher probabilities on even than odd lags. However, unlike Speaker D, their changes from lag to lag became smaller, a phenomenon called *damping*. Group 3 contained six speakers exhibiting little, or no, cyclicity. Their functions simply decreased monotonically with increased lag. Comparing Speaker K with the others in this group clearly shows that lack of cyclicity can have little relationship to degree of predictability.

These results have several implications for analysis of social interactions. First, autolags are of interest in their own right. Their magnitude and cyclicity may have interpretations useful for categorizing individuals (or different behaviors of a single person) as to social roles, styles, or other psychological attributes. Second, autocontingency imposes strong restrictions on the opportunity for other events to occur.

Over all autolags, Speaker N (Figure 2) followed himself with an average probability of 29.8%. But, his data accounted for only 2.3% of the 1506 speakerships. Given that N spoke, the chance for others to follow is much lower than that expected from unconditional probabilities. Because N followed himself 29.8% on lags 2-10, other people could only speak on 70.2% of these lags. However, the unconditional probabilities for these 15 other people sum to 97.7%. Speaker N autocontingency has therefore restricted the chance of others following him by 97.7-70.2 = 27.5%!

Autolag cyclicity also restricts chance. At excited levels of a cyclic function other events will occur by chance below their unconditional probabilities. At inhibited levels of a cycle, other events will occur by chance above their unconditional probabilities because the autocontingent event does not fulfill its own unconditional probability. For example (Figure 2), other people will have difficulty gaining the floor on even lags after Speaker D. His average probability of 37% on even lags is 30.2% over his unconditional probability of 6.8%. However, on odd lags the D average probability is 9.8%, allowing others a much better chance to talk. If D had dropped below 6.8% on odd lags, others would have a better chance to talk than expected from their unconditional probabilities.

In sum, high autolag magnitude and cyclicity make simple unconditional probabilities inadequate expected values for relationships between an autocontingent event and other events. In fact, an apparently significant crosslag dependency may actually be a spurious relationship caused by autocontingency of the criterion. Excited autolag probabilities will yield too few significant crosslags and inhibited autolag probabilities too many significant crosslags when unconditional probabilities are used as expected values. An answer to this problem involves generating models

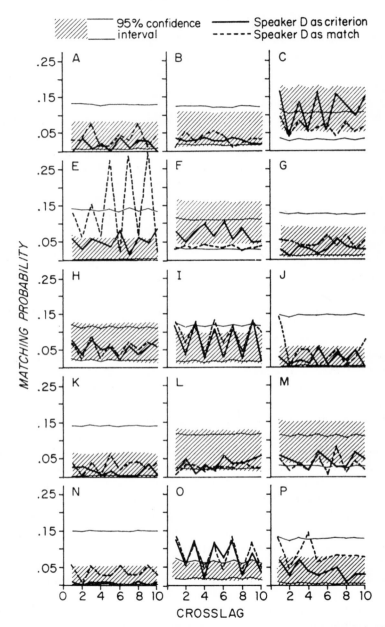

FIGURE 3. Crosslag functions for Speaker D as criterion (leader) and match (follower) with each of the 15 other conference participants.

of specific processes that may underlie observed contingencies—and doing away with the traditional unconditional probability model. Full treatment of this topic is beyond the scope of this paper. However, a method to determine whether autocontingency is, or is not, having an effect on crosslag probabilities will be detailed below.

Display of Crosslags

Figure 2 displayed only nine of the 309 lag dependencies generated for Speaker D. The remaining 300 are plotted in Figure 3. Each panel illustrates dependencies between D as both criterion (leader) and match (follower) with one other person. These crosslag functions show whether (1) D excites or inhibits each person, and (2) D is excited or inhibited by them. In experiments with behavior-subject sampling involving one person, this display could show all lag contingencies between a single response and all other measured behaviors of that person. In studying a target behavior of one subject related to behaviors by another, this display could show all contingencies between the target and the complete behavioral repertoire of the other person. These crosslag functions reveal several types of relationships.

The functions for D with Speakers I and O are extremely symmetrical. When D speaks, I and O are excited on even lags and inhibited on odd lags. When I or O speak, D is excited on even and inhibited on odd lags. This synchrony suggests that D engages in conversations with I and O of the "I talk-You talk" variety. D is also in synchrony with B,G,K,L, and N—but in a very different way. When D speaks, these people are generally inhibited over all 10 crosslags. When they speak, D is inhibited over all lags. The remaining eight people are not as symmetrically related to D; that is, they do not have as similar effects on each other.

These relationships can also be seen in Figure 4, which plots the Z values corresponding to the Figure 3 probabilities. Values above zero are relatively excited, with those at or beyond 1.96 significant (2-tailed .05 level). Values below zero are relatively inhibited, with those at or below −1.96 significant. Figure 4 displays the same functions as Figure 3, but uses *only two* curves to picture both contingency direction and statistical significance. The Z display also makes asynchronous relationships easy to visualize.

For example, when D speaks, J is immediately excited but is then inhibited on most remaining lags. When J talks, D is not excited for four lags, then has an excited-inhibited cycle for the remaining lags. The asyn-

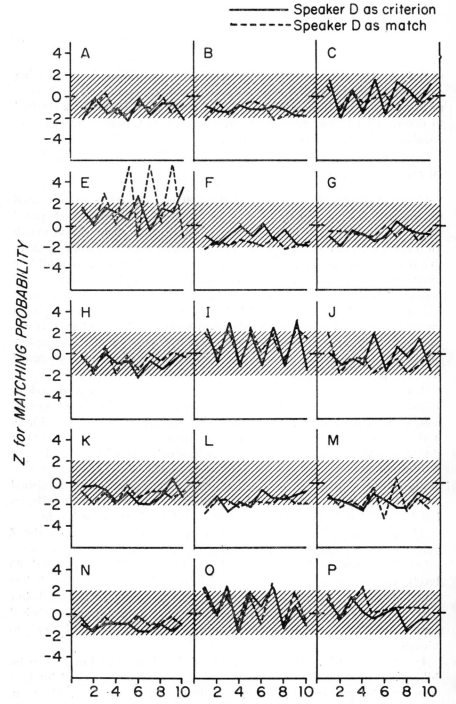

FIGURE 4. Z scores for the crosslag probabilities in figure 3. The display reduces, from 90 to 30, the number of curves needed to view all dependency relationships between Speaker D and every other person.

chrony between D and E is especially interesting. When E talks, D is relatively quiet for two lags. Then D goes into a very strong cycle of excitation and relative inhibition. When D talks, E also follows with relatively excited probabilities, but this excited relationship is much weaker than when E is the criterion. Thus, although D and E mutually excite each other, D is much more highly contingent on E as criterion than the converse.

Figure 4 also shows that, as either criterion or match, D relationships are generally inhibitory. Only a few speakers are excited by D, and these are usually the same people that excite him. We also see that not many of the 300 probabilities are significant. However, 51 were reliable, although we expect only 15 to be so by chance (2-tailed .05 level). The binomial probability of this outcome is less than .0001, suggesting that these D contingencies as a whole are real.

Reducing Lag Contingencies to Fewer Numbers

Displays such as Figures 3 and 4 can be understood, given sufficient motivation and study. However, they do deal with 300 probabilities for a single target event. The crosslags for all speakers in this study involve 4800 probabilities and plotting them requires 16 displays. What we need is a measure summarizing information in these probabilities in fewer numbers. Ideally, these numbers could be used for statistical tests of correlation, within and between subject similarities and differences, and effects of specific independent variables. Such a measure was described by Cochran (1954), and used by Bobbitt and her colleagues (1969) to study mother-infant interactions in pigtail monkeys.

Cochran's technique is based on the principle that the sum of a number (N) of independent Z scores is normally distributed, with a mean of zero and a standard deviation of the square root of N. We will refer to the statistic $\Sigma^n_1 Z / \sqrt{n}$ as a Zsum. These Zsums can (1) test for homogeneity within a conditional probability set; (2) measure general trends over lags, behaviors, or individuals; and (3) index dependency in a group of individuals or a total experiment. Let us examine some properties of Zsums using the Speaker D relationships in row 1, bottom section, Figures 3 and 4. These values are summed over all 10 lags with D as criterion (Table 3) and match (Table 4) against each of the 15 other people.

With D as criterion against Speaker A (Table 3, column 1) all Z scores were negative, although only three (lags 1, 5, 10) achieved signifi-

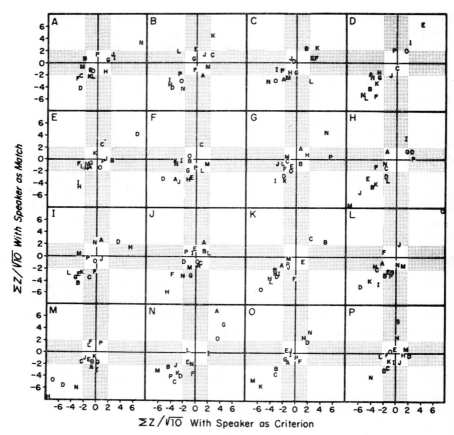

FIGURE 5. Scattergrams showing Zsum measures for each of the 16 speakers (A-P) as criterion and match with each of the 15 other people. Points in the central square are not statistically reliable. Points in the outer rectangles are reliable on only one axis. Points in the outer squares are relationships in which the target speaker has a statistically significant relationship with the other person as both discussion leader (criterion) and follower (match). Mutually excitatory dependencies are found in *Quadrant I* (upper right), the target speaker inhibits the other person while the other person excites the target in *Quadrant II* (upper left), mutually inhibitory relationships are found in *Quadrant III* (lower left), and the target speaker excites the other person while the other person inhibits the target in *Quadrant IV*.

cance. The value for $\Sigma Z/\sqrt{10}$ was -4.11. Given the null hypothesis that these Z values are independent and randomly distributed about a mean of zero, reference to the normal distribution indicates significance of this Zsum beyond the .001 level. Thus, this set of 10 lag probabilities shows a reliable trend with Speaker A inhibited following D. When D is the match against Speaker A (Table 4, column 1) eight of the 10 Z values are inhibited and none reach significance. However, the Zsum value of −2.94 indicates homogeneity among these negative values reliable beyond the .01 level.

The 30 Zsums in Tables 3 and 4 have reduced 300 crosslag probabilities to a set of 30 numbers measuring the relationship between Speaker D as a discussion leader and follower with 15 other people. What can we learn from these Zsums?

When D was the *criterion*, 11 crosslag Zsums were negative, nine significantly so beyond the .01 level. Among the four positive Zsums, two were reliable beyond the .01 level. When D was the *match*, nine of 11 negative Zsums were significant and all four positive Zsums were reliable at or beyond the .05 level. These relationships are plotted in the upper right corner of Figure 5. This graph reduces the information in Figure 4 from 300 data points to 15!

Figure 5 is a scattergram, showing the overall relationships as criterion and match between each speaker and everyone else. Points in the central squares of each graph fail to achieve statistical significance. These are interpreted as a random relationship between that speaker and the other person. Points in the arms radiating from the central squares are significant on one dimension—either criterion or match—but not on the other axis. A point in the outer squares is reliable for both criterion and matching relationship of that speaker with another person.

Each quadrant in Figure 5 represents a psychologically different relationship between the speaker and another person. *Quadrant I* (upper right) represents mutually excitatory dependency. Other people follow the speaker above expected probability, and the speaker follows them above expected probability. Speakers E, I, and O show this relationship with D (upper right graph), the E and I dependencies being significant on both axes. *Quadrant II* (upper left) represents an asymmetrical dependency in which the speaker inhibits the other person, but the other person excites the speaker. Only one such dependency appeared for Speaker D. Speaker P reliably excited D, but D had a very weak non-reliable inhibitory effect on P. *Quadrant III* (lower left) represents mutually inhibitory dependency. Following the speaker the other person is inhibited, and following the other person the speaker is inhibited. Ten people had this relationship with speaker D, seven showing jointly reliable inhibition. *Quadrant IV* (lower right) represents an asymmetrical dependency in which the speaker excites the other person, but the other person inhibits the speaker. Speaker C had the single nonreliable relationship with D in this quadrant.

Figure 5 has reduced 4800 crosslag probabilities to a set of 240. We can visualize (1) the overall relationship of any among 16 people with each of 15 others, (2) the general relationship of any given person with all of the others, and (3) the overall trend in the experiment as a whole. We see that Speaker D had mutually excitatory relationships with E and I, but E and I had mutually inhibitory relationships with each other. Speaker N had mutually excitatory relationships with A, G, and O; the latter did not have any statistically reliable relationships with each other; but O had a very strong excitatory relationship with L. The trend for the total experiment was mutually negative, 141 of 240 points lying in Quadrant III.

It is not too surprising that a conference involving formal presentations would produce most inhibitory contingencies. Furthermore, the cyclic autocontingency patterns of most speakers limit the extent to which others can follow a particular speaker. However, if this method was applied to settings such as group therapy or the homes of apparently normal children, a Quadrant II outcome could be of theoretical and practical value. Even these data could be more interesting if names had been attached to the speakers, or if variables such as sex, professional stature, or an interesting personality measure were studied. Unfortunately, names cannot be made available; only one female was present; all participants were eminent; and I possess no personality measures for these people. However, to further illustrate Zsum uses we can look at one interesting attribute of these scientists.

The 16 participants can be categorized by their total speakerships (Table 3, row 1). Speakers C, F, M, H, and L had the most speakerships, and will be called the *Talkers*. Speakers N, J, E, K, and A had the fewest, and to be polite will be called the *Thinkers* (the shy, the bored, the asleep?). My favorite, Speaker D, was intermediate in overall speaking, and I wondered if his relationships were different with Talkers than Thinkers.

Table 5 presents the Zsums relating Speaker D to each group as both criterion and match. The mean Zsums with Talkers were negative, indicating mutual inhibition. D as a leader of Thinkers was also inhibitory. But, as a follower of Thinkers, D was much less inhibited. These data resemble the design for a repeated measure analysis of variance, with Talkers versus Thinkers as an uncorrelated dimension and criterion versus matching role as a correlated variable. This analysis was performed, but neither the main effects nor interaction were significant (all $p > .20$). So, I had no evidence that Speaker D differentially affected, or was differentially affected by, the overall speaking frequency of other people.

Refusing to give up, the Talker-Thinker parameter was summarized in another way. I calculated the average Zsum, as criterion and as match, for each person paired with the four others in the same group and with the five others in the opposite group. For example, Speaker C as *criterion* had Zsums of 3.0, −1.0, −1.1, and 2.2 with F, M, H, and L—the other four Talkers. The mean of these, +0.78, indexes the overall C dependency with Talkers. With Thinkers N, J, E, K, and A, Speaker C had Zsums of −4.6, −1.0, 2.4, 3.2, and −2.2 as criterion. This yields a mean of −0.44 for the overall C dependency with Talkers.

Table 6. Relationships between Talkers (people with the most speakerships) and Thinkers (people with the least speakerships) illustrating one use of Zsums for inferential statistical tests. Scores are the average Zsums for each speaker as criterion and as match with the 4 people in the same and 5 in the opposite group. Data are arranged for analysis of variance with Talkers vs. Thinkers as independent groups, type of pairing relationship and criterion vs. match role as repeated measures. Total speakerships are in parentheses.

Group	Speaker	Paired with Talkers			Paired with Thinkers		
		As Criterion	As Match	Mean	As Criterion	As Match	Mean
TALKERS	C (170)	.78	-0.98	-0.10	-0.44	0.88	0.22
	F (151)	.75	-0.70	0.03	-2.72	-2.48	-2.60
	M (139)	-2.80	-1.55	-2.18	-1.48	-2.56	-2.02
	H (113)	-3.20	-3.45	-3.33	-3.42	-2.28	-2.85
	L (113)	-1.58	-0.80	-1.19	-1.22	-1.52	-1.37
	Mean (137)	-1.21	-1.50	<u>-1.35</u>	-1.86	-1.59	<u>-1.72</u>
THINKERS	N (35)	-1.36	-2.60	-1.98	-0.63	0.17	-0.23
	J (40)	-1.54	-2.20	-1.87	0.05	-0.23	-0.09
	E (46)	-1.98	-1.06	-1.52	-0.35	-0.33	-0.34
	K (48)	-1.70	-1.82	-1.76	-1.10	-1.45	-1.28
	A (63)	-1.74	-1.82	-1.78	1.63	0.33	0.98
	Mean (46)	-1.66	-1.90	<u>-1.78</u>	-0.08	-0.30	<u>-0.19</u>

Table 6 presents these indices for each Talker and Thinker. A repeated measure analysis of variance, with speaking frequency group as uncorrelated variable and type of pairing and role as repeated measures, was performed. The Group X Pairing interaction was the only reliable effect ($p = .02$). Means for this effect are shown in italics. Talkers had inhibitory dependencies with both Talkers (-1.35) and Thinkers (-1.72). They were somewhat, but not reliably ($p > .25$), less inhibited with other Talkers. Thinkers were also inhibitory with Talkers (-1.78). However, they were much less inhibitory with other Thinkers ($p < .05$). The mean of $-.19$ for Thinkers paired with Thinkers was close to zero. This suggests that these people had random dependencies with each other—being neither excited nor inhibited on the average.

More on Zsums: Assessing Autocontingency Effects
and Group Differences

Tables 3 and 4 will be visited for a final time, looking at the last two rows. These Zsums measure dependency on the five odd and five even crosslags of Speaker D with the other people. We already know that D has very strong cyclic autocontingency. This gives others a poor chance of matching D on even lags, and an excellent chance of matching on odd lags. Most of the other people also exhibited cyclic autocontingency. Therefore, D has the same disadvantages and advantages when matched against them. The difference between odd and even Zsums can index the degree to which autocontingency has biased the crosslag dependencies.

Over all 10 lags (column 1, overall Zsum, Tables 3 and 4) Speakers D and A have reliable mutually inhibitory dependencies. This occurs on both odd and even lags, although D matched against A as criterion is not quite significant on even lags. Mutual inhibition also occurs between D and Speakers B, F, K, L, M, and N. These mutually negative dependencies also appear when autocontingencies are either excited (even lag) or inhibited (odd lags). This suggests that these relationships are essentially independent of autolag patterns.

The overall Speaker D Zsums revealed excitatory relationships with E and I. When D was the criterion, the mutually excitatory relationship with E held on both odd and even lags. Thus, this relationship did not depend on the *D* autolag function. However, when E was the criterion, D was excited only on the odd lags. This relationship was affected by the *E* autolag function. When D was both criterion and match with I, odd

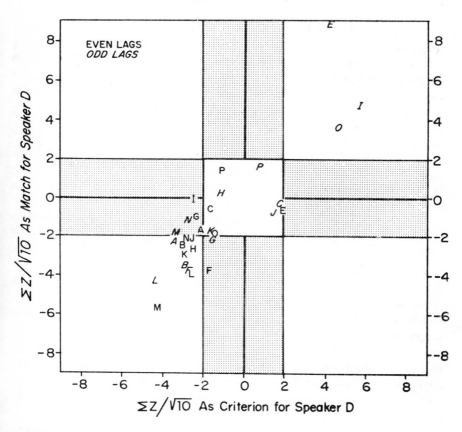

FIGURE 6. Zsums for Speaker D on odd lags (D autocontingency near chance) and even lags (D autocontingency strongly excited) as criterion and match with each of the 15 other people. Markedly discrepant points for a particular person indicate that Speaker D autocontingency has an effect on crosslag probabilities between D and the other person.

lag Zsums were positive and even lag values were negative. Thus, the D and I crosslag functions were both influenced by autocontingency. All odd and even lag Zsums for Speaker D as criterion and match with each of the 15 other people are shown in Figure 6. When the two points plotted for an individual are not discrepant, the relationship shown is largely unaffected by autocontingency (e.g., F, L, A, N, G). Pairs of points that are far apart identify relationships that are affected by autocontingency (e.g., E, I, O, J).

The basic issue of autocontingency has not been addressed by students of social interaction. Unfortunately, autocontingency does affect the degree to which crosslag dependencies can occur. In some instances, apparent crosscontingencies may be a total artifact of strong autolag functions. The Zsum technique presented here can be used to study this problem in any observational data measuring behavior sequentially.

Suppose that a target behavior such as "Infant-Looks-At-Mother" is studied as criterion in relation to 10 maternal behaviors over a maximum lag of 10 sequential steps. Suppose further that this target behavior is autocontingent—excited on lags 2, 3, 5, and 9, and inhibited on lags 4, 6, and 10. Whether this autolag function influences crosslag probabilities is assessed by calculating Zsums for looking as criterion and match against each maternal behavior on the four excited and three inhibited lag sets. Relationships having markedly different excited-inhibited Zsums are at least partially confounded by autocontingency, and might be totally spurious. Those showing little or no variation are not affected by autocontingency. If differences only occur when the target is criterion, then target autocontingency is having an influence. If differences only occur when the target is a matching behavior, then autocontingency of the maternal behavior is having an effect. Excited-inhibited Zsum discrepancies when the target is *both* criterion and match suggest that target and maternal behavior autolag functions are influencing crosslag probabilities.

Group Differences. In addition to using Zsums for studying autocontingency, these statistics can be used to assess group differences. Returning to speakership data, suppose that individual Z scores are available for the lag 1 relationship between a male speaker and 10 others. Suppose further that five subjects are males, with Z scores of −4, −2, −3, −1, and −.5, and the other five are females with scores of −.5, .5, 1, 1, and 3. Overall, $\Sigma Z / \sqrt{10}$ is −1.74, a nonsignificant result indicating heterogeneity between the 10 dependencies. However, the male Zsum of −4.70 reveals strong inhibition following the male speaker, while that of +2.24 for females indicates an excitatory relationship following the speaker. As in analysis of variance, we have partitioned an overall dependency into component parts assessing the differential effects of two groups of subjects. In the same fashion, we could partition a variable with more than two groups of subjects into separated Zsums for each group.

Final Data Reduction: Angles of Sequential Significance

We have progressed a long way in shrinking 4800 lag probabilities to smaller set of numbers. Probably, this is as far as we should, or need, o. Other techniques such as information theory (Gottman & Bakeman, 978) are viable, and perhaps even preferable, alternatives to the data ompression methods presented here. Nevertheless, having expended much time and energy on one additional scheme, I feel compelled to present it along with some assumptions about measuring social interactions.

Social interaction concerns joint relationships between two or more individuals. It is an easier concept to talk about than to measure. In an interaction, the behavior of Person A influences that of Person B, and B's behavior then influences A in a feedback or reciprocity relationship. This is quite different from a relationship in which Person A influences Person B, but B's behavior does not affect A (i.e., a unidirectional relationship). In this view there is a minimum condition which data must meet to provide evidence of actual interaction. Two or more people must have statistically reliable mutual dependencies. In lag analysis language, if the interacting people are not mutually excitatory, mutually inhibitory, or one excitatory and the other inhibitory, they are not involved in an interactive relationship.

Given this model, relationships like those in Figure 5 identify the occurrence and direction of an interaction. For example, Speaker D did not interact with C because both criterion and matching Zsums were not statistically significant. Speaker D did have a reliable relationship with H when he was the criterion, but it was not an interactive relationship because there was no reliable dependency when D was the match. By this rule, speakers J, O, and P also did not interact with D, but the remaining 10 people did have interaction with Speaker D.

A dramatically different example is seen in the graph for Speaker P. Only one of 15 relationships revealed interaction, and that was mutually inhibitory with Speaker H. Eight points were nonsignificant on both axes, and most of the remaining points were near zero on one axis. Thus, Speaker P was an almost completely noninteractive conference participant.

Because there were only 16 different events (speakers) in the conference data, the dependency relationships were fairly easy to identify from the lag analyses. However, if 100 or more events had been possible, even

TABLE 7. Calculation of vectors and angles from Speaker D Zsums. These values measure dependency relationships in polar coordinates of D with each of the other speakers and for the total conference (bottom section).

Speaker	Overall Zsums		Relationship Quadrant	Polar Coordinate Values		
	Criterion(x)	Match(y)	Q (origin)	Vector Radius (R)	Arcsin θ	Vector Angle (θ)
A	-4.11	-2.94	III (+180)	5.05	35.6	215.6
B	-4.17	-4.24	III (+180)	5.94	45.6	225.6
C	0.14	-.062	IV (-360)	0.64	75.6	284.4
E	4.31	6.29	I (0)	7.62	55.6	55.6
F	-3.24	-5.42	III (+180)	6.31	59.2	239.2
G	-2.68	-2.14	III (+180)	3.43	38.6	218.6
H	-2.74	-1.72	III (+180)	3.23	32.2	212.2
I	2.35	3.36	I (0)	4.10	55.0	55.0
J	-0.76	-2.06	III (+180)	2.19	70.2	250.2
K	-3.15	-3.27	III (+180)	4.54	46.1	226.1
L	-4.92	-5.79	III (+180)	7.60	49.6	229.6
M	-5.48	-5.28	III (+180)	7.61	43.9	223.9
N	-3.88	-2.37	III (+180)	4.55	31.4	211.4
O	1.41	1.98	I (0)	2.71	46.9	46.9
P	-0.33	2.11	II (-180)	2.14	80.3	99.6

Quadrant	N	Radius		Angle	
		Mean	SD	Mean	SD
I (Mutually Excitatory)	3	4.8	2.5	52.5	4.9
II (Criterion Inhibits Match Escites)	1	2.1	---	99.6	---
III (Mutually Inhibitory)	10	5.9	1.8	225.2	12.2
IV (Criterion Escites Match Inhibits)	1	0.6	---	284.4	---

Radius = $\sqrt{x^2 + y^2}$ Angle = Quadrant Origin $\pm$ Arcsin Y/R the data reduction of Figure 5 would be too complicated to handle by inspection. We now turn to a technique that can reduce these data still more, while retaining their essential information.

Vectors and Angles

Pairs of Zsums like those in Figure 5 can be represented in polar (circular) coordinates as a vector and an angle. In the Speaker D graph of Figure 5, consider Quadrant I as containing the angles of a circle from 0-90 degrees, Quadrant II 91-180 degrees, Quadrant III 181-270 degrees, and Quadrant IV 271-360 degrees. Each data point lies at one of these angles, and each point is at some distance from the middle 0,0 Zsum coordinate. This distance is the length of a vector projecting at that angle, and measures relative dependency strength in Zsum units. Considering the criterion Zsum as an X value and the match Zsum as a Y value, the vector length (radius) of each point is $\sqrt{X^2 + Y^2}$. Each angle is related to the arcsin of Y/radius.

The Speaker D data of Figure 5 are transformed to polar coordinates in Table 7. Each criterion (X) and match (Y) Zsum is squared and added together. The square root of each addition yields the vector radius (R). The arcsin of Y/R is then computed. If the data point is in QI (mutually excitatory), the arcsin value itself is the vector angle (θ). If the point is in QII, the angle is 180 degrees minus the arcsin value. For points in QIII the angle is 180 degrees plus the arcsin. In QIV, the angle is 360 degrees minus the arcsin.

The radii in Table 7 reduce 300 crosslag probabilities to 15 numbers measuring relative dependency strength between Speaker D and the 15 other people. The mean of these values, 4.51 ($SD = 2.18$) provides a single number indexing Speaker D's influence on the conference as a whole. The angles in Table 7 measure dependency directions between Speaker D and the other people. Each angle places D and one other person in a relationship quadrant. If the angle lies on a quadrant diagonal (45, 135, 225, and 315 degrees), the relationship is exactly equal in strength between D and the other person. Off-diagonal angles indicate that Speaker D has a different strength of dependency than the other person.

The bottom of Table 7 gives the *N*, mean, and standard deviation for radii and angles in each relationship quadrant. The four mean radii and angles, with their corresponding sample sizes and variabilities, index the average dependency relationships between D speakerships and those of

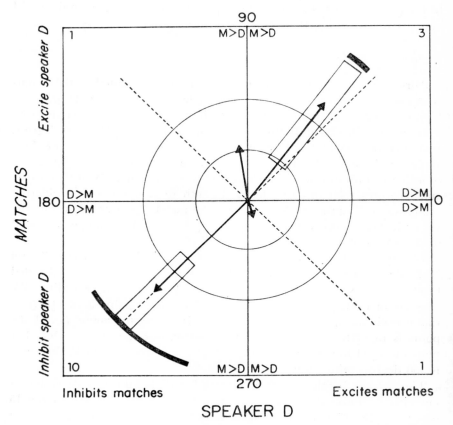

FIGURE 7. Polar graph of Speaker D average Zsum vectors and angles with all other people. In the right half D as criterion *is followed by* other people at probabilities above expected values (excitatory dependency), while in the left half D *is followed by* others less than expected (inhibitory dependency). In the upper half Speaker D *follows* other people more than expected, while in the lower half D follows others less than expected. The number of people involved in each relationship type are shown in the quadrant corners. Arcs near the corner measure the range of vector angles over the N individuals in each quadrant (no arc with $N = 1$). Vector lengths measure average strength of relationship in Zsum units (inner circle $= 2$, outer circle $= 4$). Rectangles give the standard deviation of vector length. In areas 45 degrees above and below the 0-180 plane, the Speaker D contribution to the relationship is stronger than that of other people. In areas 45 degrees to the right and left of the 90-270 plane the Speaker D contribution is weaker than that of other people.

all participants. Figure 7 graphs these indices in polar coordinates that I have called "Angles of Sequential Significance."

The X and Y axes of Figure 7 are angles from 0-360 degrees. From angles 271-90, Speaker D excites other people. From 91-270 degrees, D inhibits others. From 0-180 degrees, Speaker D is excited by other people. From 181-360 degrees, D is inhibited by other people. Mean vector lengths radiate, in Zsum units, from the center of the graph. The inner circle measures two Zsum units; the outer measures four Zsum units. The rectangles around each vector point are standard deviations of vector length. The arcs near the corners indicate the range of angles in the quadrant. Alternatively, the standard deviation of angles in the quadrant could be shown by these arcs. Sample size appears in each quadrant corner.

The relative dependency strength for the target speaker as criterion versus match is indicated by off-diagonal angles. Areas in which Speaker D dependency is stronger as criterion than match are indicated by D > M along the 0-180 degree plane. Areas indicating stronger dependency as match than criterion are shown by M > D along the 90-270 degree plane.

We can describe the information in Figure 7 as follows: (1) Ten of the 15 relationships were mutually negative (QIII) and of equal strength when Speaker D was criterion or match. (2) Three mutually positive dependencies (QI) had about the same average strength as the mutually negative ones, but were somewhat more variable. All three angles were above the QI diagonal, indicating that the other people excited D somewhat more than D excited them. (3) There were only two nonmutual relationships (QII, QIV). In the QII relationship, the match excited Speaker D more than D inhibited him. The QIV vector is too short to even discuss.

Go on to Figure 8 if you have not been completely stunned or overwhelmed by the Angles of Sequential Significance. Otherwise, go back to Figures 5, 4, or 3; or to complex probability diagrams showing only lag 1 relationships with circles and arrows going in all directions; or perhaps you have been convinced not to study sequential dependencies.

Figure 8 summarizes the complete set of Zsum relationships from Figure 5 for each conference participant. Here we see the average dependencies indexing the impact of each person on the conference as a whole. There are large individual differences in angle variability and vector lengths. Speaker P has mainly weak relationships covering the full 360 degrees. This suggests that P has essentially random relationships with little or no interaction. Speakers D, K, and N have strong mutual relationships

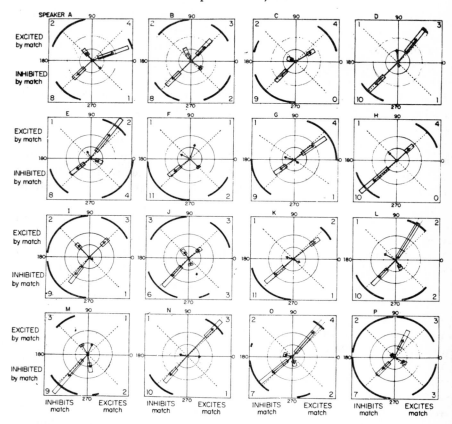

FIGURE 8. Polar graph showing the relationships between each of the 16 speakers (A-P) averaged over all 15 of the other conference participants. The symbols, vectors, and angles have the same meanings as in figure 7.

showing little variability and many interactions. Using a vector length less than two Zsum units (inner circle) to indicate lack of interaction, Speaker M is the only person failing to achieve any mutually excitatory interactions. However, Speaker M does have some dependency strength with fairly low variability in Quadrants II and IV revealing the presence of nonmutual interactions.

By now these lag probabilities have been "milked" for much more than they seem worth. However, one final data reduction step is shown in Figure 9, which compresses the essential information from 4800 probabilities into eight numbers. The graph plots the averages of sample size,

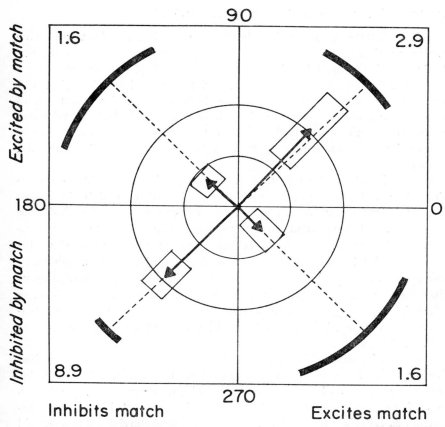

FIGURE 9. Polar graph of the dependency relationships averaged over all speakers for the conference as a whole. The display reduces 4800 original lag probabilities to 4 mean vectors and their associated sample sizes and variability. The symbols, angles, and vector lengths have the same interpretations as in figure 7. Arcs show standard deviations of the 16 mean angles entering into calculation of each vector; rectangles show standard deviations of the 16 mean vector lengths yielding each vector.

mean vector length and *SD*, and mean vector angle and *SD* from Figure 8. This display summarizes the speakership dependencies for the total conference. It shows that (1) most relationships are mutually inhibitory and of equal strength as criterion and match; (2) some relationships are mutually excitatory, of about equal strength to the mutually inhibitory dependencies, and slightly stronger for the match than the criterion dependency; and (3) the few nonmutual dependencies are quite weak.

A Research Paradigm and Statistical Analysis Plan

The Angles of Sequential Significance provide numbers measuring the interaction patterns of individual dyads, triads, or larger groups. The basic data for an individual set of subjects consist of four repeated measures—the four quadrants of mutual and nonmutual relationships. The five potential dependent measures are the number or the percentage of relationships, mean vector length and its standard deviation, and mean vector angle and its standard deviation in each quadrant. The use of this design for developmental experiments is illustrated by the following example problem.

Sameroff (1975) suggests that social interaction over time—transaction—is a major determinant of abnormal behavior in high risk infant humans. Transactions form a system in which infant behaviors influence caregivers, and consequent caregiver behaviors in turn influence the developing infant. Transactional failures over time produce deviant behavior by the infant, the caregiver, or both. Unfortunately, Sameroff's theory does not specify which transactions are important, how transactions can be measured, criteria for identifying abnormal transactions, or when in development transaction failures will result in relatively permanent anomalies. The research model presented next can be used to address these issues.

Groups of presumably high and low risk infants would be studied during social interactions in their home environments. Interaction between the infant and its caregivers would be measured for target behaviors of interest. Lag probabilities would be calculated for infant behaviors as criteria and matches against caregiver behaviors. These would be transformed to polar coordinates, and evidence for interaction would appear directly from vector lengths, with relationship quality indicated by vector angles. Repeated measures would be taken, perhaps in one-month intervals over the first two years of life. Polar graphs for a specific criterion behavior, pooled behaviors of the same general class, or all behaviors combined would show (1) whether any transactions actually occurred and (2) how they changed over two years.

Normative development, risk group differences, and risk group X time block interaction could be assessed by repeated measure analyses of variance. Risk Group would be an uncorrelated variable, and Month of Age and Relationship Quadrant would be repeated measures. The dependent variables would be vector lengths and angles calculated from the Zsums of infant behaviors as criterion and match against caregiver behaviors.

Potential confounding effects of group differences in number of relationships in each quadrant and in vector variability could be controlled using multiple regression with standard deviations and number of relationships per quadrant as covariates and vector lengths and angles as dependent variables.

The contribution of noninteractive behavior to group differences in transactions could be assessed by studying the magnitude and cyclicity of autocontingency. Zsums would be calculated separately for each dependency relationship under study on lags showing excited and inhibited

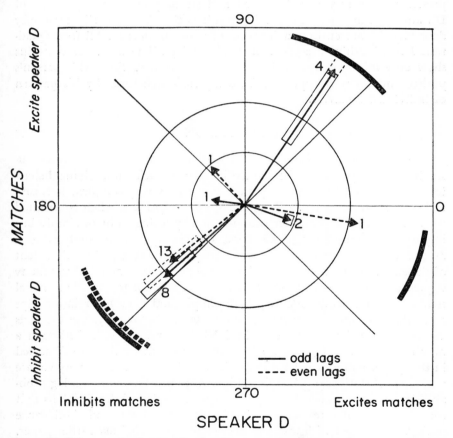

FIGURE 10. Polar graphs showing Speaker D average dependency relationships with all other speakers on odd (near chance autocontingency) and even (strongly excited autocontingency) lags. Note that mutually excitatory relationships are completely absent on even lags.

autocontingency for each infant. Polar coordinates would be generated for each Zsum set when the infant was the criterion and when it was the match. Excited versus Inhibited lags would be a third repeated measure in the basic analysis with Time Block and Quadrant. Statistical interaction of this autolag variable with effects containing the risk group factor will measure the degree to which autocontingency has influenced the observed transactional patterns.

Figure 10 shows an example of this approach using the speakership data. The graph plots Speaker D relationships on odd and even lags representing the relatively inhibited and strongly excitatory portions of D's autolag function. The striking result is that D's mutually excitatory dependencies are entirely a function of autocontingency. All four Quadrant I relationships disappear on the even lags. The other relationships show only minor variation due to autocontingency. Thus, this person's positive interactions appear to be completely structured by his pattern of individual behavior.

CONCLUSION

The generation and analysis of social interaction data are time-consuming and expensive. The sequential dependencies underlying behavioral transactions between people are potentially very complex. It is easy to become buried in trivia (e.g., the Speakership Data) when confronted with mountains of computer output, thereby losing sight of simple but important determinants of behavior. Conversely, simple analyses such as one-step contingency relationships may fail to reveal the full extent of dependencies that occur over long time periods or extend across many sequential events. This paper represents one attempt to provide a model that can, in principle, identify both simple and complex relationships and allow for study of their determinants. Unfortunately, the methods are largely untried in any meaningful behavioral research. Although a number of assumptions underlying use of these methods were discussed in this paper and an earlier one (Sackett, 1978), the methods may violate a number of statistical principles unknown to me. Furthermore, lag probabilities and Zsum statistics may have known statistical distributions that could greatly enhance their utility for data reduction and significance testing. I will close with the same statement that ended my earlier paper. Those of us interested in sequential analysis should recruit a friend in the local Statistics Department to help us pursue statistical problems in sequential dependency analysis at the theoretical level.

Part VI

OVERVIEW AND INTEGRATION OF CURRENT PERSPECTIVES ON PSYCHOSOCIAL RISK AND INFANT DEVELOPMENT

In this final chapter, Arnold J. Sameroff has used his thinking about transactional models of development and about models of parent approaches to infants as a framework for the review and integration of current issues in psychosocial risk in infants. Many of these issues have been dealt with in the other chapters of this volume. This overview by Sameroff provides a nice kind of closure for the variety of issues presented throughout this volume and from other recent research and theory. Sameroff's creative thinking about problems in infant development accomplishes this task masterfully.

341

15

Issues in Early Reproductive and Caretaking Risk: Review and Current Status

ARNOLD J. SAMEROFF

University of Illinois at Chicago Circle

and Illinois Institute for Developmental Disabilities

Over the past decade there has been a quiet revolution in developmental research. Academic stereotypes of ivory tower research have increasingly been displaced by investigations of real people in real life situations. But, surprisingly, this shift from laboratory to field has not produced the usual lack of objectivity associated with applied research, but rather an increase in objectivity. How is it possible to move from the "controlled" conditions of the laboratory to the "uncontrolled" hodgepodge which is the real world and be able to do better scientific research? The answer to that question can be found in the contents of this volume. In this review I will try to pull the threads together of what has been presented and make the following points:

(1) The developmental process is by definition dynamic and represents an interplay between an individual's characteristics and his or her experiences, both of which change over time.

(2) An individual's experience is mediated by a social surround which also engages in the dynamic developmental interplay such that both individual and surroundings are affected by their experiences with each other.

(3) Isolation and assessment of characteristics of either the individual or the environment have shown little value in explaining the developmental processes.

343

(4) The definition and assessment of developmental risk can only occur within a matrix which includes the characteristics of the child, the experiences of the child, and the social environment in which that child is reared.

I would like to begin and end the discussion with the fourth point, initially to document that developmental risk cannot be predicted where all these factors are not included, and finally to review how research can be done which does include all these influences.

A number of years ago I was asked to write a review of the role of perinatal factors in developmental deviancy. I was eager in the task because I was engaged in a research project which attempted to find the roots of serious mental disturbances, especially schizophrenia, in the perinatal period. I began both the research and the review expecting to find clear indications from early assessments which would show straightforward linkages with later disorders. I was quite surprised to find that these indicators were not evident in past research (Sameroff & Chandler, 1975) nor in my research (Sameroff & Zax, 1978; Zax, Sameroff, & Babigian, 1977).

Whenever a perinatal risk factor was hypothesized to be related to later dysfunction, prospective studies found no greater incidence of disorder in the risk population than in control populations without the risk factor. Whether the risk was related to preterm birth, low birth weight, anoxia, or neurological signs, few causal chains were found when appropriate control populations were studied. The most important variable that needed to be controlled was socioeconomic status. Where later deficits were associated with perinatal factors, it was generally in combination with an economically deprived environment. Where birth status showed little relation to later outcome, it was generally in combination with a better economic situation. The reason these birth factors were thought to be important in the past was that high percentages of infants with reproductive complications had poor intellectual outcomes (Pasamanick & Knobloch, 1966). However, the confounding factor was that most children who had these complications were from the poorer segments of society (Birch & Gussow, 1970). The review of these findings led us to propose a continuum of caretaking casuality (Sameroff & Chandler, 1975). At one end of the continuum the caretaking environment was sufficiently supportive and adaptive to compensate for almost any biological complication so that it was not transformed into later intellectual or emotional problems. At the other end of the continuum the caretaking environment had neither the educational, emotional nor economic resources to deal with even the slightest perinatal problem. Thus, the child, if allowed to survive, would maintain deficits into later stages of intellectual and emotional growth.

Models of Development

At the conclusion of our review, Chandler and I proposed three models which had been used to explain the relation between risk factors and poor developmental outcomes—a single factor model, an additive interactional model, and a transactional model. In the single factor model, it was proposed that there were clear sequences of linear causality between risk status and outcome. In the interactional model it was proposed that constitutional risk factors interacted additively with environmental support such that the effects of the risk could be augmented or reduced by better or worse environments. The transactional model was proposed to compensate for the static quality of the other two models. In the transactional model, development was hypothesized to result from a continual interplay between a changing child and a changing environment as the child entered into higher levels of cognitive and social functioning. Within this model, the only reason a deviance is perpetuated into more mature levels of functioning is because the environment perpetuated that deviancy. The environment is the mediator that perpetuates any developmental outcome, be it for better or worse.

In other writings (Sameroff, 1975a) I have continued to emphasize the necessity for using complex models for studying and explaining development. However, it must be noted that although complex models of development, such as a transactional model, are necessary for encompassing all developmental possibilities, the restrictions of a particular universe can produce effects which would justify the use of single factor or interactional models. For example, if we hypothesize a universe in which language and communication only occur in the visual modality, a blind child will not learn language in any environment within that universe. In that universe, blindness will be a single risk factor which will predict later intellectual deficits. Within our own universe, where there are other communication channels than visual, blindness is not linearly related to later cognitive deficit. If we hypothesize a universe where the only communication is vocal, deafness will be seen to have an additive interactive effect with environment. Deaf children raised in supportive environments where lip-reading is taught will do better intellectually than deaf children without such training, but in all such communicative settings, the deaf children will do more poorly than hearing children in the same environments. In our universe, language can be gestural as well as vocal. Deaf children, reared in environments where signing is encouraged and accepted, need show no intellectual deficits in comparison with hearing children reared in the same environments. In short, a transactional model is needed to explain development in environments that are sensitive to and can compensate for early deviancies so that they are not transformed into later deficits. However, when the range of environments is restricted, either through ignorance or choice, outcomes can be found which appear to be additive or produced by single risk factors taken alone.

Biological Precursors

These points can become more concrete if we move from the hypothetical to the empirical. The papers in this volume by Willerman and Hunt address the complications in using a genetic model to predict development. As Willerman points out, current controversies in genetics are not over whether environment has a role but, rather, over the percentage of variance contributed by the environment. Where cloning can be used, as in some botanical studies, it is possible to observe the same genotype developing in a range of environments so that a range of reaction can be calculated and estimates of heritability made. However, in the case of humans in which, except for monzygotic twins, all genotypes are unique, there is a major confound between genotype and environment. Willerman accepts the validity of a heritability approach but emphasizes the major role of environment in developmental outcome. He sees the importance of genetic studies less in the areas of intelligence where the links are so obscure, and more in understanding the biological processes which produce children with severe neurological damage. However, in the latter case one is not looking at risk factors for later deviances, but at the deviances themselves.

Hunt makes a more fundamental attack on the heritability-based arguments that genetic variation is a major contributor to intellectual outcome. He argues that heritability calculations are based on achievement scores in a set of particular known environments. These calculations are irrelevant to educability since educability is an issue of potential, not one of achievement. Previously untapped potentials may be revealed in an environment in which new childrearing practices have been devised. Hunt has devoted himself to the creation of new environments that make previous estimates of developmental potential obsolete. When a risk factor can be properly diagnosed developmentally so that we know how it relates to a later problem, new interventions can be designed to break the causal connection. Only where the deviance is not seen in its developmental matrix can linear causality still be found. Hunt makes another interesting point. In contrast to the standard position of geneticists that if rearing environments are similar, genetic variation will be maximized, Hunt reviews evidence that phenotypic variation is reduced in homogeneous environments relative to heterogeneous environments. An interesting question is how the child-caretaker interface operates in these homogeneous environments. Is the kind of environment to which Hunt refers a transactional or an interactional one? That is, is it an environment which operates dynamically to provide a final common outcome, or one in which each genotype must find its own developmental path through a passive surround?

The dynamic interplay between child and caretaking environment is best captured in Hawkins' review (this volume) of the relation between infantile obesity and later overweight. Hypotheses related to early measures, such as number of fat cells or overnutrition, only explain small portions of the variance in later overweight. However, an analysis of child-caretaker interactions produced evidence that asynchronies in the parent-child feeding schedule have the strongest relation to obese outcomes. Hawkins concludes that whatever the initial physical state of the infant, it is the child's history of being fed in hunger vs. hunger-free states that will be decisive in the production of later obesity. Thus, both the cause and the cure of overweight are seen to be transactional processes between child and environment.

The Caretaking Environment

It has been well documented that the environment plays a major role in initiating and maintaining behavior (Skinner, 1969). This documentation also extends to both normal and deviant social behavior. For example, Patterson's (1973) work with aggressive boys has demonstrated that family members provide both the initiating circumstances for aggressive behavior in each other (e.g., teasing by a sibling), and the positive reinforcement for these behaviors (e.g., laughter by a parent). This type of analysis has provided a clear rationale for intervention programs which are designed to modify deviant behavior in one member of the family by modifying the behavior of other family members, especially the parents. However, these efforts have met with only limited success. Patterson attributes such failures to a lack of knowledge of the factors which maintain the behavior of the parent.

One source of this problem is in the inaccuracy of parental reports of their children's behavior. The inaccuracy of retrospective reports (Yarrow, Campbell, & Burton, 1970) can be simply understood as poor or selective recall. However, how does one explain the inaccuracy of reports of concurrent behavior (Smith, 1958)? In one study of behavior change in children, Walker (1971) found that in a control group where observations of the target deviant behavior showed a slight *increase* during the experimental period, parents reported a major *decrease*. Patterson (1973) concludes that parental reports are under the control of variables other than just a desire to accurately describe the behavior of the child.

Some of these variables have been the focus of recent work on attribution theory in social psychology. Individuals filter their experience through a net of expectations and attributions such that similar events are reported as being different by people with different cognitive sets. From this perspective, inaccurate parental reports need not arise from an effort to deceive, but rather from a different evaluation of the observed behavior. For example, the more global the judgments asked of parents the more likely that their reports will be inaccurate.

Walker's contribution to this volume emphasizes the complexity of analysis necessary to predict behavior, in general, and parental behavior, in specific. Using Fishbein's (Fishbein & Ajzen, 1975) model, Walker sees overt parental behavior as the sum of intentions, attitudes, personal norms, social norms, and motivation. Assessments of parental attitudes alone have been notoriously unpredictive of actual parent behavior or of the behavior of their children (Becker & Krug, 1965). Parke's chapter documents the separation between competencies and performance in parental behavior. When the caretaking skills and interaction of fathers with their infants were compared to those of mothers, few differences were found. However, during triadic interactions, in which the father, mother and baby were all present, the father and mother assumed different roles and had differing exchanges with the baby. Parke concludes that where fathers are as competent to interact with their infants as mothers are, they may not do so because of social norms, roles, and expectations.

Attitudes, personal norms, and social norms generally do not exist in isolation but tend to be organized. The clearest evidence of organization can be seen in social norms. Each culture is an organized system of values and behavior expectations which influence the behavior of individuals within that culture. For example, deVries and deVries (1977), in a study of East African cultures, found that differences in estimates of infant competence were tied to the onset of education. The Digo believed that infants were competent at two months of age and began sensori-motor training such that toilet training was frequently completed in the first six months and the children were walking soon after. The Kikuyu, who are of the same Nilo-Hamitic genetic origins, believed that children were incompetent until one year of age and backpacked the swaddled infants until after their first birthday.

Within cultures, social classes differ in norms and expectations. Kohn (1969) found strong differences in childrearing value systems between high and low social classes in both the United States and Italy. Working class parents valued conformity and they rated neatness and good manners as important childrearing goals. Upper class parents valued self-direction in their children and they emphasized curiosity and self-control as developmental goals. Kohn found that these social class differences in values were reflected in corresponding differences in child-rearing behavior and life experiences.

On a more individual level Pharis and Manosevitz (this volume) postulated parental models which included a set of images, fantasies, attitudes, and ideas related to their infants, their parenting roles, and how life changes following the birth of a baby. These models include ideas about what constitute good and bad babies, good and bad parents, the expected rate of development of babies and whether life in the future can be expected to improve or get worse. Pharis and Manosevitz expect that such complex assessments of parents' attitudes and expectations will operationalize psychosocial adaptation during pregnancy so that better predictions can be made about parental behavior after the birth of the child. In a series of studies they found that mothers and fathers differed in their models. Moreover, women expecting a baby differed in their models from women of the same social class who were college students. Thus, in addition to culture, social class, and sex, one's own status in the life cycle is a determinant of parental models.

Another approach to understanding the organization of parental thinking is to analyze the level of abstraction utilized by parents to understand development (Sameroff, 1975a). Research on the cognitive development of the child has shown that the infant must go through a number of stages before achieving the logical thought processes that characterize adulthood (Piaget, 1950). Similarly, parents may use different levels in thinking about their relationship with the child. Furthermore, parents, whose understanding of the child is restricted to more primitive levels, may have great difficulty in dealing with what appear to be deviant children.

Piaget's stages of development can be used as a framework for the description of these cognitive levels of parental conceptions of development. Although, on the surface, this may appear to be a farfetched analogy, these stages represent the best current description of how one goes from the immediacy of perceptual experience to successively removed levels at which abstractions are made. Therefore, my attempt to formulate the stages in the mother's construction of the child specifies four levels analogous to Piaget's sensorimotor, preoperational, concrete operational, and formal operational stages of development. These hypothesized levels are (1) the symbiotic, (2) the categorical, (3) the compensating, and (4) the perspectivistic.

At the *symbiotic* level, the mother is concerned primarily with her immediate relationship to the child. She responds in a here-and-now fashion to the child's behavior. Her emotional response is directly related to how successful she is at ministering to the child. In a sense she does not see herself as separate from the child since she interprets the child's behavior as being directly tied to her own activity. The skin-to-skin contact in breast-feeding, the eye-to-eye contact in looking, the infant's cessation of crying and then smiling in response to the mother's caretaking, all are interpreted as consequences of the mother's efforts and serve to produce a positive affectional bond between mother and child.

There are no problems for parents who function at the symbiotic level as long as they can sense the effect of their efforts. However, when the infant does not produce the responses the parent expects, serious problems can arise. If the child vomits during breast-feeding, sleeps rather than looks, cries constantly with few smiles despite the mother's hugging and rocking, the parent who is restricted to this level of cognizing the infant will become very distressed. The animal literature is replete with reports of parents who will reject offspring who do not produce the appropriate responses to their mothers (Sameroff, 1975b). A similar fate occurs to human offspring with mothers limited to sensorimotor functioning. Luckily, however, humans have alternative modes of such social cognition.

At the second level, the *categorical* level, parents are able to see their children and themselves as separate entities, such that the children's actions can be viewed as being intrinsic characteristics of the child and not exclusively the result of the parents' activity. A consequence of objectification of the world is that objects are placed into categories. The mother who has had a successful experience with her child assigns positive labels, for example, the good child, the pretty child, the bright child. Once labels are assigned, however, they are thought to belong to the object. Just as the young child thinks that the label "cup" belongs to a particular object in the same way as its color or shape, so the categorical mother thinks that the child is "the good child" in the same way that he has blue eyes or brown hair. This device can be very adaptive, for when the good child occasionally acts badly, such as crying too much, breaking a few dishes, or throwing a tantrum, the mother will still think of her child as the good one. On the other hand, this device can be very maladaptive as in the case where the mother, because of the negative early experiences she may have had with the child, comes to label him as the difficult child, the bad child, or the ugly one. Even though this infant may outgrow the behavior which caused him to be labeled as difficult in the first place, the perceptions and reactions of the parent restricted to the categorical level will always be dominated by the original classification.

At the third level, the *compensating* level, parents are able to view their child as having an existence not only apart from the parents' activities, as at the symbiotic level, but also apart from their labels as at the categorical level. For example, the behavior of the child can now be related to his age. Infants cry, toddlers are hyperactive, while adolescents brood. The positive achievement at this higher level is that the behavior of the infant which could have given him a life-long label of "difficult" is seen as age-specific, and, moreover, that the child will probably behave quite differently at later ages. The parent is able to use a much broader context for valuing the child. Beauty can compensate for brains and vice versa. No single label can typify the entire range of the child's behavior. However, even at this advanced level, which typifies the majority of parents, there are limitations. Although the hyperactivity of the two year old is seen in the context of an age-specific behavior which need not typify the child at 10 years, if the same child at 10 is found to be hyperactive, the child will then be regarded as a deviant child. At this compensating level, the normative behavior at each age is considered a characteristic of human development which finds its source in the child. It takes an advance to the next level for the parent to appreciate the full relationship between the behavior of the child and the way he or she was reared.

Additional context is attained by the few parents who can view their child from the fourth level, the *perspectivistic* level. At this level the particular child and his particular caretaking situation can be placed in a hypothetical context of any child in any caretaking situation. The concrete situation at hand is only one of a multitude of possibilities. Parents are able to see children's behavior as stemming from individual experiences with specific environments. If those experiences had been different, the children's characteristics would be different. At this level deviances in the child are viewed as deviancies in the relation of a particular child to a particular environment, rather than as concrete expressions of the essential nature of the child. Remediation can be proposed by altering the experience of the child through environmental changes. The achievement of this level of cognizing the child is to free both elements in the child-caretaker system from their concrete context and to place them into a generalized hypothetical structure.

To summarize, the way parents interpret their child's behavior is related to the parents' level of cognizing development. At advanced levels the parent is able to place the elements of the interaction into an increasingly broader context, from the most simple level of here-and-now interaction with the child, to being able to separate the child from their labels, and eventually to being able to take perspective and separate the child from the particular life circumstance in which he or she was raised. If that circumstance had been, or would become different, a child with different characteristics would be produced.

A questionnaire was devised to test this model and given to several samples of women in England (Sameroff, 1975c) and in the United States (Sameroff & Feil, 1980). We found differences among parents in their level of understanding, with the majority functioning at the preoperational categorical level. More interesting was the content of the categorical thought. The main dichotomy in conceptions was between those parents who felt that the environment was the primary determinant of development as opposed to those who saw constitutional factors as the primary determinant. Just as in the professional nature-nurture controversies, the position of individual parents on this issue would have an important influence on how they deal with their children. For example, Patterson (1973) notes that in programs designed to modify children's behavior, the first step must be to convince parents that behavior is controlled by contingencies. If parents believe that children's behavior is inherent in their nature, then there is little point in asking the parents to change the environment.

Parental Perspectives

Assessments of young children's environments must cover a broad set of factors that are mediated by parents. These factors can be encompassed under the general rubric of parental perspectives and can be divided into four sub-categories: (1) the developmental model, (2) the socio-cultural model, (3) the personal model, and (4) interactional resources.

The developmental model is the understanding of how children grow up. It includes knowledge about the timing of normative events and the factors which move development along. It includes knowledge from the local textbook of child development and the cognitive complexity with which this knowledge is organized.

The socio-cultural model incorporates the norms of a particular culture for social roles and the characteristics children must have to fill those roles. It also identifies acceptable modes of socialization and limits the variability of childrearing in individual families within a given society. Subcultural varieties of the model define roles, behavior and deviancy. For example, retardation, mental illness and handicaps are defined quite differently in different socio-cultural contexts.

The personal model is the contribution made by the parent's own personality and includes much of what Pharis and Manosevitz (this volume) incorporate in their parental model. In addition to the parent's developmental stage, sex, and role in family and society, it includes mental health as well. The clinical literature is full of reports where distortions in parent-child relationships resulted from earlier distortions in the parent's own childrearing. The children of these parents may then become subject to aberrant behavior such as abuse or the deviant communications of a schizophrenic.

The last category deals with interactional resources such as time and motivation. Parents may have excellent developmental, social, and personal models, but because of an impoverished economic circumstance may have no time to care for their child. On the other hand the time may be available but the parents' motivations are tied more to their own needs than their children's needs. Clearly all these categories are intertwined and must be understood in their interconnectedness if individual developmental predictions are to be successful.

Observing Development

The interaction between biological roots and parental perspectives comes into play with the birth of the child. If the roots of later deviancy cannot be found in either aspect taken alone, then they must be assessed together. The observation of early mother-infant interaction has been an area of great activity in recent years. Penticuff in this volume discusses the importance of this early interaction and the potential hazards when the mother's initial contacts with her infant are disrupted or delayed. Klaus and Kennell (1976) have argued vigorously that early separations, either of the prolonged variety due to the placement of a preterm baby in a special care nursery for several weeks or the typical short 12-hour separation of the full-term infant from its mother, impede the establishment of emotional bonds between mother and infant. Consequently, the emotional development of the child is also impaired. Assertions about long-term negative effects of these separations are controversial, but the notion that the establishment of positive emotional ties between parent and infant is important is not controversial.

The definition of positive emotional ties is the topic of a number of papers on mother-infant interaction in this volume. Tronick and Thoman (this volume) are concerned with the synchrony of behavior between mother and child. If such synchrony exists, then it is assumed that the infant is giving off interpretable cues to a responsive caretaker. If asynchronies exist, it is because either the infant or the mother is behaving in an unusual way. Thoman presents the case of the unusual baby who becomes irritable rather than soothed when cuddled, thus violating the normal expectancies of his mother. On the other side, Tronick presents a study were an appropriately interacting mother becomes still and expressionless, thus violating the interactional expectancies of her infant. In both cases the partner was at a loss to continue an appropriate interaction.

The work of Field (this volume) and Bakeman and Brown (this volume) moves from individual cases to the study of groups of infants for whom interaction patterns are thought to be different; in this case, preterm and postterm babies. Indeed, when comparisons are made between the interaction patterns of these groups of infants and those of full-term infants many differences are found. Preterm babies were found to be less active and viewed by their mothers as less responsive and less organized. The mothers of preterm infants appeared to compensate for the lower responsivity of their offspring by becoming more active themselves.

These studies seem to indicate that infants at different levels of maturity behave differently, thereby producing different interaction patterns. Sex differences in infants also produce different interaction patterns (Moss, 1974), but it is not clear that this effect is due to differences in infants' behavior. While few studies have shown replicable sex differences in newborn behavior, there are many differences in the relation of early to later behavior for the two sexes. The tenuousness of these correlations can be seen in Yang's (this volume) contribution which reviews not only his own longitudinal research but the previous work of Bell, Weller, and Waldrop (1971). Even though the two longitudinal studies were from the same laboratory, seemingly minor alteration in procedure produced major changes in the resulting data. Longitudinal studies which replicate each other are a rare commodity in the developmental literature. One of the directions explored by Yang is a hierarchical conception of newborn behavior which can serve to cluster a variety of behaviors into meaningful dimensions.

Sackett (this volume) in his contribution also applied himself to identifying more meaningful ways of summarizing developmental data. In order to capture the dynamic nature of interactions one must produce variables which include the behavior of all the participants. Standard statistical models are not designed for dynamic systems. As a consequence, in attempts at scientific validity, researchers have forced their developmental data into nondevelopmental statistical designs such as analysis-of-variance. Rather than design research to fit the available statistics, researchers must identify models for which the appropriate statistics will have to be designed. As Sackett has shown, interaction research is one of the research areas most in need of new models.

A common theme emphasized by the authors of this interaction research is that the behavior of the mother and infant cannot be analyzed out of context but must be seen as part of a dynamic system. The interactive system tends to stabilize around a level of mutual behavior in which there is temporal stability and a turntaking quality. If one partner is less responsive, as in the case of preterm infants, the other partner takes up the slack.

These analyses further advance our understanding of the developmental process and move us towards making better predictions of psychosocial risk. It is no longer simply an issue of whether an infant is preterm or not or whether a mother is responsive or not, but rather whether the interaction as a dynamic system is functioning or not. A mother, whose behavioral tempo would be judged normal if she was interacting with a full-term infant, would now be judged as inadequate if she was interacting with a preterm infant. Field is most explicit in combining risk factors suggested by the continuum of reproductive casualty (Pasamanick & Knobloch, 1961) and the continuum of caretaking casualty (Sameroff

& Chandler, 1975) in an attempt to make better developmental predictions. The problem she runs into is that while these continua can be defined in principle, in practice they are usually confounded and compounded. Premature babies who are presumed to have a high reproductive risk are more frequently born to teenage, lower class mothers who have a high caretaking risk. As a consequence the causes for poor developmental outcomes from such children can never be clearly differentiated.

The Context of Development

Environmental influences have been seen as major factors in development, but in recent times have been taken for granted and thus neglected. Both scientific and political reasons have caused this neglect. As Hunt (this volume) points out, the scientific negligence can be attributed to an emphasis on individual differences in intelligence rather than achievement. The question is not whether children are intelligent, but rather which ones are more intelligent and which ones are less intelligent. Similarly, genetic studies focus not on the complex transactions between genes and bio-chemical environmental regulators that produce an organ such as an eye, but rather whether the eye will be brown or blue, i.e., its variability. Historically, the focus on individual differences is related to a conception of continuous development which sees IQ scores as reflecting quantitative rather than qualitative differences in performance (Riegel, 1972). Wohlwill (1973) has written eloquently about how the use of age as a developmental function masks the real developmental processes which underlie achievement. Willerman (this volume) points out, as well, that the same quantitative IQ scores at age six and age eight are attained from qualitatively different items on the Stanford-Binet. In order to produce a common IQ metric, intelligence tests have had to conceal the fact that different skills are tested at different ages.

Piaget's central importance in the history of developmental psychology may be less for the actual cognitive structures he claims for children than for the refocusing of the field on the qualitative structure of intelligence. If intelligence is seen as having an organized structure, concepts of education and assessment must be different. Structure implies a wholistic approach. The reason a child will acquire and maintain knowledge is not by the memorization of facts, but by how these facts are related to other facts the child already knows. Educational programs that center on memorization, such as that of Bereiter and Engelmann (1966), show the largest declines in IQ following termination (Karnes, Teska, & Hodgins, 1969).

The curious fact is that most children grow up to think, speak, and act like human adults. These are complex achievements which science is just beginning to acknowledge. How can children continue to reach mature adulthood without scientists and educators understanding how they do it? The simple answer is that while we as scientists tinker with bits and pieces of the system over short periods of time, society as a whole has spent eons evolving the system. It is a common biological characteristic of all surviving species that they must have a developmental agenda which produces adults. This agenda need not be planned nor reflected upon. It evolved over generations in which the changes in rearing conditions always had to produce a viable endproduct. These historic processes are what we as scientists and educators have had to grapple with. When one imposes an intervention or even a deprivation, these are usually only nuances in the grand developmental scheme. It is only the concern with individual differences that converts these nuances into the central theme of educational accountability. Educational systems are not evaluated on the basis of whether or not they produce viable adults, but rather whether these adult products are better than the adult products of other educational systems.

The production of a better product is not to be depreciated, especially in a society where individual differences rule supreme. However, if one desires ultimately to understand human development, one should not and cannot view these differences as reflecting basic psychological differences.

In sum, human development is a biosocial phenomenon which has evolved over many thousands of years. Except for children who are significantly biologically impaired or environments which are designed to abuse rather than rear children, children will grow to be socially and intellectually competent adults.

Educational and remediational programs must be seen in this light if they are to be ultimately effective. Without understanding the basic processes of development, one can never appreciate the relative success or failure of the cosmetic jobs in which we are currently engaged.

Morality, Aspirations and Effectiveness

Let me return to the earlier discussion of parental perspectives. I had outlined a series of developmental perspectives differing in level of cognitive complexity from the sensorimotor to the formal. At each level certain children are judged to be deviant if they do not fit the perspective. At the sensorimotor, symbiotic level, a child who does not satisfy the parent's needs for interaction is rejected as deviant. At the preoperational, categorical level, a child who looks or behaves atypically is categorized as deviant. Only at the formal operational, perspectivistic level are these variations in the performance of children understood as historical outcome of a unique child-environment interaction.

Why would parents be limited to lower levels of cognizing development? One of the limiting factors is the level at which their particular culture cognizes development. If the society functions preoperationally, as the Spartans did in letting female babies die or nomadic tribes do in destroying sets of twins because they are considered evil omens, then it is difficult for individual members of that society to function at higher levels.

The morality debate between Friedlander (this volume) and his respondents is an excellent example of such an issue. The issue is whether a society which gives minimal support to the psychological and economic needs of parents who must raise a deviant child can demand that the parents take responsibility for raising that child; that is, not permitting the parents to desert or kill the child. Roskies (1972) in her extraordinary book on the experience of parents of thalidomide babies discusses the conflicting demands of society and parents on these issues.

We are observing the two sides of a dialectical contradiction between two egalitarian principles. On one side is the dictum that all humans have an equal right to life. On the other hand is the dictum that all humans should enjoy a satisfying happy life. If one allows a seriously deviant child to live, one is obeying the first dictum but not the second. If one permits the child to die, one is obeying the second but not the first. But a dialectical contradiction need not be a dead end; it can be a source of development (Sameroff & Harris, 1979).

The first premise to be questioned is whether the parents and deviant child need to suffer an inequitable life. Certainly that has been the situation in the past where society not only has failed to help with the care or support of such children, but has placed a social stigma on individuals who look or behave differently. These stigmata have not been reserved for the handicapped but have been liberally applied to minority groups, women, and the elderly. More recently, society has been making significant advances from its preoperational, categorical past where a person's label was synonymous with his or her destiny. As our understanding of humanity has improved, we are less likely to evaluate individuals on any unitary standard.

Equally important is society's responsibility to support the family of the handicapped child. As Roskies pointed out in the case of the thalidomide babies, when the government began to provide social and economic support, the parents no longer felt the same isolation and stigmatization, but instead felt legitimized in the care and nurturance of their child. When support is provided, the parent need not carry the burden alone. If a society demands that one should not take a human life, then it is that society's responsibility to participate in the maintenance of that life.

The second premise to be questioned is the definition and understanding of deviancy. The contributors to this volume have made their greatest impact in this regard. By viewing the current set of developmental outcomes as only some of the possibilities, instead of all of the possibilities, the future is open for new combinations of reproductive and caretaking forces. The impact of genetic factors (Willerman), institutionalization (Hunt), feeding asymmetrics (Hawkins), prematurity (Brown & Bakeman, Field), and temperament (Thoman) have been shown to be mediated by caretaking milieus. As the significant parameters of these milieus become understood, new developmental outcomes become possible for children previously defined as deviant.

However, there is yet a great gap between the understanding of the possibilities and the achievement of the actuality. The reworking of parental perspectives requires the reworking of society's values as a whole. The failure of Head Start in the past is well discussed by Hunt (this volume). The current public school mainstreaming of handicapped individuals is another case in point. The potential failure of the mainstreaming is not because of the inadequacies of the handicapped child, but because of the inadequacies of the environment to accept these children.

The definition of psycho-social risk is not going to be an easy task. On the child's side it requires an increasingly sophisticated understanding of the mechanisms of development. On the environment's side it requires a greatly expanded view of the relevant dimensions of parental behavior. Our understanding of the sources of developmental risk is and should be an expanding one. When we limit the definition of these sources to the child's characteristics, we legitimize existing family and social environments. If, instead, we open the definition of risk to include characteristics of the family and society as well, the possibility arises for reforming the whole developmental system. The effects of such reformations on the development of our children are yet to be discovered.

Part VII

A TAXONOMY OF PSYCHOSOCIAL RISK
FACTORS IN INFANCY:
A GUIDE TO RECENT RESEARCH

One major aim of the symposia series and this edited volume was to compile a "taxonomy" of psychosocial risk factors in infancy to serve as a guide for research and as a resource in the formation of social policy. The concluding section of the volume comprises this taxonomy of citations and a bibliography of the full references for the taxonomy and the chapters in this volume.

Consistent with our operational definition of psychosocial risk in infancy, the major taxonomic categories include *Environmental Factors* (fetal environment, labor and delivery, postnatal social environment), *Infant Developmental Status at Birth and Early Characteristics*, and *Infant by Environment "Interaction."* In addition, *Developmental Outcomes* of psychosocial risks are included as a major category. The full outline of the taxonomic categories is presented in Table 1.

The bibliography of infant psychosocial risks consists of over 900 references for scientific and clinical studies appearing for the most part between 1970 and the summer of 1978. In some instances references from earlier periods were included to provide some long range perspective on the changes that have occurred in the conceptualization and methodologies for the study of infant risks. The bibliography also contains some entries not cited in the taxonomy, which were, however, referenced by the authors contributing chapters to the volume.

The reader may use two strategies for accessing the literature in the area of psychosocial risks in infancy. First, the pertinent taxonomic category may be located in the outline (Table 1) and the citations for the relevant studies found in the corresponding section of the taxonomy. Second, the reader may peruse the bibliography itself to find references of interest which are cross-indexed to the categories in the taxonomic outline.

Table 1

Table 1

Outline of Taxonomy of Psychosocial Risks in Infancy

I. Environmental Factors

    A. Fetal environment

        1. mother's physical health
        2. mother's psychological health
        3. nutritional status
        4. teratogens
        5. medication
        6. drug abuse

    B. Labor and delivery

        1. mother's physical health
        2. mother's psychological health
        3. parity
        4. delivery environment and procedures
        5. obstetrical medication
        6. iatrogenic effects

    C. Postnatal social environment

        1. socioeconomic status, cultural and other demographic variables
        2. mother's and father's psychological health
        3. mother's and father's physical health
        4. family composition
        5. parents' relationship
        6. maternal caretaking and affectional behavior
        7. paternal caretaking and affectional behavior
        8. maternal and paternal attitudes
        9. parent-infant separation
      10. other family events
      11. environmental deprivation or overstimulation
      12. assessment and intervention

II. Infant developmental status at birth and early characteristics

    A. Physical condition and characteristics
    B. Perceptual-cognitive development and functioning
    C. Temperament and social behavior

III. Infant by environment "interaction"

IV. Outcomes (criterion variables)

    A. Infant and young child
    B. Family functioning (social environment)
    C. Parenting behaviors

A TAXONOMY OF PSYCHOSOCIAL RISKS IN INFANCY

I. *Environmental Factors*
  A. *Fetal Environment*

Butler, N. R., 1974. Goldstein, K. M., Caputo, D. V., & Taub, H. B., 1976.
Lester, B. M., Emory, E. K., Huffman, S. L., & Eitzman, D. V., 1976.

1. *Mother's physical health*

Adams, B. N., Brownstein, C. A., Rennalls, I. M., & Schmitt, M. H., 1976.
Davies, D. P., Gray, O. P., Ellwood, P. C., & Abernethy, M., 1976.
Edwards, L. E., Dickes, W. F., Alton, J. R., & Hakanson, E. Y., 1978.
Field, T. M., Dabiri, C., Hallock, N., & Shulman, H. H., 1977.
Frommer, E. A., & O'Shea, G., 1973.
Hanson, J. W., Streissguth, A. P., & Smith, D. W., 1978.
Heinstein, M. I., 1967.
Henry, M., Ouellette, E., & Rosett, L., 1977.
Himwich, W. A., Hall, J. S., & MacArthur, W. F., 1977.
Jones, K. L., Smith, D. W., Streissguth, A. P., & Myrianthopoulos, N. C., 1974.
Jones, K. L., Smith, D. W., Ulleland, C. N., & Streissguth, A. P., 1973.
Landeeman-Dwyer, S., Keller, L. S., & Streissguth, A. P., 1978.
Little, R. E., Schultz, F., & Mandell, W., 1976.
Little, R. E., & Streissguth, A. P., 1978.
Martin, J., Martin, D., Lund, C., & Streissguth, A., 1977.
Mulvihill, J., Klimas, J., Stokes, D., & Risenberg, H., 1976.
Osofsky, H. J., 1974.
Osofsky, H. J., 1975 (b).
Osofsky, H. J., & Kendall, N., 1974.
Rosett, H., Ouellette, E., & Weiner, L., 1976.
Russell, M., 1977.
Sander, L., Snyder, P., Rosett, H., Lee, A., Gould, J., & Ouellette, E., 1977.
Semmens, J. P., & Lamers, W. M., Jr., 1968.
Stewart, K. R., 1976.
Streissguth, A. P., 1977.
Streissguth, A. P., 1977.
Wallace, H. M., Gold, E. M., Goldstein, H., & Oglesby, A. C., 1973.
Warner, R. H., & Rosett, H. L., 1975.
Whitelaw, A. G. L., 1976.

2. *Mother's psychological health*

Abernethy, V., & Abernethy, G. L., 1974.
Abernethy, V., Robins, D., Abernethy, G. L., Grunebaum, H., & Weiss, J. L., 1975.
Adams, B. N., Brownstein, C. A., Rennalls, I. M., & Schmitt, M. H., 1976.
Bibring, G. L.. 1959.
Bibring, G. L., Dwyer, T. F., Huntington, D. S., & Valenstein, A. F., 1961.
Caplan, G., 1951.
Caplan, G., 1959.
Ferreira, A. J., 1960.
Friederich, M. A., 1977.
Frommer, E. A., & O'Shea, G., 1973.
Gordon, R. E., & Gordon, K., 1959.
Grimm, E., & Venet, W. R., 1966.
Heinstein, M. I., 1967.
Krone, C. H., 1977.
Leifer, M., 1977.
Loesch, J. G., & Greenberg, N. H., 1962.
Newton, N., 1963.
Nuckholls, K. B., Cassell, J., & Kaplan, B. H., 1972.

Pines, D., 1972.
Pitt, B., 1977.
Pollitt, E., Eichler, A. W., & Chan, C. K., 1975.
Rossi, A., 1968.
Rubin, R., 1970.
Rubin, R., 1975.
Sameroff, A. J., & Zax, M., 1973.
Semmens, J. P., & Lamers, W. M., Jr., 1968.
Shaffer, D., Pettigrew, A., Wolking, S., & Zajicek, E., 1978.
Shereshesky, P. M., & Yarrow, L. J., 1974.
Singer, G., Stern, Y., & van der Spery, H. I. J., 1976.
Stewart, K. R., 1976.
Streissguth, A. P., 1977.
Wallace, H. M., Gold, E. M., Goldstein, H., & Oglesby, A. C., 1973.
Williams, C. C., Williams, R. A., Griswold, M. J., & Holmes, T. H., 1975.
Willmuth, R., 1975.
Yang, R., Zweig, A. R., Douthit, T. C., & Federman, E. J., 1976.
Zax, M., Sameroff, A. J., & Babigian, H. M., 1977.

3. *Nutritional status*
Davies, D. P., Gray, O. P., Ellwood, P. C., & Abernethy, M., 1976.
Edwards, L. E., Dickes, W. F., Alton, J. R., & Hakanson, E. Y., 1978.
Garn, S. M., 1976.
Gruenwald, P., 1974.
Hager, A., 1977.
Hanson, J. W., Streissguth, A. P., & Smith, D. W., 1978.
Hawkins, R. C., II, 1977.
Kaplan, B. J., 1972.
Knittle, J. L., & Hirsch, J., 1968.
Miller, H. C., 1973.
Miller, H. C., 1974.
Naeye, R. L., Blane, W., & Blane, P. C., 1973.
Osofsky, H. J., 1974.
Osofsky, H. J., 1975 (a)
Osofsky, H. J., 1975 (b)
Osofsky, H. J., & Kendall, N., 1974.
Philipps, C., & Johnson, N. E., 1977.
Russell, M., 1977.
Salans, L. B., Cushman, S. W., & Weissman, R. E., 1973.
Shearman, R. P., Shutt, D. A., & Smith, T. G., 1974.
Stein, Z., & Susser, M., 1976.
Streissguth, A. P., 1977.
Tizard, J., 1974.
Warren, N., 1973.

4. *Teratogens*
Butcher, R. E., Hawver, K., Burbacher, T., & Scott, W., 1975.
Davies, D. P., Gray, O. P., Ellwood, P. C., & Abernethy, M., 1976.
Martin, J., Martin, D., Lund, C., & Streissguth, A., 1977.

5. *Medication*
Anan, M. J., 1976.
Hollstedt, C., Olsson, O., & Rydberg, W., 1977.

6. *Drug Abuse*
Anan, M. J., 1976.
El-Gwebaly, N., & Offord, D. R., 1977.

Green, H. G., 1974.
Hanson, J. W., Streissguth, A. P., & Smith, D. W., 1978.
Harper, R. G., Solish, G., Purow, G. L., Sang, H. M., & Panepinto, W. C., 1974.
Henry, M., Ouellette, E., & Rosett, L., 1977.
Himwich, W. A., Hall, J. S., & MacArthur, W. F., 1977.
Hollstedt, C., Olsson, O., & Rydberg, W., 1977.
Jones, K. L., Smith, D. W., Streissguth, A. P., & Myrianthopoulos, N. C., 1974.
Jones, K. L., Smith, D. W., Ulleland, C. N., & Streissguth, A. P., 1973.
Landeeman-Dwyer, S., Keller, L. S., & Streissguth, A. P., 1978.
Little, R. E., Schultz, F., & Mandell, W., 1976.
Little, R. E., & Streissguth, A. P., 1978.
Martin, J., Martin, D., Lund, C., & Streissguth, A., 1977.
Mulvihill, J., Klimas, J., Stokes, D., & Risenberg, H., 1976.
Rosett, H., Ouellette, E., & Weiner, L., 1976.
Russell, M., 1977.
Sander, L., Snyder, P., Rosett, H., Lee, A., Gould, J., & Ouellette, E., 1977.
Singer, A., 1974.
Streissguth, A. P., 1976.
Streissguth, A. P., 1977.
Streissguth, A. P., 1978.
Streissguth, A. P., Herman, C. S., & Smith, D. W., 1978 (a).
Streissguth, A. P., Herman, C. S., & Smith, D. W., 1978 (b).
Warner, R. H., & Rosett, H. L., 1975.
  B. *Labor and Delivery*
    Goldstein, K. M., Caputo, D. V., & Taub, H. B., 1976.
    1. *Mother's physical health*
      Gottfried, A. W., 1973.
    2. *Mother's psychological health*
      Bibring, G. L., 1959.
      Bibring, G. L., Dwyer, T. F., Huntington, D. S., & Valenstein, A. F., 1961.
      Block, C., Block, R., & Shrock, P., 1975.
      Leifer, M., 1977.
      Lewis, E., 1976.
      Lynch, M. A., & Roberts, J., 1977.
      Lynch, M. A., Roberts, J., & Gordon, M., 1976.
      Pines, D., 1972.
      Pollitt, E., Eichler, A. W., & Chan, C. K., 1975.
      Rossi, A., 1968.
      Rubin, R., 1975.
      Sameroff, A. J., & Zax, M., 1973.
      Singer, G., Stern, Y., & van der Spery, H. I. J., 1976.
      Willmuth, R., 1975.
    3. *Parity*
    4. *Delivery environment and procedures*
      Block, C., Block, P., & Shrock, P., 1975.
      Brackbill, Y., et al., 1974.
      Gottfried, A. W., 1973.
      Hunter, R. S., Kilstrom, N., Kraybill, E. N., & Loda, F., 1978.
      Kopf, R. C., & McFadden, E. L., 1974.
      Lawson, K., Daum, C., & Turkewitz, G., 1977.
      Lynch, M. A., & Roberts, J., 1977.

Lynch, M. A.. Roberts, J., & Gordon, M., 1976.
Melber, R. S., 1968.
Nunnally, D., & Aguiar, M., 1974.
Oppe, T. E., 1975.
Parmelee, A. H., Kopp, C. B., & Sigman, M., 1976.
Sugarman, M., 1977.
Wente, A. S., & Crockenberg, S. B., 1976.
5. *Obstetrical medication*
Aleksandrowicz, M. K., 1974.
Aleksandrowicz, M. K., & Aleksandrowicz, D. R., 1974.
Brazelton, T. B., 1971.
Federman, E. J., & Yang, R. K., 1976.
Korner, A. F., 1974 (a).
Parmelee, A. H., Kopp, C. B., & Sigman, M., 1976.
Standley, K., Soule, A. B. III, Copans, S. A., & Duchowny, M. S., 1974.
Yang, R., Zweig, A. R., Douthit, T. C., & Federman, E. J., 1976.
6. *Iatrogenic effects*
Korner, A. F., 1974 (a).
Parmelee, A. H., Kopp, C. B., & Sigman, M., 1976.
Pasamanick, B., & Knobloch, M., 1966.
C. *Postnatal Social Environment*
1. *Socioeconomic status, cultural and other demographic variables*
Ainsworth, M. D. S., 1967.
Bee, H. L., VanEgeren, L. F., Streissguth, A. P., Nyman, B. A., & Lockie, M. S., 1969.
Brazelton, T. B., Robey, J. S., & Collier, G. A., 1969.
Brazelton, T. B., Tronick, E., Lechtig, A., Lasky, R. E., & Klein, R. E., 1977.
Brown, J. V., Bakeman, R., Snyder, P. A., Frederickson, W. T., Morgan, S. T., & Hepler, R., 1975.
Deutsch, C. P., 1973.
Draper, H. H., 1977.
Ferguson, C. A., 1964.
Field, T. M., 1979c.
Freedman, D. G., & Freeman, N., 1969.
Gewirtz, H. B., & Gewirtz, J. L., 1969.
Golden, M., & Birns, B., 1976.
Goldstein, K. M., Taub, H. B., Caputo, D. V., & Silberstein, R. M., 1976.
Hess, R. D., 1970.
Holden, R. H., & Willerman, L., 1972.
Hunt, J. McV., Mohandessi, K., Ghodssi, M., & Akiyama, M., 1976.
Hunt, J. McV., Paraskevopoulos, J., Schickedanz, D., & Uzgiris, I. C., 1975.
Kagan, J., 1969.
Kagan, J., 1973.
Kagan, J., & Klein, R. E., 1975.
Kilbride, H. W., Johnson, D. L., & Streissguth, A. P., 1977.
Klein, R. E., Lasky, R. E., Yarbrough, C., Habicht, J. P., & Sellers, M. J., 1977.
Lally, J. R., & Honig, A. S., 1975.
Lewis, M., & Wilson, C. D., 1972.
de Lissovoy, V., 1973.
Lopata, H. Z., 1971.
Mack, R. W., & Johnston, F. E., 1976.
Moss, H. A., & Jones, S. J., 1977.

Nadelson, C. C., 1975.
Osofsky, H. J., 1974.
Osofsky, H. J., 1975 (b).
Osofsky, H. J., & Kendall, N., 1974.
Papajohn, J., & Spiegel, J., 1975.
Paraskevopoulos, J., & Hunt, J. McV., 1971.
Rising, S. S., 1974.
Sawin, D. B., & Parke, R. D., 1976.
Scarr, S., & Weinberg, R. A., 1976.
Scott, N. T., 1974.
Streissguth, A. P., 1977.
Sugar, M., 1976.
Tulkin, S. R., 1977.
Veevers, J. E., 1973.
deVries, M. W., & deVries, M. R., 1977.
Wachs, T. D., Uzgiris, I. C., & Hunt, J. McV., 1971.
Willerman, L., Broman, S. H., & Fiedler, M., 1970.
Zegiob, L., & Forehand, R., 1975.
Zuk, G. H., Miller, R. L., Bartram, J. B., & Kling, F., 1961.
2. *Mother's and father's psychological health*
Alvy, K., 1975.
Anthony, E. J., & Benedek, T., 1971.
Banks, M. J., 1977.
Benedek, T., 1956
Bibring, G. L., 1959.
Bibring, G. L., Dwyer, T. F., Huntington, D. S., & Valenstein, A. F., 1961.
Blake, A., Stewart, A., & Turcan, D., 1975.
Carey, W. B., 1968.
Choi, M. A., 1975.
Cohler, B., Grunebaum, H., & Weiss, J., 1970.
Cohler, B. J., Grunebaum, H. U., Weiss, J. L., Hartman, C. R., & Gallant, D. H., 1976.
Gelles, R. J., 1975.
Gilman, R., & Knox, D., 1976.
Goldstein, J., 1975.
Gordon, R. E., Kapostins, E. E., & Gordon, K. K., 1965.
Greenberg, N. H., & Hurley, J., 1971.
Gutton, P., 1977.
Hock, E., 1978.
Kestenberg, J. S., 1959.
Lamb, M. E., 1976 (a).
Leifer, M., 1977.
LeMasters, E. E., 1965.
Lynch, M. A., Roberts, J., & Gordon, M., 1976.
Mannino, F. V., 1974.
McGowan, M. N., 1977.
Mercer, R. T., 1977.
Pollitt, E., Eichler, A. W., & Chan, C. K., 1975.
Prugh, D., 1953.
Reich, W. T., & Smith, H., 1973.
Rossi, A., 1968.
Rowe, J., Clyman, R., Green, C., Mikkelsen, C., Haight, J., & Ataide, L., 1978.

Rubin, R., 1972.
Rubin, R., 1975.
Rubin, R., 1977.
Sameroff, A. J., & Zax, M., 1973.
Sandgrund, A., Gaines, R., & Green, A., 1974 (c).
Schwartz, B. K., 1974.
Semmens, J. P., & Lamers, W. M., Jr., 1968.
Shaver, B. A., 1973.
Singer, G., Stern, Y., & van der Spery, H. I. J., 1976.
Sperber, Z., & Weiland, I. H., 1973.
Strom, R., & Greathouse, B., 1975.
Waleko, K., 1974.
3. *Mother's and father's physical health*
Goldstein, J., 1975.
Hamburg, D. A., Moos, R. F., & Yalom, I. D., 1968.
McGowan, M. N., 1977.
Sandgrund, A., Gaines, R., & Green, A., 1974 (c).
4. *Family composition*
Carey, W. B., Lipton, L., & Myers, R. A., 1974.
Cicirelli, V. G., 1978.
Cohen, D. J., Dibble, E., Grawe, J. M., & Pollin, W., 1973.
Cohen, S. E., & Beckwith, L., 1977.
Eldred, C., Rosenthal, D., Wender, P. H., Kety, S. S., Schulsinger, F., Weiner, J., & Jacobsen, B., 1976.
Goldstein, K. M., Taub, H. B., Caputo, D. V., & Silberstein, R. M., 1976.
Hollender, J. W., 1973.
Jacobs, B. A., & Moss, H. A., 1976.
Kellam, S. G., Emsinger, M. E., & Turner, R. J., 1977.
Kilbride, H. W., Johnson, D. L., & Streissguth, A. P., 1977.
Mannino, F. V., 1974.
Marjonibanks, K., 1976.
Mech, E. V., 1973.
Rising, S. S., 1974.
Scarr, S., & Weinberg, R. A., 1976.
Senn, M. J. E., & Hartford, C., 1968.
Thoman, E. B., Barnett, C. R., & Leiderman, P. H., 1971.
Thoman, E. B., Turner, A. M., Leiderman, P. H., & Barnett, C. R., 1970.
Yando, R., Zigler, E., & Litzinger, S., 1975.
5. *Parents' relationship*
Blake, A., Stewart, A., & Turcan, D., 1975.
Mannino, F. V., 1974.
Rising, S. S., 1974.
6. *Maternal caretaking and affectional behavior*
Ackerman, N. W., 1956.
Adams, M., 1963.
Ainsworth, M. D. S., 1967.
Ainsworth, M. D. S., 1969.
Ainsworth, M. D. S., 1973.
Ainsworth, M. D. S., & Bell, S. M., 1969.
Ainsworth, M. D. S., & Bell, S. M., 1974.
Ainsworth, M. D. S., & Bell, S. M., 1977.
Ainsworth, M. D. S., Bell, S., & Stayton, P., 1974.
Aleksandrowicz, M., & Aleksandrowicz, D. R., 1974.

Ashton, P. T., 1978.
Bakeman, R., & Brown, J. V., 1977.
Bee, H. L., VanEgeren, L. F., Streissguth, A. P., Nyman, B. A., & Lockie, M. S., 1969.
Bell, S. M., & Ainsworth, M. D. S., 1972.
Bernal, J., 1974.
Birns, B., Blank, M., & Bridger, W. H., 1966.
Blake, A., Stewart, A., & Turcan, D., 1975.
Blehar, M. C., Lieberman, A. F., & Ainsworth, M. D. S., 1977.
Carlsson, S. J., Faderberg, H., Hornemann, L., Hwang, C. P., Larsson, K., Rodholm, M., Schaller, J., Danielson, B., & Gundewall, C., 1978.
de Chateau, P., 1976.
Clarke-Stewart, K. A., 1973.
Cohen, D. J., Dibble, E., & Krane, J. M., 1977.
Cohen, E. S., & Beckwith, L., 1976.
Cohen, E. S., & Beckwith, L., 1977.
Cohler, B. J., Grunebaum, H. U., Weiss, J. L., Hartman, C. R., & Gallant, D. H., 1976.
Crawley, S. B., Rogers, P. P., Friedman, S., Jacobson, M., Criticos, A., Richardson, L., & Thompson, M. A., 1978.
David, M., & Appell, G., 1969.
Dietrich, K. N., & Starr, R. H., 1978.
Dunbar, J., 1977.
Dunn, J. B., 1975.
Dunn, J. B., 1976.
Dunn, J. B., 1977 (a).
Dunn, J. B., 1977 (c).
Dunn, J. B., & Richards, M. P. M., 1977.
Dunn, J. B., Wooding, C., & Hermann, J. B., 1977.
Field, T. M., 1977 (c).
Forrest, T., 1974.
Freese, M. P., & Thoman, E. B., 1978.
Gauthier, V., Fortin, C., Drapeau, P., Breton, J. J., Gosselin, J., Quintal, L., Weisnagel, J., Tetreault, L., & Pinard, E., 1977.
Goldstein, K. M., Taub, H. B., Caputo, D. V., & Silberstein, R. M., 1976.
Gutton, P., 1977.
Hanson, J. W., Streissguth, A. P., & Smith, D. W., 1978.
Harper, L. V., 1972.
Hawkins, R. C. II, 1977.
Helfer, R., 1974.
Hofer, M. A., 1975.
Hollender, J. W., 1973.
Jacobs, B. A., & Moss, H. A., 1976.
Jones, S. J., & Moss, H. A., 1971.
Kaye, K., 1977.
Kellam, S. G., Emsinger, M. E., & Turner, R. J., 1977.
Kennedy, J., 1973.
Kennell, J. H., Jerauld, R., Wolfe, H., Chester, D., Kreger, N. C., McAlpine, W., Steffa, M., & Klaus, M. H., 1974.
Kennell, J. H., Trause, M. A., & Klaus, M. H., 1974.
Kennell, J. H., Trause, M. A., & Klaus, M. H., 1975.
Klaus, M. H., 1970.
Klaus, M. H., Jerauld, R., Kreger, N. C., McAlpine, W., Steffa, M., &

Kennell, J. H., 1972.
Klaus, M. H., & Kennell, J. H., 1976.
Klaus, M. H., & Kennell, J. H., 1978.
Klaus, M. H., Trause, M. A., & Kennell, J. H., 1975.
Kolejkova, A., 1977.
Korner, A. F., 1973 (b).
Korner, A., & Thoman, E. B., 1970.
Lamb, M. E., 1976 (a).
Lamb, M. E., 1977 (a).
Landau, R., 1976.
Leiderman, P. H., Leifer, A. D., Seashore, M. J., Barnett, C. R., & Grobstein, R., 1973.
Lynch, M. A., & Roberts, J., 1977.
Lynch, M. A., Roberts, J., & Gordon, M., 1976.
Maccoby, E. E., & Masters, J., 1970.
Mahler, M. S., 1974.
Martin, B., 1975.
Massie, H. N., 1975.
Massie, H. N., 1977.
Massie, H. N., 1978.
McGowan, M. N., 1977.
Mercer, R. T., 1974.
Moss, H. J., & Jones, S. J., 1977.
Osofsky, J. D., 1976.
Osofsky, J. D., & Danzger, B., 1974.
Overton, W. P., 1973.
Parke, R. D., & O'Leary, S. E., 1976.
Pawlby, S., & Hall, F., 1979.
Perry, J. C., & Stern, D. N., 1975.
Pollitt, E., Eichler, A. W., & Chan, C. K., 1975.
Powell, L. F., 1974.
Richards, M. P. M., & Bernal, J. F., 1971.
Ringler, N. M., Kennell, J. H., Jarvella, R., Navojosky, B. J., & Klaus, M. H., 1975.
Robson, K. S., & Moss, H. A., 1967.
Rosenblum, L. A., 1974.
Rubenstein, J., 1967.
Rubin, R., 1975.
Sander, L. W., 1969.
Sandgrund, A., Gaines, R., & Green, A., 1974 (c).
Schachter, J., Elmer, E., Ragins, N., Wimberly, F., & Lachin, J. M., 1977.
Schaffer, R., 1977.
Scott, N. T., 1974.
Seashore, M. J., Leifer, A. D., Barnett, C. R., & Leiderman, P. H., 1973.
Seegmiller, B. R., & King, W. L., 1975.
Serafica, F. C., 1978.
Shaver, B. A., 1973
Shereshesky, P. M., & Yarrow, L. J., 1974.
Solkoff, N., & Matuszak, D., 1975.
Strom, R., & Greathouse, B., 1975.
Thoman, E. B., Korner, A. F., & Beason-Williams, L., 1977.
Thompson, W. R., & Grusec, J., 1970.
Tizard, B., & Rees, J. A., 1974.

Tulkin, S. R., & Cohler, B. J., 1973.
Walberg, H., & Marjonibanks, K., 1979.
Waters, E., 1978.
White, B. L., 1971.
White, B. L., 1975.
White, B. L., 1978.
White, B. L., Kaban, B., Shapiro, B., & Attanucci, J., 1977.
White, B. L., & Watts, J. C., 1973.
Whitelaw, A. G. L., 1976.
Williams, T. H., 1974.
Yarrow, L. J., Pedersen, F. A., & Rubenstein, J., 1977.
Yarrow, L. J., Rubenstein, J. L., & Pedersen, F. A., 1975.
Zaslow, R. W., & Berger, L., 1969.
Zegiob, L., & Forehand, R., 1975.

7. *Paternal caretaking and affectional behavior*
Ashton, P. T., 1978.
Bernal, J., 1974.
Biller, H. B., 1974.
Blake, A., Stewart, A., & Turcan, D., 1975.
Clarke-Stewart, K. A., 1978 (b).
Cohen, D. J., Dibble, E., & Krane, J. M., 1977.
Cummings, S. T., 1976.
Field, T. M., 1978 (b).
Greenberg, M., & Morris, N., 1974.
Hofer, M. A., 1975.
Hollender, J. W., 1973.
Kotelchuck, M., 1976.
Lamb, M. E., 1976 (a).
Lamb, M. E., 1976 (b).
Lamb, M. E., 1977 (a).
Lewis, M., & Weintraub, M., 1976.
Lynch, M. A., Roberts, J., & Gordon, M., 1976.
Martin, B., 1975.
Orthner, D., Brown, T., & Ferguson, D., 1976.
Parke, R. D., 1979.
Parke, R. D., & O'Leary, S. E., 1976.
Parke, R. D., & Sawin, D. B., 1976.
Parke, R. D., & Sawin, D. B., 1977 (a).
Parke, R. D., & Sawin, D. B., 1977 (b).
Rebelsky, F., & Hanks, C., 1971.
Rendina, I., & Dickerscheid, J. D., 1976.
Rubin, R., 1977.
Sandgrund, A., Gaines, R., & Green, A., 1974 (c).
Sawin, D. B., & Parke, R. D., 1976.
Shereshesky, P. M., & Yarrow, L. J., 1974.
Spelke, E., Zelazo, P., Kager, J., & Kotelchuck, M., 1973.

8. *Maternal and paternal attitudes*
Becker, W., & Krug, R., 1965.
Bidder, R. T., Crowe, E. A., & Gray, O. P., 1974.
Blake, A., Stewart, A., & Turcan, D., 1975.
Brazelton, T. B., 1973 (a).
Broussard, E. R., 1976.
Broussard, E. R., & Hartner, M. S. S., 1970.

Broussard, E. R., & Hartner, M. S. S., 1971.
Choi, M. A., 1975.
Cohen, D. J., Dibble, E., & Krane, J. M., 1977.
Cohler, B., Grunebaum, H., & Weiss, J., 1970.
Cohler, B. J., Grunebaum, H. U., Weiss, J. L., Hartman, C. R., & Gallant, D. H., 1976.
Coleman, R. W., Kris, E., & Provence, S., 1953.
Cropley, C., Lester, P., & Pennington, S., 1976.
Davids, A., & Holden, R., 1970.
Deutsch, H., 1945.
Doty, B., 1967.
Fletcher, J., 1974.
Goldstein, K. M., Taub, H. B., Caputo, D. V., & Silberstein, R. M., 1976.
Hanes, M. L., & Dunn, S. K., 1978.
Hock, E., 1978.
Kestenberg, J. S., 1959.
Lamb, M. E., 1976 (a).
Moss, H. A., & Jones, S. J., 1977.
Newton, N. R., & Newton, M., 1950.
Parke, R. D., & Sawin, D. B., 1977 (b).
Pines, D., 1972.
Rubin, J. Z., Provenzano, F. J., & Luria, Z., 1974.
Schaefer, E. S., & Bell, R., 1958.
Tulkin, S. R., & Kagan, J., 1972.
Veevers, J. E., 1973.
Will, J. A., Self, P. A., & Datan, N., 1976.
Zemlick, M. J., & Watson, R. I., 1953.
Zuk, G. H., Miller, R. L., Bartram, J. B., & Kling, F., 1961.
9. *Parent-infant separation*
Barnard, M. U., 1976.
Barnett, C. R., Leiderman, R. H., Grobstein, R., & Klaus, M., 1970.
Biller, H. B., 1974.
Clark, A. M., & Clarke, A. D. B., 1976.
Greenberg, M., & Rosenberg, I., 1973.
Hales, D. J., Lozoff, B., Sopa, R., & Kennell, J. H., 1977.
Harrell, J. E., & Ridley, C. A., 1975.
Hock, E., 1978.
Hunter, R. S., Kilstrom, N., Kraybill, E. N., & Loda, F., 1978.
Jansen, A. R., & Garland, M., 1976.
Kennedy, J., 1973.
Kennell, G., Gordon, D., & Klaus, M., 1970.
Kennell, J. H., Jerauld, R., Wolfe, H., Chester, D., Kreger, N. C., McAlpine, W., Steffa, M., & Klaus, M. H., 1974.
Kennell, J. H., Trause, M. A., & Klaus, M. H., 1974.
Kennell, J. H., Trause, M. A., & Klaus, M. H., 1975.
Klaus, M. H., 1970.
Klaus, M. H., Jerauld, R., Kreger, N. C., McAlpine, W., Steffa, M., & Kennell, J. H., 1972.
Klaus, M., & Kennell, J., 1970.
Klaus, M. H., & Kennell, J. H., 1977.
Klaus, M. H., & Kennell, J. H., 1978.
Klaus, M. H., Trause, M. A., & Kennell, J. H., 1975.
Leiderman, P. H., 1978.

Leiderman, P. H., Leifer, A. D., Seashore, M. J., Barnett, C. R., & Grobstein, R., 1973.
Leifer, A. D., Liederman, P. H., Barnett, C. R., & Williams, J. A., 1972.
Lewis, M., & Lee-Painter, S., 1974.
Mercer, R. T., 1977.
Rau, J. H., & Kaye, H., 1977.
Reynolds, E. O. R., & Stewart, A. L., 1977.
Ringler, N. M., Kennell, J. H., Jarvella, R., Navolosky, B. J., & Klaus, M. H., 1975.
Rosenzweig, M. R., & Bennett, E. L., 1977.
Rubenstein, J. L., Pederson, F. A., & Yarrow, L. L., 1977.
Rubin, R., 1977.
Rutter, M., 1974.
Salk, L., 1977.
Schlesinger, E. R., 1973.
Seashore, M. J., Leifer, A. D., Barnett, C. R., & Leiderman, P. H., 1973.
10. *Other family events*
Harrell, J. E., & Ridley, C. A., 1975.
Hock, E., 1978.
Kellam, S. G., Emsinger, M. E., & Turner, R. J., 1977.
Liptak, G. S., Hulka, B. S., & Cassell, J. C., 1977.
Mannino, F. V., 1974.
Marjonibanks, K., 1976.
Pawlby, S., & Hall, F., 1979.
Rising, S. S., 1974.
11. *Environmental deprivation or overstimulation*
Ainsworth, M. D. S., & Bell, S. M., 1969.
Biron, P., Mongeau, J. G., & Bertrand, D., 1977.
Brackbill, Y., 1973.
Brackbill, Y., 1975.
Bradley, R., & Caldwell, B., 1976.
Brazelton, T. B., Tronick, E., Lechtig, A., Lasky, R. E., & Klein, R. E., 1977.
Brook, C. D. G., Huntley, R. M. C., & Slack, J., 1972.
Bruch, H., 1973.
de Chateau, P., 1976.
Clark, A. M., & Clarke, A. D. B., 1976.
Dennis, W., 1960.
Dennis, W., 1973.
Dietrich, K. N., & Starr, R. H., 1978.
Eid, E. K., 1970.
Elardo, R., Bradley, R., & Caldwell, B. M., 1977.
Fanaroff, A. A., Kennell, J. H., & Klaus, M. H., 1972.
Field, T. M., 1977 (a).
Fomon, S. J., 1974.
Garn, S. M., 1976.
Greenberg, M., & Rosenberg, I., 1973.
Hartz, A., Giefer, E., & Rimm, A., 1977.
Hawkins, R. C. II, 1977.
Hollenbeck, A. R., 1978.
Hunt, J. McV., 1976 (b).
Hunt, J. McV., 1979.
Hunt, J. McV., Mohandessi, K., Ghodssi, M., & Akiyama, M., 1976.
Hunt, J. McV., Paraskevopoulos, J., Schickendanz, D., & Uzgiris, I. C., 1975.

Kellam, S. G., Emsinger, M. E., & Turner, R. J., 1977.
Klein, R. E., Lasky, R. E., Yarbrough, C., Habicht, J. P., & Sellers, M. J., 1977.
Korner, A. F., 1973 (b).
Landau, R., 1976.
Light, R., 1973.
Mack, R. W., & Kleinhenz, M. E., 1974.
Marjonibanks, K., 1976.
Mayer, J., 1968.
Mellbin, T., & Vuille, J. C., 1976.
Neuman, C. G., & Alpaugh, M., 1976.
Osofsky, H. J., 1975 (a).
Papousek, H., & Bernstein, P., 1969.
Perry, J. H., & Freedman, D. A., 1973.
Poskitt, E. M. E., 1977.
Poskitt, E. M. E., & Cole, T. J., 1978.
Ramey, C., Mills, P., Campbell, F., & O'Brien, C., 1975.
Richardson, S. A., Birch, H. G., & Hertzog, M. E., 1973.
Rose, H. E., & Mayer, J. 1968.
Rutter, M., 1974.
Solkoff, N., & Matuszak, D., 1975.
Sveger, T., Lindberg, T., Weilbull, B., & Ollson, V. L., 1975.
Taitz, T. S., 1971.
Thompson, W. R., & Grusec, J., 1970.
Tizard, J., 1974.
Tizard, B., & Rees, J., 1974.
Tizard, J., & Tizard, B., 1974.
Wachs, T. D., 1979.
Wachs, T. D., Uzgiris, I. C., & Hunt, J. McV., 1971.
Walberg, H., & Marjonibanks, K., 1973.
White, B. L., 1971.
White, B. L., 1975.
White, B. L., 1978.
White, B. L., Kaban, B., Shapiro, B., & Attanucci, J., 1977.
White, B. L., & Watts, J. C., 1973.
Wiel, A., 1975.
Yarrow, L. J., Rubenstein, J. L., & Pedersen, F. A., 1975.

12. *Assessment and intervention*

Ackerman, N. W., 1956.
Alvy, K., 1975.
Ames, M. D., & Schut, L., 1972.
Badger, E. D., 1971 (a).
Badger, E. D., 1971 (b).
Bennett, V. C., & Bardon, J. I., 1977.
Bradley, R. H., & Caldwell, B. M., 1977.
Brazelton, T. B., 1973 (b).
Brazelton, T. B., 1973 (c).
Bromwick, R. M., 1976.
Bronfenbrenner, U., 1975.
Broussard, E. R., 1976.
Call, J., 1974.
Campos, J. J., 1977.
Caplan, G., 1951.

Caplan, G., 1959.
Chilman, C. S., 1973.
Cicirelli, V. G., et al., 1969.
Clarke-Stewart, K. A., 1978 (a).
Colen, B. D., 1974.
Cornell, E. H., & Gottfried, A. W., 1976.
Cropley, C., Lester, P., & Pennington, S., 1976.
Diamond, J. M., 1978.
Duff, R. S., & Campbell, A. G. M., 1976.
Eldred, C. A., Grier, V. V., & Berliner, N., 1974.
Ellis, H. L., 1974.
Fletcher, J., 1975.
Fost, N., 1976.
Fraiberg, S., 1975.
Freeman, J. M., 1973.
Goldfarb, J. L., Mumford, D. M., Schum, D. A., Smith, P. P., Flowers, C., & Schum, C., 1977.
Greenberg, N. H., & Hurley, J., 1971.
Harper, R. G., Solish, G., Purow, G. L., Sang, H. M., & Panepinto, W. C., 1974.
Hayden, A. H., & Dmitriev, V., 1975.
Hollenbeck, A. R., 1978.
Honzik, M. P., 1976.
Horowitz, F. D., & Paden, L. Y., 1973.
Hunt, J. McV., 1975 (a).
Hunt, J. McV., 1976 (a).
Janson, A. R., & Garland, M. J., 1976.
Johnson, D. L., 1975.
Johnson, R. H., 1974.
Johnston, R. B., & Magrab, P. R., 1976.
Kaback, M. M., 1977.
Karnes, M. B., 1973.
Karnes, M. B., Teska, J. A., Hodgins, A. A., & Badger, E. D., 1970.
Kraemer, H. C., & Korner, A. F., 1976.
Lally, J. R., & Honig, A. S., 1975.
Van Leeuwen, G., 1972.
Littman, B., et al., 1976.
Lorber, J., 1972.
Lorber, J., 1973.
Lubs, H. A., & de la Cruz, F., 1977.
Lynch, A., 1975.
Macintyre, M. N., 1977.
Meier, J. H., 1975.
Melber, R. S., 1969.
Nadelson, C. C., 1975.
Newton, N., 1950.
Nielsen, G., Collins, S., Meisel, J., Lowry, M., Engh, H., & Johnson, D., 1975.
Ounsted, C., Oppenheimer, R., & Lindsay, J., 1974.
Ounsted, C., Oppenheimer, R., & Lindsay, J., 1975.
Page, E. B., 1975.
Papousek, H., & Papousek, M., 1977.
Parmelee, A. H., Kopp, C. B., & Sigman, M., 1976.

Provence, S., Naylor, A., & Patterson, J., 1977.
Rachels, J., 1975.
Robertson, J. A., & Fost, N., 1976.
Rynders, J. E., & Horrobin, J. M., 1975.
Sander, L. W., Stechler, G., Julia, H., & Burns, P., 1976.
Schaefer, E. S., & Bell, R. Q., 1958.
Schneider, C., Hoffmeister, J. K., & Helfer, R. E., 1976.
Schwartz, J. C., Strickland, R. G., & Krolick, G., 1974.
Shapiro, V., Fraiberg, S., & Adelson, E., 1976.
Shaw, M. W., 1977.
Slade, C. I., Redl, O. J., & Manguten, H. H., 1977.
Sosa, R., Kennell, J. H., Klaus, M., & Urrutia, J. J., 1976.
Stein, S. C., Schut, L., & Ames, M. D., 1974.
Swanson, J., 1978.
Tanguay, P. E., 1973.
Tjossen, T. D., 1976.
Wallace, H. M., Gold, E. M., Goldstein, H., & Oglesby, A. C., 1973.
Weikart, D. P., Epstein, A. S., Schweinhart, L., & Bond, J. T., 1978.
Wright, L., 1971.

II. *Infant Developmental Status at Birth and Early Characteristics*
Gordon, I. J., 1975.

A. *Physical Condition and Characteristics*

Adelson, E., & Fraiberg, S., 1974.
Ainsworth, M. D. S., & Bell, S. M., 1969.
Als, H., Tronick, E., Adamson, L., & Brazelton, T. B., 1976.
Ames, M. D., & Schut, L., 1972.
Anders, T. F., 1974.
Ashton, R., 1973.
Ashton, R., 1976.
Beckwith, L., Cohen, S. E., Kopp, C. B., Parmelee, A. H., & Marcy, T. G., 1976.
Beckwith, L., Sigman, M., Cohen, S. E., & Parmelee, A. H., 1977.
Benfield, D. G., Lieb, S. A., & Reuter, J., 1976.
Benfield, D. G., Leib, S. A., & Vollman, J. H., 1978.
Berger, M., Lezine, I., Harrison, A., & Boisselier, F., 1973.
Bergman, A. B., 1974.
Berkson, G., 1974.
Bidder, R. T., Crowe, E. A., & Gray, O. P., 1974.
Blake, A., Stewart, A., & Turcan, D., 1975.
Brazelton, T. B., Tronick, E., Lechtig, A., Lasky, R. E., & Klein, R. E., 1977.
Brown, J. V., & Bakeman, R., 1978.
Buckhalt, J. A., Rutherford, R. B., & Goldberg, K. E., 1978.
Caplan, G., Mason, E., & Kaplan, D. M., 1965.
Caputo, D. V., 1974.
Carey, W. B., 1968.
Charney, E., Goodman, H. C., McBride, M., Lyon, B., & Pratt, R., 1976.
Choi, M., 1975.
Cicchetti, D., & Sroufe, L. A., 1978.
Clark, A. L., & Alfonso, D. D., 1976.
Clark, A. M., & Clarke, A. D. B., 1976.
Cohen, E. S., & Beckwith, L., 1977.
Colen, B. D., 1974.
Condon, W. S., 1978.

Condon, W. S., & Ogston, W. D., 1967.
Condon, W. S., & Sander, L. W., 1974.
Cornell, E. H., & Gottfried, A. W., 1976.
Crook, C. K., 1976.
Cummings, S. T., 1976.
Desmond, M. M., Franklin, R. R., Vallbona, C., Hill, R. M., Plumb, R., Arnold, H., & Watts, J., 1963.
Diamond, J. M., 1978.
Diamond, M. C., 1977.
Dietrich, K. N., & Starr, R. H., 1978.
DiVitto, B., & Goldberg, S., 1978.
Dreyfus-Brisac, C., 1974.
Drillien, C. M., 1964.
Drotan, D., Baskiewitz, A., Irwin, N., Kennell, J., & Klaus, M., 1975.
Dubowitz, V., 1974.
Duff, R. S., & Campbell, A. G. M., 1976.
Dugdale, A. E., 1975.
Dunlap, W. R., & Hollingsworth, J. S., 1977.
Ellingen, R. J., Dutch, S. J., & McIntire, M. S., 1974.
Elliott, K., & Knight, J., 1974.
Ellis, H. L., 1974.
Elmer, E., & Gregg, C. S., 1967.
Emde, R. N., Katz, E. L., & Thorpe, J. K., 1978.
Fanaroff, A. A., Kennell, J. H., & Klaus, M. H., 1972.
Field, T. M., 1978 (a).
Field, T. M., 1979 (b).
Field, T. M., Goldberg, S., Stern, D., & Sostek, A., 1979.
Field, T. M., Hallock, N., Ting, G., Dempsey, J., Dabiri, C., & Shuman, H. H., 1978.
Fisch, R. O., Bilek, M. K., & Ulstrom, R., 1975.
Fitzhardinge, P. M., 1976.
Fletcher, J., 1974.
Fletcher, J., 1975.
Fost, N., 1976.
Francis-Williams, J., & Davies, P. A., 1974.
Freeman, J. M., 1973.
Gauthier, V., Fortin, C., Drapeau, P., Breton, J. J., Gosselin, J., Quintal, L., Weisnagel, J., Tetreault, L., & Pinard, E., 1977.
Goldberg, S., Brachfeld, S., & DiVitto, B., 1978.
Goldstein, K. M., Caputo, D. V., & Taub, H. B., 1976.
Gottfried, A. W., 1973.
Graham, F. K., Matarazzo, R. C., & Caldwell, B. M., 1956.
Hansen, E., & Bjerre, I., 1977.
Hardy, J. B., 1973.
Heider, G. M., 1971.
Heymann, P. B., & Holtz, S., 1975.
Hildebrandt, K. A., & Fitzgerald, H. E., 1979.
Holden, R. H., & Willerman, L., 1972.
Hunt, J. McV., & Rhodes, L., 1977.
Jansen, A. R., & Garland, M. J., 1976.
Jones, O. H. M., 1977.
Jones, O., 1978.
Jones, S. J., & Moss, H. A., 1971.

Jansen, A. R., & Garland, M., 1976.
Kaback, M. M., 1977.
Kappelman, M. M., 1971.
Kennedy, J., 1973.
Kennell, J., Slyter, H., & Klaus, M., 1970.
Klaus, M. H., & Kennell, J. H., 1976.
Klaus, M. H., & Kennell, J. H., 1978.
Klein, M., & Stern, L., 1971.
Kogan, K. L., 1978.
Kopp, C. B., 1974.
Korner, A. F., 1970.
Korner, A. F., 1973 (a).
Korner, A. F., 1974 (a).
Kubicek, L., 1978.
Lee, A. H., 1977.
Leiderman, P. H., Leifer, A. D., Seashore, M. J., Barnett, C. R., & Grobstein, R., 1973.
Lester, B. M., 1975.
Lipsitt, L. P., 1978.
Lorber, J., 1972.
Lorber, J., 1973.
Lubchenco, L. O., Horner, F. A., Reed, L. H., Hix, L. E. Jr., Metcalf, D. R., Cohig, R., Elliott, N. C., & Bours, M., 1963.
Macintyre, M. N., 1977.
Mack, R. W., & Johnston, F. E., 1976.
Mack, R. W., & Kleinhenz, M. E., 1974.
Massie, H. N., 1975.
Massie, H. N., 1977.
Massie, H. N., 1978.
Mayer, J., 1968.
McAndrew, L., 1976.
Mellbin, T., & Vuille, J. C., 1976.
Mercer, R. T., 1974.
Moss, H. A., 1967.
Moss, H. A., 1974.
Neuman, C. G., & Alpaugh, M., 1976.
Nielsen, G., Collins, S., Meisel, J., Lowry, M., Engh, H., & Johnson, D., 1975.
Nolan-Haley, J. H., 1976.
Osofsky, J. D., 1976.
Osofsky, J. D., & Danzger, B., 1974.
Pape, K. E. Buncic, R. J., Ashby, S., & Fitzhardinge, P. M., 1978.
Parke, R. D., & Collmer, C. W., 1975.
Pasamanick, B., & Knobloch, M., 1966.
Pollitt, E., & Eichler, A., 1976.
Pollitt, E., Eichler, A. W., & Chan, C. K., 1975.
Poskitt, E. M. E., 1977.
Powell, L. F., 1974.
Prechtl, H. F. R., 1974.
Prechtl, H., & Beintema, D., 1964.
Rachels, J., 1975.
Reich, W. T., & Smith, H., 1973.
Reynolds, E. O. R., & Stewart, A. L., 1977.
Robertson, J. A., & Fost, N., 1976.

Rosenblum, L. A., 1974.
Roskies, E., 1972.
Rowe, J., Clyman, R., Green, C., Mikkelsen, C., Haight, J., & Ataide, L., 1978.
Rubin, J. Z., Provenzano, F. J., & Luria, Z., 1974.
Rubin, R., Rosenblatt, C., & Balow, B., 1973.
Sameroff, A. J., & Zax, M., 1973.
Sander, L. W., Stechler, G., Burns, P., & Julia, H., 1970.
Sander, L. W., Stechler, G., Burns, P., & Lee, A., 1979.
Sander, L. W., Stechler, G., Julia, H., & Burns, P., 1976.
Scanlon, J. W., & Alper, M. H., 1974.
Scarr-Salapatek, S., & Williams, M. L., 1973.
Schlesinger, E. R., 1973.
Serrano, C. V., & Puffer, R. R., 1975.
Shaheen, E., Alexander, D., Truskowsky, M., & Barbero, G., 1968.
Shapiro, V., Fraiberg, S., & Adelson, E., 1976.
Shaver, B. A., 1973.
Slade, C. I., Redl, O. J., & Manguten, H. H., 1977.
Smith, D. W., 1976.
Solkoff, N., & Colten, C., 1975.
Solkoff, N., & Matuszak, D., 1975.
Stein, S. C., Schut, L., & Ames, M. D., 1974.
Stern, L., 1973.
Stewart, S. L., & Reynolds, E. O. R., 1974.
Streissguth, A. P., 1976.
Streissguth, A. P., 1978.
Streissguth, A. P., 1977.
Streissguth, A. P., Herman, C. S., & Smith, D. W., 1978 (a).
Streissguth, A. P., Herman, C. W., & Smith, D. W., 1978 (b).
Taub, H. B., Goldstein, K. M., & Caputo, D. V., 1977.
Tennes, K., & Carter, D., 1973.
Thoman, E. B., 1975 (a).
Thoman, E. B., 1975 (c).
Thoman, E. B., & Becker, P. T., 1979.
Thoman, E. B., Miano, V. N., & Freese, M. P., 1977.
Tjossen, T. D., 1976.
Trause, M. A., 1977.
Tronick, E., Als, H., & Brazelton, T. B., 1979.
Waechter, E. H., 1977.
Weintraub, M., & Frankel, J., 1977.
Whitelaw, A. G. L., 1977.
Widdowson, E. M., 1974.
Wiel, A., 1975.
Wiener, G., Rider, R. V., Oppel, W. C., Fischer, L., & Harper, P. A., 1965.
Will, J. A., Self, P. A., & Datan, N., 1976.
Wolff, P. H., 1959.
Wolff, P. H., 1966.
Wolff, P. H., 1971.
Wright, L., 1971.
B. *Perceptual-Cognitive Development and Functioning*
Ashton, R., 1976.
Barten, S., Birns, B., & Ronch, J., 1971.
Bruner, J., 1975.
Cicchetti, D., & Sroufe, L. A., 1978.

Connolly, K. J., & Bruner, J. S., 1974 (a).
Connolly, K. J., & Bruner, J. S., 1974 (b).
Decarie, T. G., 1978.
Fish, B., & Hagio, R., 1973.
Fraiberg, S., 1971.
Fraiberg, S., 1975.
Harmon, R. J., Morgan, G. A., & Klein, R. P., 1977.
Harnick, R. S., 1978.
Hunt, J. McV., 1975 (a).
Hunt, J. McV., 1976 (a).
Hunt, J. McV., 1979 (a).
Hunt, J. McV., Mohandessi, K., Ghodssi, M., & Akiyama, M., 1976.
Hunt, J. McV., Paraskevopoulos, J., Schickendanz, D., & Uzgiris, I. C., 1975.
Hunt, J. McV., & Rhodes, L., 1977.
Kopp, C. B., 1974.
Korner, A. F., 1970.
Lester, B. M., 1975.
Mameny, A. P. Jr., Dolan, A. B., & Wilson. R. S., 1974.
Mannino, F. V., 1974.
McCall, R. B., 1976.
McCall, R. B., 1977.
McCall, R. B., Eichorn, D. H., & Hogarty, P. S., 1977.
McCall, R. B., Hogarty, P. S., & Hurlburt, N., 1972.
Papousek, H., & Bernstein, P., 1969.
Papousek, H., & Papousek, M., 1975.
Paraskevopoulos, J., & Hunt, J. McV., 1971.
Roe, K. V., 1978.
Rosenblith, J. F., 1973, 1975.
Rosenblith, J. F., 1974.
Sameroff, A. J., Cashmore, T. P., & Dykes, A. C., 1973.
Scarr, S., & Weinberg, R. A., 1976.
Schaffer, H. R., 1974.
Seegmiller, B. R., & King, W. L., 1975.
Solkoff, N., & Colten, C., 1975.
Trevarthen, C. B., 1974.
Trevarthen, C. B., 1975.
Wulbert, M., Ingles, S., Kriegermann, E., & Mills, B., 1975.

C. *Temperament and Social Behavior*

Ainsworth, M. D. S., 1969.
Ainsworth, M. D. S., 1973.
Ainsworth, M. D. S., & Bell, S. M., 1969.
Aleksandrowicz, M., & Aleksandrowicz, D. R., 1974.
Aleksandrowicz, M. K., & Aleksandrowicz, D. R., 1976.
Ashton, R., 1973.
Bell, R. Q., 1971.
Bell, R. Q., 1975.
Bell, R. Q., Weller, G. M., & Waldrop, M. F., 1971.
Brazelton, T. B., 1974 (a).
Buss, A. H., & Plomin, R., 1975.
Carey, W. B., 1970.
Carey, W. B., 1973.
Carey, W. B., Lipton, L., & Myers, R. A., 1974.
Chess, S., 1967.

Chess, S., & Thomas, A., 1973.
Cicchetti, D., & Sroufe, L. A., 1978.
Condon, W. S., 1977.
Condon, W. S., & Ogston, W. D., 1967.
Condon, W. S., & Sander, L. W., 1974 (a).
Condon, W. S., & Sander, L. W., 1974 (b).
Connolly, K. J., & Bruner, J. S., 1974 (a).
Connolly, K. J., & Bruner, J. S., 1974 (b).
Decarie, T. G., 1978.
Donovan, W. L., Leavitt, L. A., & Balling, J. D., 1978.
Dunlap, W. R., & Hollingsworth, J. S., 1977.
Dunn, J. B., 1977 (a).
Dunn, J. B., & Richards, M. P. M., 1977.
Dunn, J. B., Wooding, C., & Hermann, J. B., 1977.
Elmer, E., & Gregg, C. S., 1967.
Emde, R. N., Katz, E. L., & Thorpe, J. K., 1978.
Ferguson, C. A., 1964.
Field, T. M., 1977 (a).
Field, T. M., 1978 (a).
Field, T. M., Goldberg, S., Stern, D., & Sostek, A., 1979.
Forrest, T., 1974.
Freedman, D. G., & Freedman, N., 1969.
Friedrich, W. N., & Boriskin, J. A., 1976.
Frodi, A. M., Lamb, M. E., Leavitt, L. A., & Donovan, W. L., 1978.
Gelles, R. J., 1975.
Gilberg, A. L., 1975.
Goldberg, S., 1977.
Goldstein, J., 1975.
Gorham, K. A., Des Jardins, C., Page, R., Pettis, E., & Schreiber, B., 1975.
Greenberg, M., & Morris, N., 1974.
Greenberg, N. H., 1971.
Gutton, P., 1977.
Hansen, E., & Bjerre, I., 1977.
Harmon, R. J., Morgan, G. A., & Klein, R. P., 1977.
Harper, L. V., 1975.
Heider, G. M., 1971.
Hildebrandt, K. A., & Fitzgerald, H. E., 1979.
Hunter, R. S., Kilstrom, N., Kraybill, E. N., & Loda, F., 1978.
Kolejkova, A., 1977.
Lamb, M. E., 1977 (a).
Lewis, M., & Rosenblum, L. A., 1974.
Lynch, M. A., & Roberts, J., 1977.
Maccoby, E. E., & Masters, J., 1970.
Mahler, M. S., 1974.
Mameny, A. P. Jr., Dolan, A. B., & Wilson, R. S., 1974.
Massie, H. N., 1975.
Massie, H. N., 1977.
Massie, H. N., 1978.
Mednick, B. R., 1973.
Mednick, S. A., Schulsinger, R., & Garfinkel, R., 1975.
Moss, H. A., 1967.
Newberger, E. H., Reed, R. B., Daniel, J. H., Hyde, J. N. Jr., & Kotelchuck, M., 1977.

Osofsky, J. D., 1976.
Osofsky, J. D., & Danzger, B., 1974.
Papousek, H., & Papousek, M., 1975.
Parke, R. D., & Collmer, C. W., 1975.
Pawlby, S., & Hall, F., 1979.
Perry, J. C., & Stern, D. N., 1975.
Rapoport, J., Pandoni, C., Renfield, M., Lake, C. R., & Ziegler, M. G., 1977.
Richards, M. P. M., & Bernal, J. F., 1971.
Rosenblith, J. F., 1974.
Ross, H. S., & Goldman, B. D., 1977.
Sander, L. W., 1969.
Sander, L. W., Stechler, G., Burns, P., & Lee, A., 1979.
Sander, L. W., Stechler, G., Julia, H., & Burns, P., 1976.
Sandgrund, A., Gaines, R., & Green, A., 1974 (c).
Schacter, J., Elmer, E., Ragins, N., Wimberly, F., & Lachin, J. M., 1977.
Seegmiller, B. R., & King, W. L., 1975.
Serafica, F. C., 1978.
Shaver, B. A., 1973.
Shaw, C., 1977.
Sostek, A. M., & Anders, T. F., 1977.
Standley, K., Soule, A. B. III, Copans, S. A., & Duchowny, M. S., 1974.
Stern, L., 1973.
Streissguth, A. P., Herman, C. S., & Smith, D. W., 1978 (a).
Streissguth, A. P., Herman, C. S., & Smith, D. W., 1978 (b).
Thoman, E. B., 1975 (a).
Thoman, E. B., 1975 (b).
Thoman, E. B., 1975 (c).
Thoman, E. B., Acebo, C., Dreyer, C. A., Becker, P. T., & Freese, M. P., 1979.
Thoman, E. B., Korner, A. F., & Kraemer, H. C., 1976.
Thomas, A., Chess, S., Birch, H. G., Hertzig, M. E., & Korn, S., 1963.
Thomas, A., & Chess, S., 1977.
Trevarthen, C. B., 1974.
Trevarthen, C. B., 1975.
Tronick, E., Als, H., & Brazelton, T. B., 1977 (a).
Tronick, E., & Brazelton, T. B., 1975.
Wiesenfield, A. R., & Klorman, R., 1978.
Wolff, P. H., 1959.
Wolff, P. H., 1966.
Wolff, P. H., 1969.
Wolff, P. H., 1973.
Yang, R. K., & Bell, R. Q., 1975.
Yang, R. K., Federman, E. J., & Douthitt, T. C., 1976.
Yang, R. K., & Halverson, C. F. Jr., 1976.
Zaslow, R. W., & Breger, L., 1969.

III. *Infant by Environment "Interaction"*

Adelson, E., & Fraiberg, S., 1974.
Ainsworth, M. D. S., 1967.
Ainsworth, M. D. S., 1973.
Aleksandrowicz, M., & Aleksandrowicz, D. R., 1974.
Alvy, K., 1975.
Anderson, B. J., 1977.
Anderson, B. J., Vietze, P., & Dokecki, P., 1977.
Bakeman, R., & Brown, J. V., 1977.

Ban, P. L., & Lewis, M., 1974.
Beckwith, L., Cohen, S. E., Kopp, C. B., Parmelee, A. H., & Marcy, T. G., 1976.
Bell, R. Q., 1971.
Bell, R. Q., 1974.
Bell, R. Q., & Harper, L. V., 1977.
Bernal, J., 1974.
Blehar, M. C., Lieberman, A. F., & Ainsworth, M. D. S., 1977.
Brazelton, T. B., 1974 (a).
Brazelton, T. B., 1974 (b).
Brazelton, T. B., Koslowski, B., & Main, M., 1974.
Brazelton, T. B., Tronick, E., Adamson, L., Als, H., & Weise, S., 1975.
Brown, J. V., & Bakeman, R., 1978.
Brown, J. V., Bakeman, R., Snyder, P. A., Frederickson, W. T., Morgan, S. T., & Hepler, R., 1975.
Bruch, H., 1973.
Buckhalt, J. A., Rutherford, R. B., & Goldberg, K. E., 1978.
Buss, A. H., & Plomin, R., 1975.
Cicirelli, V. G., 1978.
Clarke-Stewart, K. A., 1973.
Clarke-Stewart, K. A., 1978 (b).
Condon, W. S., & Sander, L. W., 1974 (a).
Condon, W. S., & Sander, L. W., 1974 (b).
Dunn, J. B., 1976.
Dunn, J. B., & Richards, M. P. M., 1977.
Elardo, R., Bradley, R., & Caldwell, B. M., 1975.
Elardo, R., Bradley, R., & Caldwell, B. M., 1977.
Escalona, S. K., 1973.
Feiring, C., & Taylor, J., 1979.
Field, T. M., 1977 (a).
Field, T. M., 1977 (c).
Field, T. M., 1978 (a).
Field, T. M., 1978 (b).
Field, T. M., 1978 (c).
Field, T. M., 1979 (b).
Field, T. M., Goldberg, S., Stern, D., & Sostek, A., 1979.
Fraiberg, S., 1971.
Friedman, S., Thompson, M. A., Crawley, S., Criticos, A. D., Iacobbo, M., Rogers, P. P., & Richardson, L., 1976.
Friedrich, W. N., & Boriskin, J. A., 1976.
Gelles, R. J., 1975.
Gewirtz, J. L., & Boyd, E. F., 1976.
Gewirtz, J. L., & Boyd, E. F., 1977.
Goldberg, S., 1977.
Goldberg, S., Brachfeld, S., & DiVitto, B., 1978.
Gunnar-Vongnechtlen, M. R., 1978.
Gutton, P., 1977.
Harnick, R. S., 1978.
Hofer, M. A., 1975.
Hollenbeck, A. R., 1978.
Jacobs, B. A., & Moss, H. A., 1976.
Kaye, K., 1977.
Kogan, K. L., 1978.
Kolejkova, A., 1977.

Korner, A. F., 1974.
Lamb, M. E., 1976 (a).
Lamb, M. E., 1977 (a).
Landau, R., 1976.
Lewis, M., & Rosenblum, L. A., 1974.
Lytton, H., 1971.
Mednick, B. R., 1973.
Mercer, R. T., 1974.
Osofsky, J. D., 1976.
Osofsky, J. D., & Danzger, B., 1974.
Overton, W. P., 1973.
Parke, R. D., & Collmer, C. W., 1975.
Parke, R. D., & O'Leary, S. E., 1976.
Parke, R. D., Power, T. G., & Gottman, J., 1979.
Parke, R. D., & Sawin, D. B., 1977 (a).
Pawlby, S., 1977.
Perry, J. H., & Freedman, D. A., 1973.
Powell, L. F., 1974.
Raguis, N., Schachter, J., Elmer, E., Preismare, R., Bower, A. E., & Harway, V., 1975.
Ramey, C., Mills, P., Campbell, F., & O'Brien, C., 1975.
Ringler, N. M., Kennell, J. H., Jarvella, R., Navojosky, B. J., & Klaus, M. H., 1975.
Ross, H. S., & Goldman, B. D., 1977.
Rubin, J. Z., Provenzano, F. J., & Luria, Z., 1974.
Sackett, G. P., 1979.
Sameroff, A. J., 1972.
Sameroff, A. J., 1975 (a).
Sameroff, A. J., 1978.
Sameroff, A. J., & Chandler, M. J., 1975.
Sandgrund, A., Gaines, R., & Green, A., 1974 (a).
Sandgrund, A., Gaines, R., & Green, A., 1974 (b).
Sandgrund, A., Gaines, R., & Green, A., 1974 (c).
Sawin, D. B., Langlois, J. H., & Leitner, E. F., 1977.
Scarr-Salapatek, S., & Williams, M. L., 1973.
Seegmiller, B. R., & King, W. L., 1975.
Serafica, F. C., 1978.
Sherrod, K. B., Friedman, S., Crawley, S., Drake, D., & Devieux, J., 1977.
Sperber, Z., & Weiland, I. H., 1973.
Sroufe, L. A., 1977.
Stern, D. N., 1971.
Stern, D. N., 1974 (a).
Stern, D. N., 1974 (b).
Stern, D. N., 1977.
Thoman, E. B., 1974.
Thoman, E. B., 1975 (b).
Thoman, E. B., 1978.
Thoman, E. B., Becker, P. T., & Freese. M. P., 1979.
Thoman, E. B., Leiderman, P. H., & Olson, J. P., 1972.
Thomas, E. A. C., & Martin, J. A., 1976.
Tronick, E., Adamson, L., Wise, S., Als, H., & Brazelton, T. B., 1975.
Tronick, E., Als, H., & Adamson, L., 1977.
Tronick, E., Als, H., Adamson, L., Wise, S., & Brazelton, T. B., 1978.
Tronick, E., Als, H., & Brazelton, T. B., 1977 (b).

Tronick, E., Als, H., & Brazelton, T. B., 1979.
Tulkin, S. R., & Kagan, J., 1972.
Waters, E., 1978.
Williams, T. H., 1974.
Wolff, P. H., 1971.
Wolff, P. H., 1973.
Wulbert, M., Ingles, S., Kriegermann, E., & Mills, B., 1975.
Yarrow, L. J., 1967.
Yarrow, L. J., & Goodwin, M., 1965.
Zegiob, L., & Forehand, R., 1975.

IV. *Outcomes (Criterion Variables)*
    A. *Infant and Young Child*
       Abramowicz, H. K., & Richardson, S. A., 1975.
       Ainsworth, M. D. S., & Bell, S. M., 1969.
       Ainsworth, M. D. S., & Bell, S. M., 1974.
       Ainsworth, M. D. S., & Bell, S. M., 1977.
       Ainsworth, M., Bell, S., & Stayton, P., 1974.
       Als, H., Tronick, E., Adamson, L., & Brazelton, T. B., 1976.
       Ambuel, G., & Harris, B., 1963.
       Ames, M. D., & Schut, L., 1972.
       Anan, M. J., 1976.
       Anthony, E. J., 1974.
       Anthony, E. J., & Benedek, T., 1971.
       Appleton, T., Clifton, R., & Goldberg, S., 1975.
       Bagg, C. E., & Crookes, T. G., 1975.
       Bavlov, B., Rubin, R., & Rosen, M., 1975.
       Ban, P. L., & Lewis, M., 1974.
       Baumrind, D., 1975.
       Beckwith, L., Cohen, S. E., Kopp, C. B., Parmelee, A. H., & Marcy, T. G., 1976.
       Bell, R. Q., 1972.
       Bell, R. Q., 1975.
       Bell, R. Q., Weller, G. M., & Waldrop, M. F., 1971.
       Bell, S. M., & Ainsworth, M. D. S., 1972.
       Bennett, V. C., & Bardon, J. I., 1977.
       Berger, M., Lezine, I., Harrison, A., & Boisselier, F., 1973.
       Biron, P., Mongeau, J. G., & Bertrand, D., 1977.
       Blake, A., Stewart, A., & Turcan, D., 1975.
       Borjeson, M., 1976.
       Bowlby, J., 1969 (a).
       Bowlby, J., 1969 (b).
       Brackbill, Y., 1973.
       Brackbill, Y., et al., 1974.
       Bradley, R., & Caldwell, B., 1976.
       Brazelton, T. B., 1971.
       Brazelton, T. B., 1973 (a).
       Brazelton, T. B., Robery, J. S., & Collier, G. A., 1969.
       Broman, S. H., Nichols, P. L., & Kennedy, W. A., 1975.
       Brook, C. D. G., Huntley, R. M. C., & Slack, J., 1972.
       Broussard, E. R., 1976.
       Broussard, E. R., & Hartner, M. S. S., 1970.
       Broussard, E. R., & Hartner, M. S. S., 1971.
       Bruch, H., 1973.

Bruner, J. S.,1969.
Bruner, J., 1971.
Buss, A. H., & Plomin, R., 1975.
Butcher, R. E., Hawver, K., Burbacher, T., & Scott, W., 1975.
Caputo, D. V., 1974.
Charney, E., Goodman, H. C., McBride, M., Lyon, B., & Pratt, R., 1976.
Clark, A., 1976.
Clark, A., & Alfonso, D. D., 1976.
Clark, A. M., & Clarke, A. D. B., 1976.
Clarke-Stewart, K. A., 1973.
Clarke-Stewart, K. A., 1978 (b).
Condon, W. S., & Sander, L. W., 1974 (a).
Condon, W. S., & Sander, L. W., 1974 (b).
David, M., & Appell, G., 1969.
Deutsch, C. P., 1973.
Dietrich, K. N., & Starr, R. H., 1978.
Draper, H. H., 1977.
Drillien, C. M., 1964.
Duff, R. S., & Campbell, A. G. M., 1976.
Dunn, J. B., 1977 (b).
Dunn, J. B., & Richards, M. P. M., 1977.
Dunn, J. B., Wooding, C., & Hermann, J. B., 1977.
Edwards, L. E., Dickes, W. F., Alton, J. R., & Hakanson, E. Y., 1978.
Eid, E. K., 1970.
Elardo, R., Bradley, R., & Caldwell, B. M., 1975.
Elardo, R., Bradley, R., & Caldwell, B. M., 1977.
Eldred, C., Rosenthal, D., Wender, P. H., Kety, S. S., Schulsinger, F., Weiner, J., & Jacobsen, B., 1976.
El-Gwebaly, N., & Offord, D. R., 1977.
Ellingen, R. J., Dutch, S. J., & Mcintire, M. S., 1974.
Elmer, E., & Gregg. C. S., 1967.
Fanaroff, A. A., Kennell, J. H., & Klaus, M. H., 1972.
Federman, E. J., & Yang, R. K., 1976.
Ferreira, A. J., 1960.
Field, T. M., 1978 (a).
Field, T. M., 1979 (b).
Field, T. M., Dabiri, C., Hallock, N., & Shuman, H. H., 1977.
Field, T. M., Goldberg, S., Stern, D., & Sostek, A., 1979.
Field, T. M., Hallock, N., Ting, G., Dempsey, J., Dabiri, C., & Shuman, H. H., 1978.
Fisch, R. O., Bilek, M. K., & Ulstrom, R., 1975.
Fish, B., & Hagio, R., 1973.
Fitzhardinge, P. M., 1976.
Fletcher, J., 1975.
Fomon, S. J., 1974.
Foss, B. M., 1969.
Fost, N., 1976.
Fraiberg, S., 1971.
Francis-Williams, J., & Davies, P. A., 1974.
Freeman, J. M., 1973.
Friedrich, W. N., & Boriskin, J. A., 1976.
Garn, S. M., 1976.
Garn, S. M., Bailey, S. M., & Higgins, I. T. T., 1976.

Gauthier, V., Fortin, C., Drapeau, P., Breton, J. J., Gosselin, J., Quintal, L., Weisnagel, J., Tetreault, L., & Pinard, E., 1977.
Gelles, R. J., 1975.
Goldberg, S., 1977.
Goldberg, S., Brachfeld, S., & DiVitto, B., 1978.
Golden, M., & Birns, B., 1976.
Goldstein, J., 1975.
Goldstein, K. M., Caputo, D. V., & Taub, H. B., 1976.
Gottfried, A. W., 1973.
Green, H. G., 1974.
Grimm, E., & Venet, W. R., 1966.
Hager, A., 1977.
Hales, D. J., Lozoff, B., Sopa, R., & Kennell, J. H., 1977.
Hanes, M. L., & Dunn, S. K., 1978.
Hansen, E., & Bjerre, I., 1977.
Hanson, D. R., Gottesman, I. I., & Meehl, P. E., 1977.
Hardy, J. B., 1973.
Harper, L. V., 1975.
Harper, L. V., 1972.
Harper, R. G., Solish, G., Purow, G. L., Sang, H. M., & Panepinto, W. C., 1974.
Hartz, A., Glefer, E., & Rimm, A., 1977.
Hawkins, R. C. II, 1977.
Heider, G. M., 1971.
Helfer, R., 1974.
Henry, M., Ouellette, E., & Rosett, L., 1977.
Hess, R. D., 1970.
Himwich, W. A., Hall, J. S., & MacArthur, W. F., 1977.
Holden, R. H., & Willerman, L., 1972.
Hollstedt, C., Olsson, O., & Rydberg, W., 1977.
Horowitz, F. D., 1978.
Hunt, J. McV., 1976 (b).
Hunt, J. McV., 1979 (a).
Hunt, J. McV., Mohandessi, K., Ghodssi, M., & Akiyama, M., 1976.
Hunt, J. McV., Paraskevopoulos, J., Schickedanz, D., & Uzgiris, I. C., 1975.
Hunt, J. McV., & Rhodes, L., 1977.
Hunter, R. S., Kilstrom, N., Kraybill, E. N., & Loda, F., 1978.
Jansen, A. R., & Garland, M. J., 1976.
Jones, K. L., Smith, D. W., Streissguth, A. P., & Myrianthopoulos, N. C., 1974.
Jones, K. L., Smith, D. W., Ulleland, C. N., & Streissguth, A. P., 1973.
Jones, S. J., & Moss, H. A., 1971.
Kaffman, M., & Elizur, E., 1977.
Kagan, J., 1969.
Kagan, J., 1971.
Kagan, J., & Klein, R. E., 1973.
Kagan, J., & Klein, R. E., 1975.
Kagan, J., & Moss, H. A., 1962.
Kaplan, B. J., 1972.
Kappelman, M. M., 1971.
Karnes, M. B., 1973.
Kaye, K., 1977.
Kellam, S. G., Emsinger, M. E., & Turner, R. J., 1977.
Kilbride, H. W., Johnson, D. L. & Streissguth, A. P., 1977.
Klaus, M. H., & Kennell, J. H., 1977.

Klaus, M. H., & Kennell, J. H., 1976.
Klaus, M. H., & Kennell, J. H., 1978.
Klein, M., & Stern, L., 1971.
Klein, R. E., Lasky, R. E., Yarbrough, C., Habicht, J. P., & Sellers, M. J., 1977.
Kopf, R. C., & McFadden, E. L., 1974.
Kopp, C. B., 1974.
Korner, A. F., 1970.
Korner, A. F., 1973 (a).
Korner, A. F., 1973 (b).
Korner, A. F., & Grobstein, R., 1967.
Korner, A., & Thoman, E. B., 1970.
Landeeman-Dwyer, S., Keller, L. S., & Streissguth, A. P., 1978.
Lee, A. H., 1977.
Leiderman, P. H., 1978.
Leonard, M. F., Rhymes, J. P., & Solnit, A. J., 1966.
Lester, B. M., Emory, E. K., Huffman, S. L., & Eitzman, D. V., 1976.
Lewis, M., & Lee-Painter, S., 1974.
Lewis, M., & Wilson, C. D., 1972.
Light, R., 1973.
Lipsitt, L. P., 1978.
Little, R. E., Schultz, F., & Mandell, W., 1976.
Little, R. E., & Streissguth, A. P., 1978.
Lorber, J., 1973.
Lubchenco, L. O., Horner, F. A., Reed, L. H., Hix, L. E. Jr., Metcalf, D. R., Cohig, R., Elliot, N. C., & Bours, M., 1963.
Lynch, M. A., & Roberts, J., 1977.
Lynch, M. A., Roberts, J., & Gordon, M., 1976.
Maccoby, E. E., & Masters, J., 1970.
Macfarlane, A., 1977.
Mack, R. W., & Johnston, F. E., 1976.
Mack, R. W., & Kleinhenz, M. E., 1974.
Magrab, P. R., 1976.
Mahler, M. S., 1974.
Mameny, A. P. Jr., Dolan, A. B., & Wilson, R. S., 1974.
Marjonibanks, K., 1976.
Martin, J., Martin. D., Lund, C., & Streissguth, A. P., 1977.
Massie, H. N., 1975.
Massie, H. N., 1977.
Massie, H. N., 1978.
Mayer, J., 1968.
McAndrew, L., 1976.
McCall, R. B., 1976.
McCall, R. B., Hogarty, P. S., & Hurlburt, N., 1972.
McGowan, M. N., 1977.
Mech, E. V., 1973.
Mednick, B. R., 1973.
Mednick, S. A., Schulsinger, R., & Garfinkel, R., 1975.
Mellbin, T., & Vuille, J. C., 1976.
Miller, H. C., 1973.
Miller, H. C., 1974.
Milner, J., & Williams, P., 1978.
Mitchell, R., 1975.
Mulvihill, J., Klimas, J., Stokes, D., & Risenberg, H., 1976.

Naeye, R. L., Blane, W., & Blane, P. C., 1973.
Neale, J. M., & Weintraub, S., 1975.
Newberger, E. H., Reed, R. B., Daniel, J. H., Hyde, J. N. Jr., & Kotelchuk, M., 1977.
Nuckholls, K. B., Cassell, J., & Kaplan, B. H., 1972.
Osofsky, H. J., 1974.
Osofsky, H. J., 1975 (a).
Osofsky, H. J., 1975 (b).
Osofsky, H. J., & Kendall, N., 1974.
Ounsted, C., Oppenheimer, R., & Lindsay, J., 1975.
Page, E. B., 1975.
Palani, P. E., 1974.
Pape, K. E., Buncic, R. J., Ashby, S., & Fitzhardinge, P. M., 1978.
Paraskevopoulos, J., & Hunt, J. McV., 1971.
Parke, R. D., & Collmer, C. W., 1975.
Parke, R. D., & Sawin, D. B., 1977 (b).
Paulson, M., 1975.
Perry, J. H., & Freedman, D. A., 1973.
Philipps, C., & Johnson, N. E., 1977.
Pollitt, E., & Eichler, A., 1976.
Poskitt, E. M. E., 1977.
Poskitt, E. M. E., & Cole, T. J., 1978.
Powell, L. F., 1974.
Raguis, N., Schachter, J., Elmer, E., Preismare, R., Bower, A. E., & Harway, V., 1975.
Ramey, C., Mills, P., Campbell, F., & O'Brien, C., 1975.
Rau, J. H., & Kaye, H., 1977.
Reynolds, E. O. R., & Stewart, A. L., 1977.
Richardson, S. A., Birch, H. G., & Hertzig, M. E., 1973.
Ringler, N. M., Kennell, J. H., Jarvella, R., Navojosky, B. J., & Klaus, M. H., 1975.
Roe, K. V., 1978.
Rose, H. E., & Mayer, J., 1968.
Rosenblith, J. F., 1973, 1975.
Rosenblith, J. F., 1974.
Rosenzweig, M. R., & Bennett, E. L., 1977.
Rosett, H., Ouellette, E., & Weiner, L., 1976.
Ross, H. S., & Goldman, B. D., 1977.
Rubenstein, J., 1967.
Rubenstein, J. L., 1977.
Rubin, R., Rosenblatt, C., & Balow, B., 1973.
Rutter, M., 1974.
Salans, L. B., Cushman, S. W., & Weissman, R. E., 1973.
Salo, K. E., 1975.
Sameroff, A. J., 1978.
Sameroff, A. J., & Chandler, M. J., 1975.
Sander, L., Snyder, P., Rosett, H., Lee, A., Gould, J., & Ouellette, E., 1977.
Sander, L. W., Stechler, G., Burns, P., & Julia, H., 1970.
Sandgrund, A., Gaines, R., & Green, A., 1974 (a).
Sawin, D. B., & Parke, R. D., 1976.
Scanlon, J. W., & Alper, M. H., 1974.
Scarr, S., & Weinberg, R. A., 1976.
Scarr-Salapatek, S., & Williams, M. L., 1973.

Schacter, J., Elmer, E., Ragins, N., Wimberly, F., & Lachin, J. M., 1977.
Schlesinger, E. R., 1973.
Schneider, C., Hoffmeister, J. K., & Helfer, R. E., 1976.
Seegmiller, B. R., & King, W. L., 1975.
Senn, M. J. E., & Hartford, C., 1968.
Serrano, C. V., & Puffer, R. R., 1975.
Shaheen, E., Alexander, D., Truskowsky, M., & Barbero, G., 1968.
Shapiro, V., Fraiberg, S., & Adelson, E., 1976.
Shearman, R. P., Shutt, D. A., & Smith, T. G., 1974.
Shereshesky, P. M., & Yarrow, L. J., 1974.
Singer, G., Stern, Y., & van der Spery, H. I. J., 1976.
Slade, C. I., Redl, O. J., & Manguten, H. H., 1977.
Solkoff, N., & Matuszak, D., 1975.
Solomon, R., & Decaire, T., 1976.
Sosa, R., Kennell, J. H., Klaus, M., & Urrutia, J. J., 1976.
Sostek, A. M., & Anders, T. F., 1977.
Spelke, E., Zelazo, P., Kager, J., & Kotelchuck, M., 1973.
Sroufe, L. A., & Waters, E., 1977.
Standley, K., & Soule, A. B., 1974.
Stein, S. C., Schut, L., & Ames, M. D., 1974.
Stein, Z., & Susser, M., 1976.
Stern, L., 1973.
Stewart, S. L., & Reynolds, E. O. R., 1974.
Streissguth, A. P., 1976.
Streissguth, A. P., 1977.
Streissguth, A. P., 1978.
Streissguth, A. P., Herman, C. S., & Smith, D. W., 1978 (a).
Streissguth, A. P., Herman, C. S., & Smith, D. W., 1978 (b).
Strom, R., & Greathouse, B., 1975.
Sugar, M., 1976.
Sveger, T., Lindberg, T., Weilbull, B., & Ollson, V. L., 1975.
Taitz, T. S., 1971.
Tanner, J. M., 1974.
Taub, H. B., Goldstein, K. M., & Caputo, D. V., 1977.
Tennes, K., & Carter, D., 1973.
Thoman, E. B., 1975 (c).
Thoman, E. B., 1978.
Thoman, E. B., & Becker, P. T., 1979.
Thoman, E. B., Korner, A. F., & Kraemer, H. C., 1976.
Thoman, E. B., Miano, V. N., & Freese, M. P., 1977.
Thomas, A., Chess, S., Birch, H. G., Hertzig, M. E., & Korn, S., 1963.
Thomas, A., & Chess, S., 1977.
Thompson, W. R., & Grusec, J., 1970.
Tizard, J., 1974.
Tizard, B., & Rees, J., 1974.
Tizard, J., & Tizard, B., 1974.
Trause, M. A., 1977.
Tronik, E., & Brazelton, T. B., 1975.
Tulkin, S. R., 1977.
Wachs, T. D., 1976.
Wachs, T. D., 1979.
Wachs, T. D., Uzgiris, I. C., & Hunt, J. McV., 1971.
Walberg, H., & Marjonibanks, K., 1973.

Walters, C. E., 1965.
Walters, C. E., 1975.
Warner, R. H., & Rosett, H. L., 1975.
Warren, N., 1973.
Waters, E., 1978.
White, B. L., 1971.
White, B. L., 1975.
White, B. L., 1978.
White, B. L., Kaban, B., Shapiro, B., & Attanucci, J., 1977.
White, B. L., & Watts, J. C., 1973.
Whitelaw, A. G. L., 1976.
Whitelaw, A. G. L., 1977.
Widdowson, E. M., 1974.
Wiel, A., 1975.
Wiener, G., Rider, R. V., Oppel, W. C., Fischer, L., & Harper, P. A., 1965.
Willerman, L., Broman, S. H., & Fiedler, M., 1970.
Williams, T. H., 1974.
Wolff, P. H., 1973.
Yang, R., Zweig, A. R., Douthit, T. C., & Federman, E. J., 1976.
Yang, R. K., & Halverson, C. F. Jr., 1976.
Yarrow, L. J., Pedersen, F. A., & Rubenstein, J., 1977.
Yarrow, L. J., Rubenstein, J. L., & Pedersen, F. A., 1975.
Zaslow, R. W., & Breger, L., 1969.
Zax, M., Sameroff, A. J., & Babigian, H. M., 1977.
B. *Family Functioning (Social Environment)*
Adelson, E., & Fraiberg, S., 1974.
Ames, M. D., & Schut, L., 1972.
Ban, P. L., & Lewis, M., 1974.
Bell, R. Q., 1972.
Benfield, D. G., Lieb, S. A., & Reuter, J., 1976.
Benfield, D. G., Leib, S. A., & Vollman, J. H., 1978.
Bennett, V. C., & Bardon, J. I., 1977.
Bergman, A. B., 1974.
Berkson, G., 1974.
Bibring, G. L., 1959.
Bibring, G. L., Dwyer, T. F., Huntington, D. S., & Valenstein, A. F., 1961.
Blake, A., Stewart, A., & Turcan, D., 1975.
Blehar, M. C., Lieberman, A. F., & Ainsworth, M. D. S., 1977.
Bowlby, J., 1969 (a).
Bowlby, J., 1969 (b).
Buss, A. H., & Plomin, R., 1975.
Caplan, G., Mason, E., & Kaplan, D. M., 1965.
de Chateau, P., 1976.
Choi, M., 1975.
Clark, A., 1976.
Clark, A. L., & Alfonso, D. D., 1976 (a).
Clark, A. L., & Alfonso, D. D., 1976 (b).
Clarke-Stewart, K. A., 1978 (b).
Cohler, B., Grunebaum, H., & Weiss, J., 1970.
Colen, B. D., 1974.
Crawley, S. B., Rogers, P. P., Friedman, S., Jacobson, M., Criticos, A., Richardson, L., & Thompson, M. A., 1978.

Cummings, S. T., 1976.
Diamond, J. M., 1978.
DiVitto, B., & Goldberg, S., 1978.
Donovan, W. L., Leavitt, L. A., & Balling, J. D., 1978.
Drotan, D., Baskiewitz, A., Irwin, N., Kennell, J., & Klaus, M., 1975.
Duff, R. S., & Campbell, A. G. M., 1976.
Dunlap, W. R., & Hollingsworth, J. S., 1977.
Dunn, J. B., 1976.
Dunn, J. B., 1977 (a).
Dunn, J. B., 1977 (b).
Dunn, J. B., 1977 (c).
Dunn, J. B., & Richards, M. P. M., 1977.
Dunn, J. B., Wooding, C., & Hermann, J. B., 1977.
Ellis, H. L., 1974.
Field, T. M., 1977 (a).
Field, T. M., Dabiri, C., Hallock, N., & Shuman, H. H., 1977.
Field, T. M., Hallock, N., Ting, G., Dempsey, J., Dabiri, C., & Shuman, H. H., 1978.
Fitzhardinge, P. M., 1976.
Fletcher, J., 1974.
Fletcher, J., 1975.
Forrest, T., 1974.
Fost, N., 1976.
Freeman, J. M., 1973.
Friedrich, W. N., & Boriskin, J. A., 1976.
Frodi, A. M., Lamb, M. E., Leavitt, L. A., & Donovan, W. L., 1978.
Frommer, E. A., & O'Shea, G., 1973.
Gewirtz, J. L., 1972.
Gilman, R., & Knox, 1976.
Goldberg, S., 1977.
Goldberg, S., Brachfeld, S., & DiVitto, B., 1978.
Goldstein, J., 1975.
Gordon, R. E., & Gordon, K., 1957.
Gorham, K. A., Des Jardins, C., Page, R., Pettis, E., & Schreiber, B., 1975.
Greenberg, M., & Morris, N., 1974.
Greenberg, N. H., 1971.
Grimm, E., & Venet, W. R., 1966.
Hales, D. J., Lozoff, B., Sopa, R., & Kennell, J. H., 1977.
Hanes, M. L., & Dunn, S. K., 1978.
Harper, L. V., 1975.
Harper, R. G., Solish, G., Purow, G. L., Sang, H. M., & Panepinto, W. C., 1974.
Harrell, J. E., & Ridley, C. A., 1975.
Helfer, R., 1974.
Heymann, P. B., & Holtz, S., 1975.
Hildebrandt, K. A., & Fitzgerald, H. E., 1979.
Hill, V., 1978.
Hobbs, D. F., 1965.
Hollender, J. W., 1973.
Horowitz, F. D., 1978.
Hunter, R. S., Kilstrom, N., Kraybill, E. N., & Loda, F., 1978.
Jansen, A. R., & Garland, M. J., 1976.
Jones, O. H. M., 1977.
Jones, O., 1978.

Jonsen, A. R., & Garland, M., 1976.
Kaback, M. M., 1977.
Kagan, J., 1977.
Kennedy, J., 1973.
Kennell, G., Gordon, D., & Klaus, M., 1970.
Kennell, J. H., Jerauld, R., Wolfe, H., Chester, D., Kreger, N. C., McAlpine, W., Steffa, M., & Klaus, M. H., 1974.
Kennell, J. H., Trause, M. A., & Klaus, M. H., 1974.
Kennell, J. H., Trause, M. A., & Klaus, M. H., 1975.
Kennell, J. H., Slyter, H., & Klaus, M., 1970.
Klaus, M. H., Jerauld, R., Kreger, N. C., McAlpine, W., Steffa, M., & Kennell, J. H., 1972.
Klaus, M. H., & Kennell, J. H., 1976.
Klaus, M. H., & Kennell, J. H., 1978.
Klein, M., & Stern, L., 1971.
Kogan, K. L., 1978.
Kolejkova, A., 1977.
Korner, A. F., 1967.
Korner, A. F., 1974 (a).
Korner, A. F., 1974 (b).
Korner, A. F., & Grobstein, R., 1967.
Kotelchuck, M., 1976.
Kubicek, L., 1978.
Lamb, M. E., 1977 (b).
Lawson, K., Daum, C., & Turkewitz, G., 1977.
Leiderman, P. H., 1978.
Leiderman, P. H., Leifer, A. D., Seashore, M. J., Barnett, C. B., & Grobstein, R., 1973.
Leifer, M., 1977.
Leifer, A. D., Liederman, P. H., Barnett, C. R., & Williams, J. A., 1972.
LeMasters, E. E., 1965.
Lewis, E., 1976.
Lewis, M., & Lee-Painter, S., 1974.
Lewis, M., & Rosenblum, L. A., 1974.
Lewis, M., & Weintraub, M., 1976.
Littman, B., et al., 1976.
Lorber, J., 1973.
Lynch, M. A., & Roberts, J., 1977.
Macfarlane, A., 1977.
Macintyre, M. N., 1977.
Magrab, P. R., 1976.
McAndrew, L., 1976.
McGowan, M. N., 1977.
Mech, E. V., 1973.
Mercer, R. T., 1974.
Mercer, R. T., 1977.
Milner, J., & Williams, P., 1978.
Mitchell, R., 1975.
Moss, H. A., 1967.
Moss, H. A., 1974.
Nolan-Haley, J. H., 1976.
Nunnally, D., & Aguiar, M., 1974.
Osofsky, H. J., 1974.

Osofsky, J. D., 1976.
Osofsky, J. D., & Danzger, B., 1974.
Ounsted, C., Oppenheimer, R., & Lindsay, J., 1974.
Ounsted, C., Oppenheimer, R., & Lindsay, J., 1975.
Papousek, H., & Papousek, M., 1975.
Papousek, H., & Papousek, M., 1977.
Parke, R. D., 1974.
Parke, R. D., & Collmer, C. W., 1975.
Parke, R. D., & Sawin, D. B., 1976.
Parke, R. D., & Sawin, D. B., 1977 (b).
Paulson, M., 1977.
Pawlby, S., & Hall, F., 1979.
Pollitt, E., Eichler, A. W., & Chan, C. K., 1975.
Rachels, J., 1975.
Ramey, C., Mills, P., Campbell, F., & O'Brien, C., 1975.
Rau, J. H., & Kaye, H., 1977.
Reich, W. T., & Smith, H., 1973.
Rexford, E. N., Sander, L. W., & Shapiro, T., 1976.
Richards, M. P. H., 1974.
Richards, M. P. M., & Bernal, J. F., 1971.
Rising, S. S., 1974.
Robertson, J. A., & Fost, N., 1976.
Robson, K. S., 1967.
Robson, K. S., & Moss, H. A., 1967.
Robson, K. S., & Moss, H. A., 1970.
Rosenblum, L. A., 1974.
Rosenthal, M., 1973.
Roskies, E., 1972.
Rowe, J., Clyman, R., Green, C., Mikkelsen, C., Haight, J., & Ataide, L., 1978.
Rubenstein, J. L., Pederson, F. A., & Yarrow, L. L., 1977.
Rutter, M., 1974.
Salk, L., 1973.
Salk, L., 1977.
Salo, K. E., 1975.
Sameroff, A. J., 1972.
Sameroff, A. J., 1975 (a).
Sameroff, A. J., 1975 (b).
Sameroff, A. J., 1978.
Sameroff, A. J., & Chandler, M. J., 1975.
Sander, L. W., 1969.
Sander, L. W., Stechler, G., Burns, P., & Julia, H., 1970.
Sander, L. W., Stechler, G., Burns, P., & Lee, A., 1979.
Sander, L. W., Stechler, G., Julia, H., & Burns, P., 1976.
Sandgrund, A., Gaines, R., & Green, A., 1974 (b).
Sandgrund, A., Gaines, R., & Green, A., 1974 (c).
Sawin, D. B., & Parke, R. D., 1976.
Schlesinger, E. R., 1973.
Seashore, M. J., Leifer, A. D., Barnett, C. R., & Leiderman, P. H., 1973.
Senn, M. J. E., & Hartford, C., 1966.
Serafica, F. C., 1978.
Shaffer, D., Pettigrew, A., Wolking, S., & Zajicek, E., 1978.
Shapiro, V., Fraiberg, S., & Adelson, E., 1976.
Shaver, B. A., 1973.

Shaw, C., 1977.
Sroufe, L. A., & Waters, E., 1977.
Stein, S. C., Schut, L. & Ames, M. D., 1974.
Sugarman, M., 1977.
Swanson, J., 1978.
Thoman, E. B., 1975 (a).
Thoman, E. B., Acebo, C., Dreyer, C. A., Becker, P. T., & Freese, M. P., 1979.
Thoman, E. B., Korner, A. F., & Beason-Williams, L., 1977.
Tronick, E., Als, H., & Brazelton, T. B., 1977 (a).
Waechter, E. H., 1977.
Walters, C. E., 1975.
Weintraub, M., 1978.
Weintraub, M., & Frankel, J., 1977.
Wente, A. S., & Crockenberg, S. B., 1976.
White, B. L., 1975.
Whiten, A., 1977.
Williams, C. C., Williams, R. A., Griswold, M. J., & Holmes, T. H., 1975.
Williams, T. H., 1974.
Wolff, P. H., 1976.
Wulbert, M., Ingles, S., Kriegermann, E., & Mills, B., 1975.
Zuk, G. H., Miller, R. L., Bartram, J. B., & Kling, F., 1961.
C. *Parenting Behaviors*
Ashton, P. T., 1978.
Bell, R. Q., 1974.
Brody, S., 1956.
Brown, J. V., & Bakeman, R., 1978.
Buckhalt, J. A., Rutherford, R. B., & Goldberg, K. E., 1978.
Carlsson, S. J., Faderberg, H., Hornemann, L., Hwang, C. P., Larsson, K., Rodholm, M., Schaller, J., Danielson, B., & Gundewall, C., 1978.
Cohen, E. S., & Beckwith, L., 1977.
Cohler, B. J., Grunebaum, H. U., Weiss, J. L., Hartman, C. R., & Gallant, D. H., 1976.
Donovan, W. L., Leavitt, L. A., & Balling, J. D., 1978.
Dreyfus-Brisac, C., 1974.
Freese, M. P., & Thoman, E. B., 1978.
Gewirtz, H. B., & Gewirtz, J. L., 1969.
Gilberg, A. L., 1975.
Greenberg, M., Rosenberg, I., 1973.
Hansen, E., & Bjerre, I., 1977.
Helfer, R., 1974.
Hock, E., 1978.
Kestenberg, J. S., 1959.
de Lissovoy, V., 1973.
Singer, A., 1974.
Sosa, R., Kennell, J. H., Klaus, M., & Urrutia, J. J., 1976.
Thoman, E. B., 1975 (b).
Thoman, E. B., Barnett, C. R., & Leiderman, P. H., 1971.
Thoman, E. B., Turner, A. M., Leiderman, P. H., & Barnett, C. R., 1970.
Tulkin, S. R., 1977.
Tulkin, S. R., & Cohler, B. J., 1973.
Wiesenfield, A. R., & Klorman, R., 1978.
Will, J. A., Self, P. A., & Datan, N., 1976.

COMPREHENSIVE BIBLIOGRAPHY

Abernethy, V., & Abernethy, G. L. Risk for unwanted pregnancy among mentally ill adolescent girls. *American Journal of Orthopsychiatry*, 1974, 44, 442-449.

Abernethy, V., Robbins, D., Abernethy, G. L., Grunebaum, H. & Weiss, J. L. Identification of women at risk for unwanted pregnancy, *American Journal of Psychiatry*, 1975, 132, 1027-1031.

Abramowicz, H. K., & Richardson, S. A. Epidemiology of severe mental retardation in children. *American Journal of Mental Deficiency*, 1975, 80, 18-39.

Ackerman, N. W. Disturbances of mothering and criteria for treatment. *American Journal of Orthopsychiatry*, 1956, 26, 252-263.

Adams, B. N., Brownstein, C. A., Rennalls, I. M., & Schmitt, M. H. The pregnant adolescent: A group approach. *Adolescence*, 1976, 11, 467-485.

Adams, M. Early concerns of primagravida mothers regarding infant care activities. *Nursing Research*, 1963, 12, 72-77.

Adelson, E., & Fraiberg, S. Gross motor development in infants blind from birth. *Child Development*, 1974, 45, 114-126.

Ainsworth, M. D. S. *Infancy in Uganda: Infant Care and the Growth of Attachment.* Baltimore: The Johns Hopkins Press, 1967.

Ainsworth, M. D. S. Object relations, dependency and attachment: A theoretical review of the infant-mother relationship. *Child Development*, 1969, 40, 969-1025.

Ainsworth, M. D. S. The development of infant-mother attachment. In B. M. Caldwell & H. N. Ricciuti (Eds.), *Review of Child Development Research*, (Vol. 3). Chicago: University of Chicago Press, 1973.

Ainsworth, M. D. S., & Bell, S. M. Some contemporary patterns of mother-infant interaction in the feeding situation. In A. Ambrose (Ed.), *Stimulation in Early Infancy.* New York: Academic Press, 1969.

Ainsworth, M. D. S., & Bell, S. M. Mother-infant interaction and the development of competence. In K. Connolly & J. Bruner (Eds.), *The Growth of Competence.* New York: Academic Press, 1974.

Ainsworth, M. D. S., & Bell, S. M. Infant crying and maternal responsiveness: A rejoinder to Gewirtz and Boyd. *Child Development*, 1977, 48, 1208-1216.

Ainsworth, M. D. S., Bell, S., & Stayton, P. Infant-mother attachment and social development: 'Socialization' as a product of reciprocal responsiveness to signals. In M. Richards (Ed.), *The Integration of a Child Into a Social World.* London: Cambridge University Press, 1974.

Ajzen, I., & Fishbein, M. The prediction of behavior from attitudinal and normative variables. *Journal of Experimental Psychology*, 1970, 6, 466-487.

Aleksandrowicz, M. K. The effect of pain relieving drugs administered during labor and delivery on the behavior of the newborn. *Merrill-Palmer Quarterly*, 1974, 20, 121-141.

Aleksandrowicz, M., & Aleksandrowicz, D. R. The molding of personality: A newborn's innate characteristics in interaction with parents' personalities. *Child Psychiatry and Human Development,* 1974, 5, 231-241.

Aleksandrowicz, M. K., & Aleksandrowicz, D. R. Obstetrical pain relieving drugs as predictors of infant behavior variability. *Child Development,* 1974, 45, 935-945.

Aleksandrowicz, M. K., & Aleksandrowicz, D. R. Precursors of ego in neonates: Factor analysis of Brazelton scale data. *Journal of the American Academy of Child Psychiatry,* 1976, 15, 257-268.

Als, H., Tronick, E., Adamson, L., & Brazelton, T. B. The behavior of the full-term but underweight newborn infant. *Developmental Medicine and Child Neurology,* 1976, 18, 590-602.

Altmann, S. A. Sociobiology of rhesus monkeys. II. Stochastics of social communication. *Journal of Theoretical Biology,* 1965, 8, 490-522.

Alvy, K. Preventing child abuse. *American Psychologist,* 1975, 30, 921-928.

Ambrose, A. (Ed.), *Stimulation in Early Infancy.* New York: Academic Press, 1969.

Ambuel, G., & Harris, B. Failure to thrive: A study of failure to grow in height or weight. *Ohio Medical Journal,* 1963, 59, 977.

Ames, M. D., & Schut, L. Results of treatment of 171 consecutive myelomeningoceles 1963-68. *Pediatrics,* 1972, 50, 466.

Anan, M. J. Side effects on fetus and infant of psychotropic drug use during pregnancy. *International Pharmacopsychiatry,* 1976, 11, 246-260.

Anders, T. F. The infant sleep profile. *Neuropediatrie,* 1974, 5, 425-442.

Anderson, B. J. Reciprocity in vocal interactions of mothers and infants. *Child Development,* 1977, 48, 1676-1681.

Anderson, B. J., & Standley, K. A methodology for observation of the childbirth environment. Paper presented to the American Psychological Association, Washington, DC, September, 1976.

Anderson, B. J., Vietze, P., & Dokecki, P. Reciprocity in vocal interactions of mothers and infants. *Child Development,* 1977, 48, 1676-1681.

Anthony, E. J. The syndrome of the psychologically invulnerable child. In E. J. Anthony & C. Koupernik (Eds.), *The Child and His Family: Children at Psychiatric Risk.* New York: John Wiley & Sons, 1974.

Anthony, E. J., & Benedek, T. *Parenthood: Its Psychology and Psychopathology.* Boston: Little, Brown & Co., Inc., 1971.

Anthony, E. J., & Koupernik, C. (Eds.), *The Child in His Family: Children at Psychiatric Risk.* New York: John Wiley, 1974.

Appleton, T., Clifton, R., & Goldberg, S. The development of behavioral competence in infancy. In F. D. Horowitz (Ed.), *Review of Child Development Research,* Vol. 4. Chicago: University of Chicago Press, 1975.

Ashby, W. R. *An Introduction to Cybernetics.* London: University Paperbacks. 1956.

Ashton, P. T. The role of the attachment bond in effective parenting. In J. S. Stevens & M. Matthews (Eds.), *Mother/Child, Father/Child Relationships.* Washington, DC: NAEYC, 1978.

Ashton, R. The state variable in neonatal research: A review. *Merrill-Palmer Quarterly,* 1973, 19, 3-20.

Ashton, R. Aspects of timing in child development. *Child Development,* 1976, 4, 622-626.

Atkin, R., Bray, R., Davison, M., Herzberger, S., Humphreys, L., & Selzer, U. Cross-lagged panel analysis of sixteen cognitive measures at four grade levels. *Child Development,* 1977, 48, 944-952.

Badger, E. D. *Teaching Guide; Infant Learning Program.* Paoli, PA: The Instructo Corporation, 1971 (a).

Badger, E. D. *Teaching Guide: Toddler Learning Program.* Paoli, PA: The Instructo Corporation, 1971 (b).

Badger, E. The infant-stimulation/mother-training project. In B. Caldwell and D.

Stedman (Eds.), *Infant Education: A Guide for Helping Handicapped Children in the First Three Years.* New York: Walker Publishing Co. pp. 45-60, 1977.

Badger, E. Mild to moderately handicapped infants: How do you assess the progress of both mother and infant. In T. Black (Ed.), *Perspectives on Measurement.* Chapel Hill, NC: TADS. pp. 39-47, 1979.

Badger, E. Maternal social risk factors as predictors of developmental outcome in early childhood. *Child Development,* submitted for publication, 1980 (a).

Badger, E. Effects of a parent-education program on teenage mothers and their offspring. In T. G. Scott, T. Fields, & E. Robertson (Eds.), *Teenage Mothers and their Offspring.* New York: Grune & Stratton, in press, 1980 (b).

Badger, E. Promoting child development: A coalition model for community-service delivery. Paper for the Vermont Conference on Primary Prevention for the Enhancement of Infant Competence, 1980 (c).

Badger, E., & Burns, D. The impact of a parent-education program on the personal development of teenage mothers. *Pediatric Psychology,* accepted for publication, 1980.

Bagg, C. E., & Crookes, T. G. The responses of neonates to noise in relation to the personalities of their parents. *Developmental Medicine and Child Neurology,* 1975, 17, 732-735.

Bakeman, R. High-risk infant: Is the risk social? Paper presented at American Psychological Association Meeting, Toronto, May, 1978.

Bakeman, R. Untangling streams of behavior: Sequential analyses of observation data. In G. P. Sackett (Ed.), *Observing Behavior,* (Vol. 2), *Data Collection and Analysis Methods.* Baltimore: University Park Press, 1978.

Bakeman, R., & Brown, J. V. Behavioral dialogues: An approach to the assessment of mother-infant interaction. *Child Development,* 1977, 48, 195-203.

Bakeman, R., & Brown, J. V. Mother-infant interaction during the first months of life: Differences between preterm and fullterm infant-mother dyads from a low income population (Tech. Rep. 5). Atlanta: Georgia State University, Infancy Laboratory, December 1977.

Bakeman, R., & Dabbs, J. M., Jr. Social interaction observed: Some approaches to the analysis of behavior streams. *Personality and Social Psychology Bulletin,* 1976, 2, 335-345.

Bakow, H., Sameroff, A., Kelly, P., & Zax, M. Relations between newborn behaviors and mother-child interaction at four months. Paper presented at the meeting of the Society for Research in Child Development, Philadelphia, PA, 1973.

Baldwin, A. The study of child behavior and development. In P. H. Mussen (Ed.), *Handbook of Research Methods in Child Development.* New York: Wiley, 1960.

Balov, B., Rubin, R., & Rosen, M. Perinatal events as precursors of reading disabilities. *Reading Research Quarterly,* 1975, 11, 36-71.

Baltes, P. B., & Schaie, K. W. On life span developmental research paradigms: Retrospects and prospects. In P. B. Baltes & K. W. Schaie (Eds.), *Life Span Developmental Psychology: Personality and Socialization.* New York: Academic Press, 1973.

Ban, P. L., & Lewis, M. Mother and father, girls and boys: Attachment behavior in the one-year-old. *Merrill-Palmer Quarterly,* 1974, 28, 195-204.

Banks, M. J. A family's over-concern about a child in the first two years of life. *Maternal-Child Nursing Journal,* 1977, 6, 187-194.

Barnard, K. E. *Nursing Child Assessment Satellite Training.* Seattle: University of Washington, 1978.

Barnard, M. U. Supportive nursing care for the mother and newborn who are separated from each other. *Maternal-Child Nursing Journal,* 1976, 1, 107-110.

Barnett, C. R., Leiderman, R. H., Grobstein, R., & Klaus, M. Neonatal separation: The maternal side of interactional deprivation. *Pediatrics,* 1970, 45, 197-205.

Barten, S., Birns, B., & Ronch, J. Individual differences in the visual pursuit of neonates. *Child Development,* 1971, 42, 313-319.

Bateson, P. P. G., & Hinde, R. A. (Eds.), *Advances in Ethology.* Cambridge: Cambridge University Press, 1978.

Baumrind, D. The contributions of the family to the development of competence in children. *Schizophrenia Bulletin,* 1975, 14, 12-37.

Bayley, N. *Bayley Scales of Infant Development Manual.* New York: The Psychological Corporation, 1969.

Becker, W., & Krug, R. The parent attitude research instrument: A research review. *Child Development,* 1965, 36, 329-365.

Beckwith, L., Cohen, E. S., Kopp, C. B., Parmelee, A. H., & Marcy, T. G. Caregiver-infant interaction and early cognitive development in preterm infants. *Child Development,* 1976, 27, 579-587.

Beckwith, L., Sigman, M., Cohen, S. E., & Parmelee, A. H. Vocal output in preterm infants. *Developmental Psychobiology,* 1977, 10, 543-554.

Bee, H. L., VanEgeren, L. F., Streissguth, A. P., Nyman, B. A., & Lockie, M. S. Social class differences in maternal teaching styles and speech patterns. *Developmental Psychology,* 1969, 1, 726-734.

Bell, R. Q. Convergence: An accelerated longitudinal approach. *Child Development,* 1953, 24, 145-152.

Bell, R. Q. Stimulus control of parent or caretaker by offspring. *Developmental Psychology,* 1971, 4, 63-72.

Bell, R. Q. Detection of cross-stage relations between transition periods in which the form of behavior differs markedly: Approaches used and findings from a longitudinal study of the newborn and preschool period. In F. J. Monks, W. H., Hartup, & J. de Wit (Eds.), *Determinants of Behavioral Development.* New York: Academic Press, 1972.

Bell, R. Q. Contributions of human infants to care-giving and social interaction. In M. Lewis & L. Rosenblum (Eds.), *The Effect of the Infant on Its Caregiver.* New York: Wiley, 1974.

Bell, R. Q. A congenital contribution to emotional response in early infancy and the preschool period. In R. Porter & M. O'Connor, *Parent-Infant Interaction* (Ciba Foundation Symposium 33). Amsterdam, The Netherlands: Associated Scientific Publishers, 1975.

Bell, R. Q. Congenital contributors to temperament in findings of the Bethesda Longitudinal Study. Paper presented at a conference at the University of Louisville, School of Medicine, September, 1978.

Bell, R. Q., & Harper, L. V. *Child Effects on Adults.* New York: Wiley, 1977.

Bell, R. Q., Weller, G. M., & Waldrop. M. F. Newborn and preschooler: Organization of behavior and relations between periods. *Monographs of the Society for Research in Child Development,* 1971, 36, (1-2, Serial No. 142).

Bell, S. M., & Ainsworth, M. D. S. Infant crying and maternal responsiveness. *Child Development,* 1972, 43, 1171-1190.

Benedek, T. Psychological aspects of mothering. *American Journal of Orthopsychiatry,* 1956, 26, 272-278.

Benfield, D. G., Lieb, S. A., & Reuter, J. Grief response of parents after referral of the critically ill newborn to a regional center. *New England Journal of Medicine,* 1976, 294, 975-978.

Benfield, D. G., Leib, S. A., & Vollman, J. H. Grief response of parents to neonatal death and parent participation in deciding care. *Pediatrics,* 1978, 62, 171-177.

Bennett, V. C., & Bardon, J. I. The effects of a school program on teenage mothers and their children. *American Journal of Orthopsychiatry,* 1977, 47, 671-678.

Bereiter, C., & Engelmann, S. *Teaching Disadvantaged Children in Preschool.* Englewood Cliffs, NJ: Prentice-Hall, 1966.

Berger, M., Lezine, I., Harrison, A., & Boisselier, F. The syndrome of the post-premature child: A study of its significance. *Early Child Development,* 1973, 2, 61-94.

Bergman, A. B. Psychological aspects of sudden unexpected death in infants and children. Review and commentary. *Pediatric Clinics of North America,* 1974, 21, 115-121.

Berkson, G. Social responses of animals to infants with defects. In M. Lewis & L. A. Rosenblum (Eds.), *The Effect of the Infant on Its Caregiver.* New York: Wiley, 1974.

Bernal, J. Attachment behavior of one-year-olds as a function of mother vs. father, sex of child, session, and toys. *Genetic Psychology Monographs,* 1974, 90, 305-324.

Bessman, S. P., Williamson, M. L., & Koch, R. Diet, genetics, and mental retardation: Interaction between phenylketonuric heterozygous mother and fetus to produce nonspecific diminution in IQ: Evidence in support of the justification hypothesis. *Proceedings of the National Academy of Science, USA,* 1978, 1562-1566.

Bibring, G. L. Some considerations of the psychological processes in pregnancy. *Psychoanalytic Study of the Child,* 1959, 14, 113-121.

Bibring, G. L., Dwyer, T. F., Huntington, D. S., & Valenstein, A. F. A study of the psychological processes in pregnancy and of the earliest mother-child relationship. *Psychoanalytic Study of the Child,* 1961, 16, 9-72.

Bidder, R. T., Crowe, E. A., & Gray, O. P. Mothers' attitudes to preterm infants. *Archives of Diseases in Children,* 1974, 49, 766-769.

Biller, H. B. *Paternal Deprivation.* Lexington, MA: Heath, 1974.

Binet, A. *Les Idees Modernes sur les Enfants.* Paris: Ernest Flamarion, 1909. (Cited from Stoddard, G. D. The IQ: Its ups and downs. *Educational Record,* 1939, 20, 44-57).

Binet, A., & Simon, T. Methodes nouvelles pour le diagnostic du niveau intellectuel des anormaux. *Annee Psychol,* 1905, 11, 191-244.

Birch, H., & Gussow, G. D. *Disadvantaged Children.* New York: Grune & Stratton, 1970.

Biron, P., Mongeau, J. G., & Bertrand, D. Familial resemblance of body weight and weight/height in 374 homes with adopted children. *Journal of Pediatrics,* 1977, 91, 555-558.

Birns, B., Blank, M., & Bridger, W. H. The effectiveness of various soothing techniques on human neonates. *Psychosomatic Medicine,* 1966, 28, 316-322.

Blake, A., Stewart, A., & Turcan, D. Parents of babies of very low birth weight: A long-term follow-up. In R. Porter & M. O'Connor (Eds.), *Parent-Infant Interaction* (Ciba Foundation Symposium 33). Amsterdam, The Netherlands: Associated Scientific Publishers, 1975.

Blehar, M. C., Lieberman, A. F., & Ainsworth, M. D. S. Early face-to-face interactions and its relation to later infant-mother attachment. *Child Development,* 1977, 48, 182-194.

Block, C., Block, R., & Shrock, P. The effect of support of the husband and obstetrician on pain perception and control in childbirth. *Birth and the Family Journal,* 1975, 2, 43-48.

Bloom, B. S. *Stability and Change in Human Characteristics.* New York: Wiley, 1964.

Bobbitt, R. A., Gourevitch, V. P., Miller, L. E., & Jensen, G. D. Dynamics of social interactive behavior: A computerized procedure for analyzing trends, patterns, and sequences. *Psychological Bulletin,* 1969, 71, 110-120.

Borjeson, M. The aetiology of obesity in children. *Acta Paediatrica Scandinavica,* 1976, 65, 279-287.

Bower, T. G. R. *A Primer of Infant Development.* San Francisco: W. H. Freeman and Co., 1977.

Bowlby, G. *Maternal Care and Mental Health.* Geneva: World Health Organization, 1951.

Bowlby, J. *Attachment and Loss (Vol. 1). Attachment.* New York: Basic Books, 1969 (a).

Bowlby, J. *Attachment and Loss (Vol. 2). Separation.* New York: Basic Books, 1969 (a).

Brackbill, Y. Introduction. In Y. Brackbill (Ed.), *Infancy and Early Childhood.* New York: Free Press, 1967.

Brackbill, Y. Continuous stimulation reduces arousal level: Stability of the effect over time. *Child Development,* 1973, 44, 43-46.

Brackbill, Y. Continuous stimulation and arousal level in infancy: Effects of stimulus intensity and stress. *Child Development,* 1975, 46, 364-369.

Brackbill, Y., et al. Obstetric premedication and infant outcome. *American Journal of Obstetrics and Gynecology,* 1974, 118, 377-384.

Bradley, R., & Caldwell, B. Early home environment and changes in mental test performance in children from 6 to 36 months. *Developmental Psychology,* 1976, 12, 93-97.

Bradley, R. H., & Caldwell, B. M. Home Observation for Measurement of the Environment: A validation study of screening efficiency. *American Journal of Mental Deficiencies,* 1977, 81, 417-420.

Brazelton, T. B. Influence of perinatal drugs on the behavior of the neonate. In J. Hellmuth (Ed.), *Exceptional Infant.* (Vol. 2) *Studies in Abnormalities.* New York: Brunner/Mazel, 1971.

Brazelton, T. B. Effect of maternal expectations on early infant behavior. *Early Child Development and Care,* 1973 (a), 2, 259-273.

Brazelton, T. B. Assessment of the infant at risk. *Clinical Obstetrics and Gynecology,* 1973 (b), 16, 361-375.

Brazelton, T. B. *Neonatal Behavioral Assessment Scale.* (Clinics in Developmental Medicine, No. 50). London: Spastics International Medical Publication in Association with Heinemann, and Philadelphia: Lippincott, 1973 (c).

Brazelton, T. B. Does the neonate shape his environment? *Birth Defects,* 1974 (a), 10, 131-140.

Brazelton, T. B. The origins of reciprocity: The early mother-infant interaction. In M. Lewis & L. Rosenblum (Eds.), *The Effect of the Infant on Its Caregiver.* New York: Wiley, 1974 (b).

Brazelton, T. B. Discussion commentary. In R. H. Porter & M. O'Connor (Eds.), *Parent-Infant Interaction* (Ciba Foundation Symposium). Amsterdam: Associated Scientific Publishers, 1975.

Brazelton, T. B., Koslowski, B., & Main, M. The origins of reciprocity: The early mother-infant interaction. In M. Lewis & L. A. Rosenblum (Eds.), *The Effect of the Infant on Its Caregiver.* New York: Wiley, 1974.

Brazelton, T. B., Robey, J. S., & Collier, G. A. Infant development in the Zinacanteco Indians of southern Mexico. *Pediatrics,* 1969, 44, 272-290.

Brazelton, T. B., Tronick, E., Adamson, L., Als, H., & Wise, S. Early mother-infant reciprocity. *Parent-Infant Interaction* (Ciba Foundation Symposium 33). Amsterdam, The Netherlands: Associated Scientific Publishers, 1975.

Brazelton, T. B., Tronick, E., Als, H., & Yogman, M. Reciprocity between adults and infants. Paper presented at the IV Biennal Conference of the International Society for the Study of Behavioral Development. Pavia, Italy, September 19-23, 1977.

Brazelton, T. B., Tronick, E., Lechtig, A., Lasky, R. E., & Klein, R. E. The behavior of nutritionally deprived Guatemalan infants. *Developmental Medicine and Child Neurology,* 1977, 19, 364-372.

Brody, S. *Patterns of Mothering.* New York: International Universities Press, 1956.

Broman, S. H., Nichols, P. L., & Kennedy, W. A. *Preschool IQ: Prenatal and Early Developmental Correlates.* Hillsdale, NJ: Lawrence Erlbaum Associates, 1975.

Bromwick, R. M. Focus on maternal behavior in infant intervention. *American Journal of Orthopsychiatry,* 1976, 46, 439-446.

Bronfenbrenner, U. The origins of alienation. *Scientific American,* 1974, 213 (2), 53-57; 60-61.

Bronfenbrenner, U. Is early intervention effective? In B. Z. Friedlander, G. M. Sterritt, & G. E. Kirk (Eds.), *Exceptional Infant.* (Vol. 3). *Assessment and Intervention.* New York: Brunner/Mazel, 1975.

Bronfenbrenner, U. The changing American family. In E. M. Hetherington & R. D. Parke (Eds.), *Contemporary Readings in Child Psychology.* New York: McGraw-Hill, 1977 (a).

Bronfenbrenner, U. Toward an experimental ecology of human development. *American Psychologist,* 1977 (b), 32, 513-531.

Brook, C. D. G. Genetic aspects of obesity. *Postgraduate Medical Journal,* 1977, 53, 93-96.

Brook, C. D. G., Huntley, R. M. C., & Slack, J. Influence of heredity and environment in determination of skinfold thickness. *British Medical Journal,* 1972, 2, 719-721.

Brook, C. D. G., Lloyd, J. K., & Wolff, O. H. Relation between age of onset of obesity and size and number of adipose cells. *British Medical Journal,* 1972, 21, 25-27.

Brooks, J., & Weinraub, M. A history of intelligence testing. In M. Lewis (Ed.), *Origins of Intelligence.* New York: Plenum Press, 1976.

Broussard, E. R. Neonatal pediction and outcome at age 10/11 years. *Child Psychiatry and Human Development,* 1976, 7, 85-93.

Broussard, E. R. Evaluation of televised anticipatory guidance to primiparas. *Community Mental Health Journal,* 1976, 12, 203-210.

Broussard, E. R., & Hartner, M. S. S. Maternal perception of the neonate as related to development. *Child Psychiatry and Human Development,* 1970, 1, 16-25.

Broussard, E. R., & Hartner, M. S. S. Further considerations regarding maternal perception of the newborn. In J. Hellmuth (Ed.), *Exceptional Infant.* (Vol. 2) *Studies in Abnormalities.* New York: Brunner/Mazel, 1971.

Brown, F., Lieberman, J., & Winson, J. Studies in choice of infant feeding by primiparas: 1. Attitudinal factors and extraneous influences. *Psychosomatic Medicine,* 1960, 22, 421.

Brown, J. V., & Bakeman, R. Mother-infant behavior codes: Birth through three months (Tech. Rep. 3). Atlanta: Georgia State University, Infancy Laboratory, June 1975.

Brown, J. V., & Bakeman, R. Relations of human mothers with their infants during the first year of life: Effects of prematurity. In R. W. Bell, & W. P. Smotherman (Eds.), *Maternal Influences and Early Behavior.* Holliswood, NY: Spectrum, 1979.

Brown, J. V., Bakeman, R., Snyder, P. A., Frederickson, W. T., Morgan, S. T., & Hepler, R. Interactions of black inner-city mothers with their newborn infants. *Child Development,* 1975, 46, 677-686.

Bruch, H. *Eating Disorders.* New York: Basic Books, 1973.

Bruch, H. *The Golden Cage: The Enigma of Anorexia Nervosa.* Cambridge, MA: Harvard University Press, 1978.

Bruner, J. S. Processes of growth in infancy. In A. Ambrose (Ed.), *Stimulation in Early Infancy.* New York: Academic Press, 1969.

Bruner, J. The growth and structure of skill. In K. J. Connolly (Ed.), *Motor Skills.* London: Academic Press, 1971.

Bruner, J. The ontogenesis of speech acts. *Journal of Child Language,* 1975, 2, 1-19.

Buckhalt, J. A., Rutherford, R. B., & Goldberg, K. E. Verbal and nonverbal interaction of mothers with their Down's syndrome and nonretarded infants. *American Journal of Mental Deficiency,* 1978, 82, 337-343.

Bugen, L. A. Control, quality of life, and the right to die. In L. A. Bugen (Ed.), *Death and Dying: Theory, Research and Practice*. Dubuque: Wm. C. Brown, 1979 (a).

Bugen, L. A. Fundamentals of bereavement intervention. In L. A. Bugen (Ed.), *Death and Dying: Theory, Research and Practice*. Dubuque: Wm. C. Brown, 1979 (b).

Bugen, L. A. Human grief: A model for prediction and intervention. *American Journal of Orthopsychiatry*, 1977, 47, 196-207.

Burt, C. The genetic determination of differences in intelligence: A study of monozygotic twins reared together and apart. *British Journal of Psychology*, 1966, 57, 137-153.

Buss, A. H., & Plomin, R. *A Temperament Theory of Personality Development*. New York: Wiley, 1975.

Butcher, R. E., Hawver, K., Burbacher, T., & Scott, W. Behavioral effects from antenatal exposure to teratogens. In N. R. Ellis (Ed.), *Aberrant Development in Infancy*. Hillsdale, NJ: Lawrence Erlbaum Associates, 1975.

Butler, N. R. Risk factors in human intrauterine growth retardation. *Size at Birth*, (Ciba Foundation Symposium). Amsterdam: Associated Scientific Publishers, 1974.

Call, J. Newborn approach behavior and early ego development. *International Journal of Psychoanalysis*, 1964, 45, 286-294.

Call, J. Helping infants cope with change. *Early Child Development and Care*, 1974, 3, 229-247.

Callaway, E. *Brain Electrical Potentials and Individual Psychological Differences*. New York: Grune & Stratton, 1975.

Campbell, D. T., & Fiske, D. W. Convergent and discriminant validation by the multitrait-multimethod matrix. *Psychological Bulletin*, 1959, 56, 81-105.

Campos, J. J. Heartrate: A sensitive tool for the study of emotional development in the infant. In L. P. Lipsitt (Ed.), *Psychobiology: The Significance of Infancy*. New York: L. Erlbaum, 1977.

Caplan, G. Mental hygiene work with expectant mothers. *Mental Hygiene*, 1951, 35, 41-50.

Caplan, G. *Concepts of Mental Health and Consultation: Their Application in Public Health Social Work*. Washington: Children's Bureau, 1959.

Caplan, G., Mason, E., & Kaplan, D. M. Four studies of crisis in parents of prematures. *Community Mental Health Journal*, 1965, 1, 149-161.

Caputo, D. V. An evaluation of various parameters of maturation at birth as predictors of development at one year of life. *Perception and Motor Skills*, 1974, 39, 631-652.

Carey, W. B. Maternal anxiety and infantile colic: Is there a relationship? *Clinical Pediatrics*, 1968, 7, 590-595.

Carey, W. B. A simplified method for measuring infant temperament. *Journal of Pediatrics*, 1970, 77, 188-194.

Carey, W. B. Measurement of infant temperament in pediatric practice. In J. C. Westman (Ed.), *Individual Differences in Children*. New York: Wiley, 1973.

Carey, W. B., Lipton, L., & Myers, R. A. Temperament in adopted and foster babies. *Child Welfare*, 1974, 53, 352-369.

Carlsson, S. J., Faderberg, H., Hornemann, L., Hwang, C. P., Larsson, K., Rodholm, M., Schaller, J., Danielson, B., & Gundewall, C. Effects of amount of contact between mother and child on the mother's nursing behavior. *Developmental Psychology*, 1978, 11, 143-150.

Carmichael, L. (Ed.), *Manual of Child Psychology*. New York: Wiley, 1954.

Causey, R. Scientific progress. *Texas Engineering and Science Magazine*, 1969, 6, 22-29.

Chapple, E. D. Experimental production of transients in human interaction. *Nature*, 1970, 228, 630-633.

Charney, E., Goodman, H. C., McBride, M., Lyon, B., & Pratt, R. Childhood antecedents of adult obesity. *New England Journal of Medicine,* 1976, 295, 6-9.

de Chateau, P. The influence of early contact on maternal and infant behavior in primiparae. *Birth and the Family Journal,* 1976, 3, 149-155.

Chess, S. Temperament in the normal infant. In J. Hellmuth (Ed.), *Exceptional Infant.* (Vol. 1) *The Normal Infant.* New York: Brunner/Mazel, 1967, 144-162.

Chess, S., & Thomas, A. Temperament in the normal infant. In J. C. Westman (Ed.), *Individual Differences in Children.* New York: Wiley, 1973.

Chilman, C. S. Programs for disadvantaged parents. In M. Caldwell & H. N. Ricciutti (Eds.), *Review of Child Development Research,* Vol. 3. Chicago: University of Chicago Press, 1973.

Choi, M. A comparison of maternal psychological reactions to premature and full-size newborns. *Maternal-Child Nursing Journal,* 1975, 45, 1-11.

Chomsky, N. The general properties of language. In F. L. Darley (Ed.), *Brain Mechanisms, Speech and Language.* New York: Grune & Stratton, 1967, 73-80.

Cicchetti, D., & Sroufe, L. A. An organizational view of affect: Illustration from the study of Down's syndrome infants. In M. Lewis & L. A. Rosenblum (Eds.), *The Development of Affect.* New York: Plenum Press, 1978.

Cicirelli, V. G., et al. *The Impact of Head Start: An Evaluation of the Effects of Head Start on Children's Cognitive and Affective Development* (Vols. 1 & 2). Bladensburg, MD: Westinghouse Learning Corporation, 1969. (Distributed by Clearinghouse for Federal Scientific and Technical Information, Springfield, VA: 22151.)

Cicirelli, V. G. Effect of sibling preference on mother-child interaction. *Developmental Psychology,* 1978, 14, 315-316.

Clark, A. Application of psychosocial concepts (to postpartum). *Childbearing: A Nursing Perspective.* Philadelphia: Davis Co., 1976.

Clark, A. L., & Alfonso, D. D. *Childbearing: A Nursing Perspective.* Philadelphia: Davis Co., 1976 (a).

Clark, A. L., & Alfonso, D. D. Infant behavior and maternal attachment: Two sides to the coin. *Maternal-Child Nursing Journal,* 1976 (b), 1, 94-99.

Clark, A. M., & Clarke, A. D. B. *Early Experience: Myths and Evidence.* New York: Free Press, 1976.

Clarke-Stewart, K. A. Interactions between mothers and their young children: Characteristics and consequences. *Monographs of the Society for Research in Child Development,* 1973, 38, 6-7.

Clarke-Stewart, K. A. Popular primers for parents. *American Psychologist,* 1978 (a), 33, 359-369.

Clarke-Stewart, K. A. And daddy makes three: The father's impact on mother and young child. *Child Development,* 1978 (b), 49, 466-478.

Clausen, J. Psychophysiology in mental retardation. In N. R. Ellis (Ed.), *International Review of Research in Mental Retardation,* 1978. New York: Academic Press, pp. 85-125.

Cochran, W. G. Some methods for strengthening the common chi square tests. *Biometrics,* 1954, 10, 417-451.

Cohen, D. B. Dark hair and light eyes in female college students: A potential biological marker for liability to psychopathology. *Journal of Abnormal Psychology,* 1978, 87, 455-458.

Cohen, D. J., Dibble, E., Grawe, J. M., & Pollin, W. Separating identical from fraternal twins. *Archives of General Psychiatry,* 1973, 29, 465-469.

Cohen, D. J., Dibble, E., & Krane, J. M. Parental style: Mothers and fathers and perceptions of their relations with twin children. *Archives of General Psychiatry,* 1977, 34, 445-451.

Cohen, E. S., & Beckwith, L. Maternal language in infancy. *Developmental Psychology,* 1976, 12, 371-372.

Cohen, E. S., & Beckwith, L. Caregiving behaviors and early cognitive development as related to ordinal position in pre-term infants. *Child Development,* 1977, 48, 152-157.

Cohen, L. B., & Salapatek, P. (Eds.), *Infant Perception: From Sensation to Cognition.* (Vols. I & II). New York: Academic Press, 1975, 1976.

Cohler, B., Grunebaum, H., & Weiss, J. Childcare attitudes and emotional disturbances among mothers of young children. *Genetic Psychology Monographs,* 1970, 82, 3-47.

Cohler, B. J., Grunebaum, H. U., Weiss, J. L., Hartman, C. R., & Gallant, D. H. Child care attitudes and adaptation to the maternal role among mentally ill and well mothers. *American Journal of Orthopsychiatry,* 1976, 46, 123-134.

Cohler, B. J., Weiss, J. L., & Grunebaum, H. U. The maternal attitude scale: A questionnaire for studying childrearing attitudes in mothers of young children. Available from Microfiche Publications, Division of Microfiche Systems Corp., 305 East 45th St., New York, NY 10017. (Order #00963).

Coleman, R. W., Kris, E., & Provence, S. The study of variations in early parental attitudes. *The Psychoanalytic Study of the Child,* 1953, 8, 20-47.

Colen, B. D. Life or death for infants. *Washington Post,* March 11, 1974.

Collipp, P. J. *Childhood Obesity.* Action, MA: Publishing Science Group, 1975.

Condon, W. S. A primary phase in the organization of infant responding. In H. R. Schaffer (Ed.), *Studies in Mother-Infant Interaction.* New York: Academic Press, 1977.

Condon, W. S. Multiple response to sound in dysfunctional children. *Journal of Autism and Childhood Schizophrenia,* 1979, 5, 37-56.

Condon, W. S., & Ogston, W. D. A segmentation of behavior. *Journal of Psychiatric Research,* 1967, 5, 221-235.

Condon, W. S., & Sander, L. W. Synchrony demonstrated between movements of the neonate and adult speech. *Child Development,* 1974 (a), 45, 456-462.

Condon, W. S., & Sander, L. W. Neonate movement is synchronized with adult speech: Interactional participation and language acquisition. *Science,* 1974 (b), 183, 99-101.

Connolly, K. J., & Bruner, J. S. Competence: Its nature and nurture. In K. J. Connolly & J. S. Bruner (Eds.), *The Growth of Competence.* New York: Academic Press, 1974 (a).

Connolly, K. J., & Bruner, J., S. (Eds.), *The Growth of Competence.* New York: Academic Press, 1974 (b).

Cook, S. W., & Selltiz, C. A multiple-indicator approach to attitude measurement. *Psychological Bulletin,* 1964, 62, 36-55.

Cornell, E. H., & Gottfried, A. W. Intervention with premature human infants. *Child Development,* 1976, 47, 32-39.

Corter, C., Trehub, S., Boukydis, C., Ford, L., Celhoffer, L., & Minde, K. Nurses' judgments of the attractiveness of premature infants. Unpublished manuscript, University of Toronto and Hospital for Sick Children, 1976.

Crawley, S. B., Rogers, P. P., Friedman, S., Jacobson, M., Criticos, A., Richardson, L., & Thompson, M. A. Developmental changes in the structure of mother-infant play. *Developmental Psychology,* 1978, 14, 30-36.

Cremin, L. A. *The Transformation of the School: Progressivism in American Education, 1876-1957.* New York: Knopf, 1962.

Cronbach, L. Coefficient alpha and the internal consistency of tests. *Psychometrika,* 1951, 16, 25-32.

Crook, C. K. Neonatal sucking: Effects of quantity of the response-contingent fluid upon sucking rhythm and heart rate. *Journal of Experimental Child Psychology,* 1976, 21, 539-548.

Crook, J. H. Social organization and the environment: Aspects of contemporary social ethology. *Animal Behavior,* 1970, 18, 197-209.

Cropley, C., Lester, P., & Pennington, S. Assessment tool for measuring maternal attachment behaviors. In L. K. McNall & J. T. Galeener, *Current Practice in Obstetric and Gynecologic Nursing,* Vol. 1. St. Louis: C. V. Mosby Co., 1976.

Cummings, S. T. The impact of a child's deficiency on the father: A study of fathers of mentally retarded and chronically ill children. *American Journal of Orthopsychiatry,* 1976, 46, 246-255.

David, M., & Appell, G. Mother-child interaction and its impact on the child. In A. Ambrose (Ed.), *Stimulation in Early Infancy.* New York: Academic Press, 1969.

Davids, A., & Holden, R. Consistency in maternal attitudes and personality from pregnancy to eight months following childbirth. *Developmental Psychology,* 1970, 2, 364-366.

Davies, D. P., Gray, O. P., Ellwood, P. C., & Abernethy, M. Cigarette smoking in pregnancy: Association with maternal weight gain and fetal growth. *Lancet,* 1976, 1, 385-387.

Davis, A. American status systems and the socialization of the child. *Personality in Nature, Society and Culture.* New York: Knopf, 1959.

Decarie, T. G. Affect development and cognition in a Piagetian context. In M. Lewis & L. A. Rosenblum (Eds.), *The Development of Affect.* New York: Plenum Press, 1978.

Dennis, W. Causes of retardation among institutional children: Iran. *Journal of Genetic Psychology,* 1960, 96, 47-59.

Dennis, W. *Children of the Creche.* New York: Appleton-Century-Crofts, 1973.

Desmond, M. M., Franklin, R. R., Vallbona, C., Hill, R. M., Plumb, R., Arnold, H., & Watts, J. The clinical behavior of the newlyborn. *Journal of Pediatrics,* 1963, 62, 307-325.

Deutsch, C. P. Social class and child development. In B. M. Caldwell & H. N. Ricciuti (Eds.), *Review of Child Development Research,* Vol. 3. Chicago: University of Chicago Press, 1973.

Deutsch, H. *The Psychology of Women* (Vol. 2) *Motherhood.* New York: Grune and Stratton, 1945.

Deutscher, I. Words and deeds: Social science and social policy. *Social Problems,* 1966, 13, 235-254.

de Vries, M. W. & de Vries, M. R. Cultural relativity of toilet training readiness: A perspective from East Africa. *Pediatrics,* 1977, 60, 170-177.

Diamond, J. M. Ethics to axes, a response to dilemmas in the nursery. *The New Physician,* 1978, 27, 18-20.

Diamond, M. C. Anatomical brain changes induced by environment. In L. Petrinovich & J. L. McGaugh (Eds.), *Knowing, Thinking, and Believing.* New York: Plenum, 1977, 215-241.

Dietrich, K. N., & Starr, R. H. Maternal handling and developmental characteristics of abused infants. In T. Field, S. Goldberg, D. Stern, & A. Sostek (Eds.), *Interactions of High-Risk Infants and Children.* New York: Academic Press, 1979.

DiVitto, B., & Goldberg, S. The effects of newborn medical status on early parent-infant interaction. In T. Field, A. Sostek, S. Goldberg, & H. H. Shuman (Eds.), *Infants Born at Risk.* New York: Spectrum, 1979.

Dohrenwend, B., & Dohrenwend, B. *Stressful Life Events: Their Nature and Effects.* New York: Wiley, 1974.

Donovan, W. L., Leavitt, L. A., & Balling, J. D. Maternal physiological response to infant signals. *Psychophysiology,* 1978, 15, 68-74.

Doty, B. Relationships among attitudes in pregnancy and other maternal characteristics. *The Journal of Genetic Psychology,* 1967, 3, 203-217.

Draper, H. H. Biological, cultural, and social determinants of nutritional status. In P. H. Leiderman, S. R. Tulkin, & A. Rosenfeld (Eds.), *Culture and Infancy: Variations in the Human Experience.* New York: Academic Press, 1977.

Dreyfus-Brisac, C. Organization of sleep in prematures: Implications for caretaking. In M. Lewis & L. A. Rosenblum (Eds.), *The Effect of the Infant on Its Caregiver.* New York: Wiley, 1974.

Drillien, C. M. *The Growth and Development of the Prematurely Born Infant.* Baltimore: Williams and Wilkins, 1964.

Drotan, D., Baskiewitz, A., Irwin, N., Kennell, J., & Klaus, M. The adaptation of parents to the birth of an infant with a congenital malformation: A hypothetical model. *Pediatrics,* 1975, 56, 710.

Dubowitz, V. The infant of inappropriate size. *Size at Birth,* (Ciba Foundation Symposium). Amsterdam: Associated Scientific Publishers, 1974.

Duff, R. S., & Campbell, A. G. M. On deciding the care of severely handicapped or dying persons: With particular reference to infants. *Pediatrics,* 1976, 57, 487.

Dugdale, A. E. Pattern of fat and lean tissue deposition in children. *Nature,* 1975, 256, 725-726.

Dunbar, J. Maternal contact behaviors with newborn infants during feedings. *Maternal-Child Nursing Journal,* 1977, 6, 209-299.

Duncan, S. Some signals and rules for taking speaking turns in conversations. *Journal of Personality and Social Psychology,* 1972, 23, 283-292.

Dunlap, W. R., & Hollingsworth, J. S. How does a handicapped child affect the family? Interpretations for practitioners. *Family Coordinator,* 1977, 26, 286-293.

Dunn, J. B. Consistency and change in styles of mothering. *Parent-Infant Interaction,* (Ciba Foundation Symposium). Amsterdam, The Netherlands: Associated Scientific Publishers, 1975).

Dunn, J. B. Continuity in patterns of interaction between mother and baby from the post-natal period. *Journal of Psychosomatic Research,* 1976, 4, 273-278.

Dunn, J. B. *Distress and Comfort.* Cambridge, MA: Harvard University Press, 1977 (a).

Dunn, J. B. Patterns of early interaction: Continuities and consequences. In H. R. Schaffer (Ed.), *Studies in Mother-Infant Interaction.* New York: Academic Press, 1977 (b).

Dunn, J. B. Changes in styles of mothering. In *Parent-Infant Interaction.* London: Ciba Foundation Symposium (New Series 33), 1977 (c).

Dunn, J. B., & Richards, M. P. M. Observations on the developing relationship between mother and baby in the neonatal period. In N. R. Schaffer (Ed.), *Studies in Mother-Infant Interaction.* New York: Academic Press, 1977.

Dunn, J. B., Wooding, C., & Hermann, J. B. Mother's speech to young children: Variation in context. *Developmental Medicine and Child Neurology,* 1977, 19, 629-638.

Dunn, L. C., *A Short History of Genetics.* New York: McGraw-Hill, 1965.

Edwards, L. E., Dickes, W. F., Alton, J. R., & Hakanson, E. Y. Pregnancy in the massively obese. Course, outcome, and obesity prognosis of the infant. *American Journal of Obstetrical Gynecology,* 1978, 131, 479-483.

Eichorn, D. H. Longitudinal research: Alternative methods and major findings. *JSAS Catalog of Selected Documents in Psychology,* 1976, 6, 95.

Eid, E. K. Follow-up study of physical growth of children who had excessive weight gain in the first six months of life. *British Medical Journal,* 1970, 2, 47-76.

Eimas, P. Speech perception in early infancy. In L. Cohen & P. Salapatek (Eds.), *Infant Perception from Sensation to Cognition,* New York: Academic Press, 1975.

Eimas, P., Siqueland, E. R., Jusczyk, P., & Vigorito, J. Speech perception in infants, *Science,* 1971, 171, 303-306.

Elardo, R., Bradley, R., & Caldwell, B. M. The relation of infants' home environments to mental test performance from 6 to 36 months: A longitudinal analysis. *Child Development,* 1975, 46, 71-76.

Elardo, R., Bradley, R., & Caldwell, B. M. A longitudinal study of the relation of infants' home environments to language development at age three. *Child Development,* 1977, 48, 595-603.

Eldred, C. A., Grier, V. V., & Berliner, N. Comprehensive treatment for heroin addicted mothers. *Social Casework,* 1974, 55, 470-477.

Eldred, C., Rosenthal, D., Wender, P. H., Kety, S. S., Schulsinger, F., Weiner, J., & Jacobsen, B. Some aspects of adoption in selected samples of adult adoptees. *American Journal of Orthopsychiatry,* 1976, 46, 279-286.

El-Gwebaly, N., & Offord, D. R. The offspring of alcoholism: A critical review. *American Journal of Psychiatry,* 1977, 134, 357-365.

Ellingen, R. J., Dutch, S. J., & McIntire, M. S. EEGs of prematures: 3-8 year follow-up study. *Developmental Psychobiology,* 1974, 1, 529-538.

Elliot, K., & Knight, J. (Eds.) *Size at Birth.* (Ciba Foundation Symposium). Amsterdam, The Netherlands: Associated Scientific Publishers, 1974.

Ellis, H. L. Parental involvement in the decision to treat spina bifada cystica. *British Medical Journal,* 1974, 1, 369-372.

Ellis, N. R. (Ed.) *Aberrant Development in Infancy: Human and Animal Studies.* Hillsdale, NJ: L. Erlbaum, 1975.

Elmer, E., & Gregg, C. S. Developmental interactions of abused children. *Pediatrics,* 1967, 40, 596.

Emde, R. N., Katz, E. L., & Thorpe, J. K. Emotional expression in infancy: II. Early deviations in Down's syndrome. In M. Lewis & L. H. Rosenblum (Eds.), *The Development of Affect.* New York: Plenum Press, 1978.

Epstein, H. T. Phrenoblysis: Special brain and mind growth periods. I. Human brain and skull development. *Developmental Psychobiology,* 1974 (a), 7, 3, 207-216.

Epstein, H. T. Phrenoblysis: Special brain and mind growth periods. II. Human mental development. *Developmental Psychobiology,* 1974 (b), 7, 3, 217-224.

Erikson, E. H. *Childhood and Society.* New York: Norton, 1950.

Escalona, S. The use of infant tests for predictive purposes. *Bulletin of the Menninger Clinic,* 1950, 14, 117-128.

Escalona, S. K., The differential impact of environmental conditions as a function of different reaction patterns in infancy. In J. C. Westman (Ed.), *Individual Differences in Children.* New York: Wiley, 1973.

Escalona, S. K. *Roots of Individuality.* Chicago: Aldine, 1968.

Ethical dilemmas in current obstetric and newborn care. Report of the 65th Ross Conference on Peditric Research, October 1973. Columbus, Ohio: Ross Laboratories, 1973.

Fanaroff, A. A., Kennell, J. H., & Klaus, M. H. Follow-up of low birth weight infants: The predictive value of maternal visiting patterns. *Pediatrics,* 1972, 49, 287-290.

Federman, E. J., & Yang, R. K. A critique of "Obstetrical pain-relieving drugs as predictors of infant behavior variability." *Child Development,* 1976, 47, 294-296.

Feiring, C., & Taylor, J. The influence of the infant and secondary parent on maternal behavior: Toward a social systems view of infant attachment. *Merrill-Palmer Quarterly,* in press.

Ferguson, C. A. Baby talk in six languages. *American Anthropologist.* 1964, 66, 103-114.

Ferreira, A. J. The pregnant woman's emotional attitude and its reflection on the newborn. *American Journal of Orthopsychiatry,* 1960, 30, 553-561.

Festinger, L. A. *A Theory of Cognitive Dissonance.* Evanston, IL: Row, Peterson, 1957.

Feuerstein, R. *The Dynamic Assessment of Retarded Performers: The Learning Potential Assessment Device, Theory, Instruments and Techniques.* Baltimore, Md.: University Park Press, 1979.

410   *Exceptional Infant*

Feuerstein, R. *Instrumental Enrichment: An Intervention Program for Cognitive Modifiability.* Baltimore, Md.: University Park Press, 1980.

Field, T. M. Effects of early separation, interactive deficits, and experimental manipulations on infant-mother face-to-face interaction. *Child Development,* 1977 (a), 48, 763-771.

Field, T. M. Maternal stimulation during infant feeding. *Developmental Psychology,* 1977 (b), 13, 539-540.

Field, T. M. Interaction behaviors of primary versus secondary caretaker fathers. *Developmental Psychology,* 1978 (a), 14, 183-184.

Field, T. M. Interactions between twins and their mothers. Unpublished manuscript, University of Miami, 1978 (b).

Field, T. M. The 3 Rs of infant-adult social interactions: Rhythms, repertoires and responsivity. *Pediatric Psychology,* 1978 (c), 3, 131-136.

Field, T. M. Games parents play with normal and high-risk infants. *Child Psychiatry and Human Development,* 1979 (a), 10, 41-48.

Field, T. M. Interaction patterns of high-risk and normal infants. In T. M. Field et al. (Eds.), *Infants Born at Risk.* New York: Spectrum, 1979 (b).

Field, T. M. Visual and cardiac responses to animate and inanimate faces by young term and preterm infants. *Child Development,* 1979 (c), 50, 188-195.

Field, T. M. Interactions of preterm infants to lower-SES, teenage mothers. In T. Field, Goldberg, S., Stern, D. & Sostek, A. (Eds.) *High-Risk Infants and Children: Adult and Peer Interactions.* New York: Academic Press, 1980.

Field, T. M., Dabiri, C., Hallock, N., & Shuman, H. H. Developmental effects of prolonged pregnancy and the postmaturity syndrome. *Journal of Pediatrics,* 1977, 90, 836-839.

Field, T. M., Goldberg, S., Stern, D., & Sostek, A. (Eds.) *High-Risk Infants and Children: Adult and Peer Interactions.* New York: Academic Press, 1980.

Field, T. M., Hallock, N., Ting, E., Dempsey. J., Dabiri, C., & Shuman, H. H. A first-year follow-up of high-risk infants: Formulation of a cumulative risk index. *Child Development,* 1978, 49, 119-131.

Field, T. M., & Pawlby, S. Early face-to-face interactions of British and American working and middle-class mother-infant dyads. *Child Development,* 1980, 51, 250-253.

Field, T. M., Sostek, A. M., Goldberg, S., & Shuman, H. H. (Eds.) *Infants Born at Risk: Behavior and Development.* New York: Spectrum, 1979.

Fisch, R. O., Bilek, M. K., & Ulstrom, R. Obesity and leanness at birth and their relation to body habits in later childhood. *Pediatrics,* 1975, 56, 521-528.

Fish, B., & Hagio, R. Visual-motor disorders in infants at risk for schizophrenia. *Archives of General Psychiatry,* 1973, 28, 900-904.

Fishbein, H. D. *Evolution, Development, and Children's Learning.* Pacific Palisades, CA: Goodyear Publishing Co., 1976.

Fishbein, M. Attitude and the prediction of behavior. In M. Fishbein (Ed.), *Readings in Attitude Theory and Measurement.* New York: Wiley, 1967 (a), 477-492.

Fishbein, M. A consideration of beliefs and their role in attitude theory and measurement. In M. Fishbein (Ed.), *Readings in Attitude Theory and Measurement.* New York: Wiley, 1967 (b), 257-266.

Fishbein, M., & Ajzen, I. *Belief, Attitude, Intention and Behavior.* Reading, MA: Addison-Wesley, 1975.

Fiske, D. W., & Maddi, S. R. *Functions of Varied Experience.* Illinois: Dorsey Press, 1961.

Fitzhardinge, P. M. Follow-up studies on the low birth weight infant. *Clinics in Perinatology,* 1976, 3, 503.

Fitzpatrick, E., Reeder, S. R., & Mastroianni, L. *Maternity Nursing*. Philadelphia: Lippincott, 1971.

Fletcher, J. Attitudes toward defective newborns. *Hastings Center Studies*, 1974, 2, 21-32.

Fletcher, J. Abortion, euthanasia, and care of defective newborns. *New England Journal of Medicine*, 1975, 292, 75-78.

Fomon, S. J. *Infant Nutrition* (Second Edition). Philadelphia: Saunders, 1974.

Forrest, T. The family dynamics of maternal violence. *Journal of the American Academy of Psychoanalysis*, 1974, 2, 215-230.

Foss, B. M. (Ed.). *Determinants of Infant Behavior*, Vols. 1-4. New York: Wiley, 1969.

Fost, N. Ethical problems in pediatrics. *Current Problems in Pediatrics*, 1976, 6, 13.

Fox, N. Attachment of kibbutz infants to mother and metapelet. *Child Development*, 1977, 48, 1228-1239.

Fraiberg, S. Smiling and stranger reaction in blind infants. In J. Hellmuth (Ed.), *Exceptional Infant* (Vol. 2), *Studies in Abnormalities*. New York: Brunner/Mazel, 1971.

Fraiberg, S. Intervention in infancy: A program for blind infants. In B. Z. Friedlander, G. M. Sterritt, & G. E. Kirk (Eds.), *Exceptional Infant* (Vol. 3), *Assessment and Intervention*. New York: Brunner/Mazel, 1975.

Francis-Williams, J., & Davies, P. A. Very low birthweight and later intelligence. *Developmental Medicine and Child Neurology*, 1974, 16, 709-728.

Freedman, D. G., & Freedman, N. Behavioral differences between Chinese-American and European-American newborns. *Nature*, 1969, 224, 1227.

Freeman, J. M. To treat or not to treat: Ethical dilemmas in the management of myelomeningocele. *Clinical Neurosurgery*, 1973, 20, 134-146.

Freese, M. P. Assessment of maternal attitudes and analysis of their role in early mother-infant interaction. Unpublished doctoral dissertation, University of Connecticut, 1975.

Freese, M. P., & Thoman, E. B. The assessment of maternal characteristics for the study of mother-infant interaction. *Infant Behavior and Development*, 1978, 1, 95-105.

Friederich, M. A. Psychological changes during pregnancy. *Contemporary Obstetrics and Gynecology*, 1977, 9, 27-34.

Friedlander, B. Z., Sterritt, G. M., & Kirk, G. E. (Eds.), *Exceptional Infant*, Vol. 3, *Assessment and Intervention*. New York: Brunner/Mazel, 1975.

Friedman, S., Thompson, M. A., Crawley, S., Criticos, A. D., Iacobbo, M., Rogers, P. P., & Richardson, L. Mutual visual regard during mother/infant play. *Perceptual and Motor Skills*, 1976, 42, 427-431.

Friedrich, W. N., & Boriskin, J. A. The role of the child in abuse: A review of the literature. *American Journal of Orthopsychiatry*, 1976, 46, 580-590.

Frodi, A. M., Lamb, M. E., Leavitt, L. A., & Donovan, W. L. Fathers' and mothers' responses to infant smiles and cries. *Infant Behavior and Development*, 1978, 1, 187-198.

Froebel, F. *The Education of Man*. (W. N. Hailman, Transl., 1826) New York: Appleton, 1892.

Frommer, E. A., & O'Shea, G. Antenatal identification of women liable to have problems in managing their infants. *British Journal of Psychiatry*, 1973, 123, 149-156.

Furstenberg, F. F., Jr. *Unplanned Parenthood*. New York: The Free Press, 1976.

Gajdusek, D. C. Environmental modification of human form and function. The problem of coding in the study of patterning in infancy of nervous system function. An approach to the study of learning. A paper presented at the First Plenary Session on Growth and Development, XII International Congress of Pediatrics, Mexico, D. F., December 1-7, 1968.

Garn, S. M. The origins of obesity. *Archives of the American Journal of Diseases of Children,* 1976, 130, 465-476.

Garn, S. M., Bailey, S. M., & Higgins, I. T. T. Fatness similarities in adopted pairs. *American Journal of Clinical Nutrition,* 1976, 29, 1067-1068.

Gauthier, V., Fortin, C., Drapeau, P., Breton, J. J., Gosselin, J., Quintal, L., Weisnagel, J., Tetreault, L., & Pinard, E. The mother-child relationship and the development of autonomy and self-assertion in young (14-30 months) asthmatic children: Correlating allergic and psychological factors. *Journal of the American Academy of Child Psychiatry,* 1977, 16, 109-131.

Geiken, K. Expectations concerning husband-wife responsibility in the home. *Journal of Marriage and the Family,* 1964, 26, 349-360.

Gelles, R. J. The social construction of child abuse. *American Journal of Orthopsychiatry,* 1975, 45, 363-371.

Gesell, A. The ontogenesis of infant behavior. In L. Carmichael (Ed.), *Manual of Child Psychology.* New York: Wiley, 1954.

Gewirtz, H. B., & Gewirtz, J. L. Caretaking settings, background events and behavior differences in four Israeli childbearing environments: Some preliminary trends. In B. Foss (Ed.), *Determinants of Infant Behavior IV.* London: Methuen, 1969, 229-252.

Gewirtz, J. L. (Ed.), *Attachment and Dependency.* New York: Wiley, 1972.

Gewirtz, J. L., & Boyd, E. F. Mother-infant interaction and its study. In H. W. Reese Ed.), *Advances in Child Development and Behaviors.* New York: Academic Press, 1976.

Gewirtz, J. L., & Boyd, E. F. Does maternal responding imply reduced infant crying? A critique of the 1972 Bell and Ainsworth report. *Child Development,* 1977, 48, 1200-1207.

Gilberg, A. L. The stresses of parenting. *Child Psychiatry and Human Development,* 1975, 6, 59-67.

Gilman, R., & Knox, D. Coping with fatherhood: The first year. *Child Psychiatry and Human Development,* 1976, 6, 134-148.

Ginsberg, B. E. Genotypic variables affecting responses to postnatal stimulation. In A. Ambrose (Ed.), *Stimulation in Early Infancy.* New York: Academic Press, 1969.

Glaser, R. Instructional technology and the measurement of learning outcomes: Some questions. *American Psychologist,* 1963, 18, 519-521.

Golani, I. Methodologies for developmental study. A paper presented at the Center for Interdisciplinary Research, University of Bielefeld, Bielefeld, West Germany: Early Development in Animals and Man, 1978.

Goldberg, S. Social competence in infancy: A model for parent-infant interaction. *Merrill-Palmer Quarterly,* 1977, 23, 163-177.

Goldberg, S., Brachfeld, S., & DiVitto, B. Feeding, fussing and play: Parent-infant interactions in the first year as a function of early medical problems. In T. Field, S. Goldberg, D. Stern, & A. Sostek (Eds.), *Interactions of High-Risk Infants and Children.* New York: Academic Press, 1978.

Goldblatt, P. B., Moore, M. E., & Stunkard, A. J. Social factors in obesity. *Journal of the American Medical Association,* 1965, 192, 1039-1044.

Golden, M., & Birns, B. Social class and infant intelligence. In M. Lewis (Ed.), *Origins of Intelligence: Infancy and Early Childhood.* New York: Plenum Press, 1976.

Goldfarb, J. L., Mumford, D. M., Schum, D. A., Smith, P. B., Flowers, C., & Schum, C. An attempt to detect "pregnancy susceptibility" in indigent adolescent girls. *Journal of Youth and Adolescence,* 1977, 60, 294-304.

Goldstein, J. The incidence and nature of child abuse. *Developmental Medicine and Child Neurology,* 1975, 17, 641-644.

Goldstein, K. M., Caputo, D. V., & Taub, H. B. The effects of prenatal and perinatal complications on development at one year of age. *Child Development*, 1976, 47, 613-621.

Goldstein, K. M., Taub, H. B., Caputo, D. V., & Silberstein, R. M. Child status and demographic variables as related to maternal child-rearing attitudes. *Perceptual and Motor Skills*, 1976, 42, 87-97.

Goldston, S. An overview of primary prevention programs: Implications for the mental health of black consumers. Presentation at the First Annual Symposium on Delivery of Mental Health Services to the Black Consumer. Milwaukee, Wisconsin, April 30, 1976.

Gordon, I. J. *The Infant Experience*. Columbus, OH: Charles E. Merrill, 1975.

Gordon, R. E., & Gordon, K. Some social-psychiatric aspects of pregnancy and child-bearing. *Journal of the Medical Society of New Jersey*, 1957, 54, 569-572.

Gordon, R. E., & Gordon, K. Social factors in the prediction and treatment of emotional disorders of pregnancy. *American Journal of Obstetrics and Gynecology*, 1959, 77, 1074-1083.

Gordon, R. E., Kapostins, E. E., & Gordon, K. K. Factors in postpartum emotional adjustment. *Obstetrics and Gynecology*, 1965, 25, 158-166.

Gorham, K. A., Des Jardins, C., Page, R., Pettis, E., & Schreiber, B. Effect on parents. In N. Hobbs (Ed.), *Issues in the Classification of Children* (Vol. 2). San Francisco: Jossey-Bass, 1975.

Gottesman, I. I., & Golden, R. R. Exploring psychiatric taxa and their validity with genetic family studies. In R. L. Spitzer & D. F. Klein (Eds.), *Critical Issues in Psychiatric Diagnosis*. New York: Raven Press, 1978, 237-247.

Gottfried, A. W. Intellectual consequences of perinatal anoxia. *Psychological Bulletin*, 1973, 80, 231-242.

Gottman, J. M., & Bakeman, R. The sequential analysis of observational data. In M. Lamb, S. Suomi, & G. Stephenson (Eds.), *Methodological Problems in the Study of Social Interaction*. Madison: University of Wisconsin Press, 1979.

Gottman, J. M., & Notarius, C. Sequential analysis of observational data using Markov chains. In T. Kratochwill (Ed.), *Strategies to Evaluate Change in Single Subject Research*. New York: Academic Press, 1976.

Graham, F. K., & Clifton, R. K. Heartrate change as a component of the orienting response. *Psychological Bulletin*, 1966, 65, 305-320.

Graham, F. K., & Jackson, J. C. Arousal systems and infant heart rate responses. In L. P. Lipsitt & M. W. Reese (Eds.), *Advances in Child Development and Behavior* (Vol. 5). New York: Academic Press, 1970, 59-117.

Graham, F. K., Matarazzo, R. C., & Caldwell, B. M. Behavioral differences between normal and traumatized newborns. *Genetic Psychology Monographs*, 1956, 70, 427.

Gray, S., & Klaus, R. An experimental preschool program for culturally deprived children. *Child Development*, 1965, 36, 887-898.

Greenberg, M., & Morris, N. Engrossment: The newborn's impact upon the father. *American Journal of Orthopsychiatry*, 1974, 44, 520-531.

Greenberg, M., & Rosenberg, I. First mothers rooming-in with their newborns: Its impact upon the mother. *American Journal of Orthopsychiatry*, 1973, 43, 783-788.

Greenberg, N. H. A comparison of infant-mother interactional behavior in infants with atypical behavior and normal infants. In J. Hellmuth (Ed.), *Exceptional Infant* (Vol. 2), *Studies in Abnormalities*. New York: Brunner/Mazel, 1971.

Greenberg, N. H., & Hurley, J. The maternal personality inventory. In J. Hellmuth (Ed.), *Exceptional Infant* (Vol. 2), *Studies in Abnormalities*. New York: Brunner/ Mazel, 1971.

Green, H. G. Infants of alcoholic mothers. *American Journal of Obstetrics and Gynecology*, 1974, 118, 713-716.

Green, M., & Solnit, A. Reactions to the threatened loss of a child: A vulnerable child syndrome. *Pediatrics,* 1964, 34, 58.

Greenough, W. T. Experimental modification of the developing brain. *American Scientist,* 1975, 63, 37-46.

Greenough, W. T. Enduring brain effects of differential experience and training. In M. R. Rosenzweig & E. L. Bennett (Eds.), *Neural Mechanisms of Learning and Memory.* Cambridge, MA: MIT Press, 1976, 255-278.

Grice, H. P. Utterer's meaning, sentence meaning and word meaning. *Foundations in Language,* 1968, 4, 1-16.

Grimm, E., & Venet, W. R. The relationship of emotional adjustment and attitudes to the course and outcome of pregnancy. *Psychosomatic Medicine,* 1966, 28, 34-49.

Grinker, J., & Hirsch, J. Metabolic and behavioral correlates of obesity. In J. Knight (Ed.), *Physiology, Emotion and Psychosomatic Illness* (Ciba Foundation Symposium). Amsterdam, The Netherlands: Associated Scientific Publishers, 1972.

Gruenwald, P. Pathology of the deprived fetus and its supply line. *Size at Birth* (Ciba Foundation Symposium). Amsterdam, The Netherlands: Associated Scientific Publishers, 1974.

Gunnar-Vongnechtlen, M. R. Changing a frightening toy into a pleasant toy by allowing the infant to control its actions. *Developmental Psychology,* 1978, 14, 157-162.

Gunther, M. Infant behavior at the breast. In B. M. Foss (Ed.), *Determinants of Infant Behavior.* New York: Wiley, 1961.

Gustafson, G. E., & Green, J. A. The infants' role in mother-infant games: A longitudinal study. Paper presented at the fifth biennial meeting of the Southeastern Conference on Human Development, Atlanta, April, 1978.

Gutton, P. Behavioral dialogues: An approach to the assessment of mother-infant interaction. *Child Development,* 1977, 48, 195-203.

Habermas, J. *Knowledge and Human Interests.* Boston: Boston Press, 1969.

Hager, A. Adipose cell size and number in relation to obesity. *Postgraduate Medical Journal,* 1977, 53, 101-110.

Hales, D. J., Lozoff, B., Sopa, R., & Kennell, J. H. Defining the limits of the maternal sensitive period. *Developmental Medicine and Child Neurology,* 1977, 19, 454-461.

Halverson, C. F., Moss, H. A., & Jones-Kearns, S. Longitudinal antecedents of preschool behaviors. Paper presented at the meeting of the Society for Research in Child Development, New Orleans, LA, 1977.

Hamburg, D. A., Moos, R. F., & Yalom, I. D. Studies of distress in the menstrual cycle and the postpartum period. In R. P. Michall (Ed.), *Endocrinology and Human Behavior.* London: Oxford University, 1968.

Hanes, M. L., & Dunn, S. K. Maternal attitudes and the development of mothers and children. In J. H. Stevens & M. Matthews (Eds.), *Mother/Child, Father/Child Relationships.* Washington, DC: NAEYC, 1978.

Hansen, E., & Bjerre, I. Mother-child relationships in low birthweight groups. *Child: Care, Health ,and Development,* 1977, 3, 93-103.

Hanson, D. R., Gottesman, I. I., & Meehl, P. E. Genetic theories and the validation of psychiatric diagnoses: Implications for the study of children of schizophrenics. *Journal of Abnormal Psychology,* 1977, 86, 575-588.

Hanson, J. W., Streissguth, A. P., & Smith, D. W. The effects of moderate alcohol consumption during pregnancy on fetal growth and morphogenesis. *Journal of Pediatrics,* 1978, 92, 457-460.

Hardy, J. B. Editorial: Birth weight and subsequent physical and intellectual development. *New England Journal of Medicine,* 1973, 289, 973-974.

Harlow, H., & Harlow, M. The effect of rearing conditions on behavior. *Bulletin of the Menninger Clinic,* 1962, 26, 213.

Harlow, H. F., Harlow, M. K., & Hansen, E. W. The maternal affectional system of rhesus monkeys. In H. Reingold (Ed.), *Maternal Behavior in Mammals*. New York: Wiley, 1963.

Harmon, R. J., Morgan, G. A., & Klein, R. P. Determinants of normal variation in infants' negative reactions to unfamiliar adults. *Journal of the American Academy of Child Psychiatry*, 1977, 16, 670-683.

Harnick, R. S. The relationship between ability level and task difficulty in producing imitation in infants. *Child Development*, 1978, 49, 209-212.

Harper, L. V. The scope of offspring effects: From caregiver to culture. *Psychological Bulletin*, 1975, 82, 784-801.

Harper, L. V. Early maternal handling and preschool behavior of human children. *Developmental Psychobiology*, 1972, 5, 61-70.

Harper, R. G., Solish, G., Purow, G. L., Sang, H. M., & Panepinto, W. C. The effects of a methadone treatment program upon pregnant addicts and their newborn infants. *Pediatrics*, 1974, 54, 300-305.

Harrell, J. E., & Ridley, C. A. Substitute child care, maternal employment and the quality of mother-infant interaction. *Journal of Marriage and Family*, 1975, 37, 556-564.

Harris, Z. J., & Shakow, D. Scatter on the Stanford-Binet in schizophrenic, normal, and delinquent adults. *Journal of Abnormal and Social Psychology*, 1938, 33, 100-111.

Hartz, A., Giefer, E., & Rimm, A. Relative importance of the effect of family environment and heredity on obesity. *Annals of Human Genetics*, 1977, 41, 185-193.

Hawkins, R. C. II. Meal initiation and meal termination: Clinical and developmental aspects of human obesity. In L. M. Barker, M. Best, & M. Domjan (Eds.), *Learning Mechanisms in Food Selection*. Waco, TX: Baylor University Press, 1977.

Hawkins, R. C. II, Setty, R. M., & Baldwin, B. Treatment manual for the Psychological Weight Control Program at The University of Texas at Austin. Unpublished manuscript, 1977.

Hayden, A. H., & Dmitriev, V. The multidisciplinary preschool program for Down's syndrome children at the University of Washington model preschool center. In B. Z. Friedlander, G. M. Sterritt, & G. E. Kirk (Eds.), *Exceptional Infant*, (Vol. 3), *Assessment and Intervention*. New York: Brunner/Mazel, 1975.

Healy, W., Bronner, A., & Bowers, A. M. *The Structure and Meaning of Psychoanalysis*. New York: Knopf, 1930.

Hebb, D. O. *Organization of Behavior*. New York: Wiley, 1949.

Heber, F. R. Sociocultural mental retardation: A longitudinal study. In D. Forgays (Ed.), *Primary Prevention of Psychopathology*, (Vol. II), *Environmental Influences*. Hanover, NH: University Press of New England, 1978, 39-62.

Heber, R., & Garber, H. The Milwaukee project: A study on the use of family intervention to prevent cultural-familial mental retardation. In B. Z. Friedlander, G. M. Sterritt, & G. E. Kirk (Eds.), *Exceptional Infant*, (Vol. 3), *Assessment and Intervention*. New York: Brunner/Mazel, 1975.

Heber, R., Garber, H., Harrington, S., Hoffman, C., & Falender, C. *Rehabilitation of Families at Risk for Mental Retardation*. Madison: Rehabilitation Research and Training Center in Mental Retardation, University of Wisconsin, 1972.

Hegmann, J. P. The response to selection for altered conduction velocity in mice. *Behavioral Biology*, 1975, 13, 413-423.

Heider, G. M. Factors in vulnerability from infancy to later age levels. In J. Hellmuth (Ed.), *Exceptional Infant*, (Vol. 2), *Studies in Abnormalities*. New York: Brunner/Mazel, 1971.

Heinstein, M. I., Expressed attitudes and feelings of pregnant women and their relations to physical complications of pregnancy. *Merrill-Palmer Quarterly*, 1967, 13, 217-236.

Helfer, R. Relationship between lack of bonding and child abuse and neglect. In M. H. Klaus, T. Leger, & M. A. Trause (Eds.), *Maternal Attachment and Mothering Disorders: A Round Table.* Sausalito, CA: Johnson and Johnson Baby Products Co., 1974.

Hellmuth, J. (Ed.) *Exceptional Infant,* (Vol. 1), *The Normal Infant.* New York: Brunner/Mazel, 1967.

Hellmuth, J. (Ed.) *Exceptional Infant,* (Vol. 2), *Studies in Abnormalities.* New York: Brunner/Mazel, 1971.

Henry, M., Ouellette, E., & Rosett, L. Adverse effects on offspring of maternal alcohol abuse during pregnancy. *New England Journal of Medicine,* 1977, 297, 528-531.

Herrnstein, R. IQ. *The Atlantic Monthly,* 1971, 228, 43-64.

Herrnstein, R. *IQ in the Meritocracy.* Boston: Little, Brown, 1973.

Hersher, L., Richmond, G., & Moore, A. Maternal behavior in sheep and goats. In H. Rheingold (Ed.), *Maternal Behavior in Mammals.* New York: Wiley, 1963.

Hess, E. H. Ethology and developmental psychology. In P. Mussen (Ed.), *Carmichael's Manual of Child Psychology,* (Vol. 1). New York: Wiley, 1970.

Hess, R. D. Social class and ethnic influences on socialization. In P. H. Mussen (Ed.), *Carmichael's Manual of Child Psychology,* (3rd Ed., Vol. 2). New York: Wiley, 1970.

Heymann, P. B., & Holtz, S. The severely defective newborn: The dilemma and the decision process. *Public Policy,* 1975, 23, 381-418.

Hildebrandt, K. A., & Fitzgerald, H. E. Facial feature determinants of perceived infant cuteness. Paper presented at the annual meeting of the Midwestern Psychological Association, Chicago, May 1977.

Hildebrandt, K. A., & Fitzgerald, H. E. Adult responses to infants varying in pereviced cuteness. *Behavioral Processes,* 1978, 3, 159-172.

Hill, V. *The Importance of Caregiver-Infant Interaction.* Seattle: Nursing Child Assessment Training, University of Washington, 1978.

Hilton, I. The dependent firstborn and how he grew. Paper presented at the meeting of the American Psychological Association, San Francisco, September, 1968.

Himwich, W. A., Hall, J. S., & MacArthur, W. F. Maternal alcohol and neonatal health. *Biological Psychiatry,* 1977, 12, 495-506.

Himmelfarb, S., & Eagly, A. H. Orientations to the study of attitudes and their change. In S. Himmelfarb & A. H. Eagly (Eds.), *Readings in Attitude Change.* New York: Wiley, 1974, 2-49.

Hirsch, J. Genetics and competence: Do heritability indices predict educability? In J. McV. Hunt (Ed.), *Human Intelligence.* New Brunswick, NJ: Transactions Books, 1972, 7-29.

Hirsch, J. Jensenism: The bankruptcy of "science" without scholarship. *United States Congressional Record, 122,* No. 73, E2671-2672; No. 74, E2693-2695; No. 75, E2703-2705, E2716-2718, E2721-2722, 1976.

Hobbs, D. F. Parenthood as a crisis: A third study. *Journal of Marriage and the Family,* 1965, 27, 367-372.

Hock, E. Working and nonworking mothers with infants: Perceptions of their careers, their infants' needs, and satisfaction with mothering. *Developmental Psychology,* 1978, 14, 37-43.

Hofer, M. A. Parent-infant interaction. Summing up. *Ciba Foundation Symposium,* 1975, 33, 309-313.

Hoffman, L. Effects of the employment of mothers on parental power relations and the division of household tasks. *Marriage and Family Living,* 1960, 22, 27-40.

Hoffman, M. L., & Hoffman, L. W. (Eds.), *Review of Child Development Research,* (Vols. 1-2). New York: Russell Sage Foundation, 1964-1966.

Holden, R. H., & Willerman, L. Neurological abnormality in infancy, intelligence, and social class. In E. P. Trapp & P. Himelstein (Eds.), *Readings on the Exceptional Child*, (2nd Ed.). New York: Appleton-Century-Crofts, Inc., 1972, 501-511.

Hollenbeck, A. R. Early infant home environments: Validation of the home observation for measurement of the environment inventory. *Developmental Psychology*, 1978, 14, 416-418.

Hollenbeck, A. R. Problems of reliability in observational research. In G. P. Sackett (Ed.), *Observing Behavior*, (Vol. II), *Data Collection and Analysis Methods*. Baltimore, MD: University Park Press, 1978.

Hollender, J. W. Interpersonal distance: Sibling structure and parental affection antecedents. *Journal of Genetic Psychology*, 1973, 123, 35-45.

Hollingshead, A. B. *Two Factor Index of Social Position*. New Haven, CT: Author, 1957, Unpublished manuscript.

Hollstedt, C., Olsson, O., & Rydberg, W. The effects of alcohol on the developing organism. Genetical, teratological and physiological aspects. *Medical Biology*, 1977, 55, 1-14.

Holmes, T., & Rahe, R. The Social Readjustment Rating Scale. *Journal of Psychosomatic Research*, 1967, 11, 213-218.

Holzinger, K. J. The relative effect of nature and nurture influences on twin differences. *Journal of Educational Psychology*, 1929, 20, 214-248.

Honzik, M. P. Value and limitations of infant tests: An overview. In M. Lewis (Ed.), *Origins of Intelligence: Infancy and Early Childhood*. New York: Plenum Press, 1976.

Horowitz, F. D. Epilogue: Safeguarding the developmental journey. In F. D. Horowitz (Ed.), *Early Developmental Hazards: Predictors and Precautions*. Boulder, CO: Westview Press, 1978.

Horowitz, F. D. The human infant and the processes of development. In F. D. Horowitz (Ed.), *Early Developmental Hazards: Predictors and Precautions*. Boulder, CO: Westview Press, 1978.

Horowitz, F. D., & Paden, L. Y. The effectiveness of environmental intervention programs. In B. M. Caldwell & H. H. Ricciuti (Eds.), *Review of Child Development Research*, (Vol. 3). Chicago: University of Chicago Press, 1973.

Hunt E. Mechanics of verbal ability. *Psychological Review*, 1978, 85, 109-130.

Hunt, J. McV. *Intelligence and Experience*. New York: Ronald Press, 1961.

Hunt, J. McV. Motivation inherent in information processing and action. In O. J. Harvey (Ed.), *Motivation and Social Interaction: The Cognitive Determinants*. New York: Ronald Press, 1963, 35-94.

Hunt, J. McV. Intrinsic motivation and its role in psychological development. In D. Levine (Ed.), *Nebraska Symposium on Motivation*, 1965, 13, 189-282. Lincoln: University of Nebraska Press, 1965.

Hunt, J. McV. The epigenesis of intrinsic motivation and the fostering of early cognitive development. In R. N. Haber (Ed.), *Current Research in Motivation*. New York: Holt, Rinehart, & Winston, 1966.

Hunt, J. McV. Toward a theory of guided learning in development. In R. H. Ojemann & K. Pritchett (Eds.), *Giving Emphasis to Guided Learning*. Cleveland, OH: Educational Research Council, 1966, 98-160.

Hunt, J. McV. *The Challenge of Incompetence and Poverty: Papers on the Role of Early Education*. Urbana: University of Illinois Press, 1969.

Hunt, J. McV. Intrinsic motivation and psychological development. In H. M. Schroder & P. Suedfeld (Eds.), *Personality Theory and Information Processing*. New York: Ronald Press, 1971.

Hunt, J. McV. Implications of sequential order and hierarchy in early psychological development. In B. Z. Friedlander, G. M. Sterritt, & G. E. Kirk (Eds.), *Exceptional Infant*, (Vol. 3), *Assessment and Intervention*. New York: Brunner/Mazel, 1975 (a).

Hunt, J. McV. Reflections on a decade of early education. *Journal of Abnormal Child Psychology,* 1975 (b), 3, 275-330.

Hunt, J. McV. Psychological development and the educational enterprise. *Educational Theory,* 1975 (c), 25 (4), 333-353.

Hunt, J. McV. Psychological assessment in education and social class. In M. L. Maehr & W. M. Stallings (Eds.), *Culture, Child, and School.* Monterey, CA; Brooks/Cole Publishing Co., pp. 132-171, 1975 (d).

Hunt, J. McV. Utility of ordinal scales derived from Piaget's observations. *Merrill-Palmer Quarterly,* 1976 (a), 22, (1), 31-45.

Hunt, J. McV. Environmental risk in fetal and neonatal life and measured infant intelligence. In M. Lewis (Ed.), *Origins of Intelligence: Infancy and Early Childhood.* New York: Plenum Press, 1976 (b).

Hunt, J. McV. *Specificity in Early Development and Experience.* Annual Lecture in Developmental Pediatrics. Omaha, Neb.: Meyer Children's Rehabilitation Institute, University of Nebraska Medical Center, 1977.

Hunt, J. McV. Language acquisition and experience. G. Stanley Hall Award Address, Meetings of the APA, San Francisco, 1979 (a).

Hunt, J. McV. Developmental psychology: Early experience. In *Annual Review of Psychology,* 1979 (b), 30, 103-143.

Hunt, J. McV. The experiential roots of intention, initiative, and trust. In H. I. Day (Ed.), *Advances in Intrinsic Motivation and Aesthetics.* New York: Plenum Publishing Corp., 1980.

Hunt, J. McV., & Kirk, G. E. Social aspects of intelligence: Evidence and issues. In R. Cancro (Ed.), *Intelligence: Genetic and Environmental Influences.* New York: Grune & Stratton, 1971.

Hunt, J. McV. Mohandessi, K., Ghodssi, M., & Akiyama, M. The psychological development of orphanage-reared infants: Interventions with outcomes (Tehran). *Genetic Psychology Monographs,* 1976, 94, 177-226.

Hunt, J. McV., & Paraskevopoulos, J. Children's psychological development as a function of the inaccuracy of their mother's knowledge of their abilities. *Journal of Genetic Psychology,* 1980, 136, 285-298.

Hunt, J. McV., Paraskevopoulos, J., Schickedanz, D., & Uzgiris, I. C. Variations in the mean ages of achieving object permanence under diverse conditions of rearing. In B. L. Friedlander, G. M. Sterritt, & G. E. Kirk (Eds.), *Exceptional Infant* (Vol. 3), *Assessment and Intervention.* New York: Brunner/Mazel, 1975.

Hunt, J. McV., & Rhodes, L. Mental development of pre-term infants during the first year. *Child Development,* 1977, 48, 204-210.

Hunter, R. S., Kilstrom, N., Kraybill, E. N., & Loda, F. Antecedents of child abuse and neglect in premature infants: A prospective study in a newborn intensive care unit. *Pediatrics,* 1978, 61, 629-635.

Jacobs, B. A., & Moss, H. A. Birth order and sex of sibling as determinants of mother-infant interaction. *Child Development,* 1976, 47, 315-322.

Jaffe, J., & Feldstein, S. *Rhythms of Dialogue.* New York: Academic Press, 1970.

Jansen, A. R., & Garland, M. J. (Eds.), *Ethics of Newborn Intensive Care.* A joint publication of Health Policy Program, School of Medicine, University of California, San Francisco and Institute of Governmental Studies, University of California, Berkeley, 1976.

Jencks, C. *Inequality: A Reassessment of the Effect of Family and Schooling in America.* New York: Basic Books, 1972.

Jenkins, G. M., & Watts, D. G. *Spectral Analysis and Its Applications.* San Francisco: Holden-Day, 1969.

Jensen, A. R. Estimation of the limits of heritability of traits by comparison of monozygotic and dizygotic twins. *Proceedings of the National Academy of Science,* 1967, 58, 149-157.

Jensen, A. R. How much can we boost IQ and scholastic achievement *Harvard Educational Review*, 1969, 39, 1-123.

Jensen, A. R. *Genetics and Education*. New York: Harper & Row, 1972.

Jensen, A. R. *Educability and Group Differences*. New York: Harper & Row, 1973.

Jensen, A. R. Let's understand Skodak and Skeels, finally. *Educational Psychologist*, 1973, 10, 30-35.

Johannsen, W. Om Arvelighed i Samfund og i rene Linier. Oversigt over det Kgl. danske videnskabernes selskabs forhandlinger #3 forelagt i modet den 6 Feb 1903. (From Peters, J. A., *Classic Papers in Genetics*. Englewood Cliffs, NJ: Prentice-Hall, 1959.)

Johannsen, W. *Elemente der exakten Erblichkeitslebre*. Jena: Fisher, 1909.

John, E. R., & Schwarz, E. L. The neurophysiology of information processing and cognition. *Annual Review of Psychology*, 1978, 29, 1-29.

Johnson, C. A., Ahern, F. M., & Johnson, R. C. Level of functioning of siblings and parents of probands of varying degrees of retardation. *Behavior Genetics*, 1976, 6, 473-477.

Johnson, D. L. The development of a program for parent-child education among Mexican-Americans in Texas. In B. Z. Friedlander, G. M. Sterritt, & G. E. Kirk (Eds.), *Exceptional Infant*, (Vol. 3), *Assessment and Intervention*. New York: Brunner/Mazel, 1975.

Johnson, R. H. An antipoverty delivery system model: Intervention strategies for families with children below the age of three years. *Birth Defects*, 1974, 10, 119-129.

Johnston, R. B., & Magrab, P. R. (Eds.). *Developmental Disorders: Assessment, Treatment, Education*. Baltimore: University Park Press, 1976.

Jones, H. E. The environment and mental development. In L. Carmichael (Ed.), *Handbook of Child Psychology*. New York: Wiley, 1954.

Jones, K. L., Smith, D. W., Streissguth, A. P., & Myrianthopoulos, N. C. Outcome in offspring of chronic alcoholic women. *The Lancet*, 1974, 1, 1076-1078.

Jones, K. L., Smith, D. W., Ulleland, C. N., & Streissguth, A. P. Pattern of malformation in offspring of chronic alcoholic mothers. *Lancet*, 1973, 1, 1267-1271.

Jones, O. H. M. Mother-child communication with pre-linguistic Down's syndrome and normal infants. In H. R. Schaffer (Ed.), *Studies in Mother-Infant Interaction*. New York: Academic Press, 1977.

Jones, O. Mother-child communication in very young Down's syndrome and normal children. In T. Field et al. (Eds.), *High-Risk Infants and Children*. New York: Academic Press, 1980.

Jones, O., & Pawlby, S. Pre-verbal mediation of the infant's social environment. Paper presented at the biennial conference of the International Society for the Study of Behavioral Development, Guildford, England, July, 1975.

Jones, S. J., & Moss, H. A. Age, state and maternal behavior associated with infant vocalizations. *Child Development*, 1971, 42, 1039-1051.

Josselyn, I. M. Cultural forces, motherliness, and fatherliness. *American Journal of Orthopsychiatry*, 1956, 26, 264-271.

Kaback, M. M. Detection of Tay-Sachs disease carriers: Lessons and ramifications. In H. A. Dubs & F. de la Cruz (Eds.), *Genetic Counseling*. New York: Raven Press, 1977.

Kaffman, M., & Elizur, E. Infants who become enuretics: A longitudinal study of 161 Kibbutz children. *Monographs of the Society for Research in Child Development*, 1977, 42, (3, Serial No. 171).

Kagan, J. Some response measures that show relations between social class and the course of cognitive development in infancy. In A. Ambrose (Ed.), *Stimulation in Early Infancy*. New York: Academic Press, 1969.

Kagan, J. *Change and Continuity in Infancy*. New York: Wiley, 1971.

Kagan, J. The child in the family. *Daedalus,* Spring, 1977, 33-56.

Kagan, J., & Klein, R. E. Cross-cultural perspectives on early development. *American Psychologist,* 1973, 28, 947-961.

Kagan, J., & Klein, R. E. Cross-cultural perspectives on early development. In B. Z. Friedlander, G. M. Sterrit, & G. E. Kirk (Eds.), *Exceptional Infant,* (Vol. 3), *Assessment and Intervention.* New York: Brunner/Mazel, 1975.

Kagan, J., & Moss, H. A. *Birth to Maturity.* New York: Wiley, 1962.

Kaplan, B. J. Malnutrition and mental deficiency. *Psychological Bulletin,* 1972, 78, 321-334.

Kappelman, M. M. Prenatal and perinatal factors which influence learning. In J. Hellmuth (Ed.), *Exceptional Infant,* (Vol. 2), *Studies in Abnormalities.* New York: Brunner/Mazel, 1971.

Karnes, M. B. Evaluation and implications of research with young handicapped and low-income children. In J. C. Stanley (Ed.), *Compensatory Education for Children, Ages 2 to 8.* Baltimore: Johns Hopkins University Press, 1973, 109-144.

Karnes, M. B., Teska, J. A., & Hodgins, A. S. A longitudinal study of disadvantaged children who participated in three different preschool programs. In *Selected Convention Papers, 47th Annual International Convention.* Arlington, VA: Council for Exceptional Children, 1969, 438-454.

Karnes, M. B., Teska, J. A., Hodgins, A. A., & Badger, E. D. Educational intervention at home by mothers of disadvantaged infants. *Child Development,* 1970, 41, 925-935.

Kaye, K. The maternal role in developing communication and language. In M. Bullowa (Ed.), *Before Speech: The Beginnings of Human Communication.* Cambridge: Cambridge University Press, 1977.

Kaye, K., & Brazelton, T. B. Mother-infant interaction in the organization of sucking. Paper presented at meeting of the Society for Research in Child Development, Minneapolis, April, 1971.

Keefer, C. A cross-cultural study of face-to-face interaction: Gusii infants and mothers. Paper presented at the Society for Research in Child Development, New Orleans, March, 1977.

Kellam, S. G., Emsinger, M. E., & Turner, R. J. Family structure and the mental health of children. *Archives of General Psychiatry,* 1977, 34, 1021-1022.

Kendon, A. Some functions of gaze direction in social interaction. *Acta Psychologica,* 1967, 26, 22-63.

Kennedy, J. The high risk maternal infant acquaintance process. *Nursing Clinics of North America,* 1973, 8, 549-556.

Kennell, G., Gordon, D. & Klaus, M. The effects of early mother-infant separation on later maternal performance. *Pediatric Research,* 1970, 4, 473-474.

Kennell, J. H., Jerauld, R., Wolfe, H., Chester, D., Kreger, N. C., McAlpine, W., Steffa, M., & Klaus, M. H. Maternal behavior one year after early and extended postpartum contact. *Developmental Medicine and Child Neurology,* 1974, 16, 172-179.

Kennell, J. H., Slyter, H., & Klaus, M. The mourning response of parents to the death of a newborn infant. *New England Journal of Medicine,* 1970, 283, 344.

Kennell, J. H., Trause, M. A., & Klaus, M. H. Evidence for a sensitive period in the human mother. *Parent-Infant Interaction,* Ciba Foundation Symposium. Amsterdam: Associated Scientific Publishers, 1974.

Kennell, J. H., Trause, M. A., & Klaus, M. H. Evidence for a sensitive period in the human mother. In R. H. Porter & M. O'Connor (Eds.), *Parent-Infant Interaction,* (Ciba Foundation Symposium 33). Amsterdam, The Netherlands: Associated Scientific Publishers, 1975.

Kessen, W. Comparative personality development. In E. F. Borgotta & W. W. Lambert (Eds.), *Handbook of Personality Theory and Research.* Chicago: Rand McNally, 1968.

Kestenberg, J. S. On the development of maternal feelings in early childhood. *Psychoanalytic Study of the Child,* 1959, 11, 257-291.

Kety, S. S., Rosenthal, D., Wender, P. H., & Schulsinger, F. Studies based on a total sample of adopted individuals and their relatives: Why they were necessary, what they demonstrated and failed to demonstrate. *Schizophrenia Bulletin,* 1976, 2, 413-428.

Kilbride, H. W., Johnson, D. L., & Streissguth, A. P. Social class, birth order, and newborn experience. *Child Development,* 1977, 48, 1686-1688.

Kinney, D. K., & Jacobsen, B. Environmental factors in schizophrenia: New adoption study evidence. In L. G. Wynne, R. L. Cromwell, & S. Mathysse (Eds.), *The Nature of Schizophrenia.* New York: Wiley, 1978, 38-51.

Kirk, G. E., & Hunt. J. McV. Social class and preschool language skill: I. Introduction. *Genetic Psychology Monographs,* 1975, 91, 281-298.

Kirk, G. E., Hunt, J. McV., and Volkmar, F. Social class and preschool language skill: VI. Child to Child communication and semantic mastery. *Genetic Psychology Monographs,* 1979, 100, 111-138.

Kitzinger, S. *The Experience of Childbirth,* New York: Penguin, 1972.

Klaus, M. H. Human maternal behavior at the first contact with her young. *Pediatrics,* 1970, 46, 187-192.

Klaus, M. H. Paper presented at Conference on Maternal-Infant Bonding. Boston, 1978.

Klaus, M. H., Jerauld, R., Kreger, N. C., McAlpine, W., Steffa, M., & Kennell, J. H. Maternal attachment, importance of the first postpartum days. *New England Journal of Medicine,* 1972, 286, 460-463.

Klaus, M., & Kennell, J. Mothers separated from their newborn infants. *Pediatric Clinics of North America,* 1970, 17, 1035.

Klaus, M. H., & Kennell, J. H. Mothers separated from their newborn infants. In J. L. Schwartz & L. H. Schwartz (Eds.), *Vulnerable Infants: A Psychosocial Dilemma.* New York: McGraw-Hill Book Company, 1977, 113-135.

Klaus, M. H., & Kennell, J. H. *Maternal-Infant Bonding.* St. Louis: The C. V. Mosby Co., 1976.

Klaus, M. H., & Kennell, J. H. Parent to infant attachment. In J. H. Stevens & M. Mathews (Eds.), *Mother/Child, Father/Child Relationships.* Washington, DC: NAEYC, 1978.

Klaus, M. H., Trause, M. A., & Kennell, J. H. Does human maternal behavior after delivery show a characteristic pattern? In R. H. Porter & M. O'Connor (Eds.), *Parent-Infant Interaction* (Ciba Foundation Symposium). Amsterdam, The Netherlands: Associated Scientific Publishers, 1975.

Klaus, R. A., & Gray S. W. The early training project for disadvantaged children: A report after five years. *Monographs of the Society for Research in Child Development,* 1968, 33 (4), No. 120.

Klein, M., & Stern, L. Low birth weight and the battered child syndrome. *American Journal of Diseases of Children,* 1971, 122, 15.

Klein, R. E., Lasky, R. E., Yarbrough, C., Habicht, J. P., Sellers, M. J. Relationship of infant/caretaker interaction, social class and nutritional status to developmental test performance among Guatemalan infants. In P. H. Leiderman, S. R. Tulkin, & A. Rosenfeld (Eds.), *Culture and Infancy: Variations in the Human Experience.* New York: Academic Press, 1977.

Klopfer, P. H., Adams, D. K., & Klopfer, M. S. Maternal "imprinting" in goats. *Proceedings of the National Academy of Sciences,* 1964, 52, 911-914.

Knittle, J. L., & Hirsch, J. Effects of early nutrition on the development of rat epididymal fat pads: Cellularity and metabolism. *Journal of Clinical Investigation,* 1968, 47, 2091.

Koch, H. L. Child psychology. *Annual Review of Psychology,* 1954, 5, 1026.

Kogan, K. L. Interaction systems between preschool aged handicapped or developmentally delayed children and their parents. In T. M. Field, S. Goldberg, D. Stern, & A. Sostek (Eds.), *Interactions of High-Risk Infants and Children.* New York: Academic Press, 1979.

Kohler, W. *The Mentality of Apes.* New York: Harcourt, Brace, 1926.

Kohn, M. L. *Class and Conformity.* Homewood, IL.: Dorsey, 1969.

Kolejkova, A. Early face-to-face interaction and its relation to later infant-mother attachment. *Child Development,* 1977, 48, 182-194.

Koluchová, J. A report on the further development of twins after severe and prolonged deprivation. In A. M. Clarke & A. D. B. Clarke, *Early Experience: Myth and Evidence.* New York: The Free Press, 1976, 58-66.

Kopf, R. C., & McFadden, E. L. Nursing inervention in the crisis of newborn illness. *Journal of Nursing Midwifery,* 1974, 18, 11.

Kopp, C. B. Fine motor abilities of infants. *Developmental Medicine and Child Neurology,* 1974, 16, 629-636.

Korner, A. F. Some hypotheses regarding the significance of individual differences at birth for later development. In J. Hellmuth (Ed.), *Exceptional Infant,* (Vol. 1), *The Normal Infant.* New York: Brunner/Mazel, 1967.

Korner, A. F. Visual alertness in neonates: Individual differences and their correlates. *Perceptual and Motor Skills,* 1970, 31, 499-509.

Korner, A. F. Sex differences in newborns with special reference to differences in the organization of oral behavior. *Journal of Child Psychology and Psychiatry,* 1973 (a), 14, 19-29.

Korner, A. F. Early stimulation and maternal care as related to infant capacities and individual differences. *Early Child Development and Care,* 1973 (b), 2, 307-327.

Korner, A. F. The effect of the infant's state, level of arousal, sex and ontogenetic stage on the caregiver. In M. Lewis & L. Rosenblum (Eds.), *The Effect of the Infant on Its Caregiver.* New York: John Wiley, 1974 (a).

Korner, A. F. Individual differences at birth: Implications for child care practice. *Birth Defects,* 1974 (b), 10, 51.

Korner, A. F., & Grobstein, R. Individual differences at birth: Implications for mother-infant relationships and later development. *Journal of the American Academy of Child Psychiatry,* 1967, 6, 676-690.

Korner, A., & Thoman, E. B. Visual alertness in neonates as evoked by maternal care. *Journal of Experimental Child Psychology,* 1970, 10, 76-78.

Kotelchuck, M. The infant's relationship to the father: Experimental evidence. In M. E. Lamb (Ed.), *The Role of the Father in Child Development.* New York: Wiley, 1976.

Kraemer, H. C., & Korner, A. F. Statistical alternatives in assessing reliability, consistency and individual differences for quantitative measures: Application to behavioral measures of neonates. *Psychological Bulletin,* 1976, 83, 914-921.

Krone, C. H. Mental health needs of women during pregnancy: The mental health nurse in obstetrics. *Michigan Nurse,* 1977, 50, 4-7.

Kubicek, L. Mother interactions of twins: An autistic and non-autistic twin. In T. M. Field, S. Goldberg, D. Stern, & A. Sostek (Eds.), *Interactions of High-Risk Infants and Children.* New York: Academic Press, 1979.

Kuo, Z. Y. Ontogeny of embryonic behavior in aves: IV. The influence of embryonic movements upon the behavior after hatching. *Journal of Comparative Psychology,* 1932, 14, 109-122.

Lally, J. R., & Honig, A. S. Education of infants and toddlers from low income and low education backgrounds: Support for the family's role and identity. In B. Z. Friedlander, G. M. Sterritt, & G. E. Kirk (Eds.), *Exceptional Infant,* (Vol. 3), *Assessment and Intervention.* New York: Brunner/Mazel, 1975.

Lamb, M. E. Effects of stress and cohort in mother- and father-infant interaction. *Developmental Psychology*, 1976 (a), 12, 435-443.

Lamb, M. E. The role of the father: An overview. In M. E. Lamb (Ed.), *The Role of the Father in Child Development*. New York: Wiley, 1976 (b).

Lamb, M. E. Father-infant and mother-infant interaction in the first year of life. *Child Development*, 1977 (a), 48, 167-181.

Lamb, M. E. A re-examination of the infant social world. *Human Development*, 1977 (b), 20, 65-85.

Landau, R. Extent that the mother represents the social stimulation to which the infant is exposed: Finding from a cross-sectional study. *Developmental Psychology*, 1976, 12, 399-405.

Landeeman-Dwyer, S., Keller, L. S., & Streissguth, A. P. Naturalistic observations of newborns, effects of maternal alcohol intake. *Alcoholism* (N. Y.), 1978, 2, 171-177.

Langman, J. *Medical Embryology*. Baltimore: Williams & Wilkins, 1975.

LaPiere, R. T. Attitudes versus actions. *Social Forces*, 1934, 13, 230-237.

Larsen, V. L., Brodsack, D. C., Dungley, L., Evans, T., Harmon, J., Hixson, A., Johnson, H., Liddane, M. J., Main, D., Martin, L., & Tallent, D. *Prediction and Improvement of Postpartum Adjustment*. (Children's Bureau Research Grant: H-66) Fort Steilacoom, WA: Division of Research, 1968.

Lashley, K. S. The problem of serial order in behavior. In L. A. Jeffress (Ed.), *Cerebral Mechanisms in Behavior: The Hixon Symposium*. New York: Wiley, 1951, 112-146.

Lasko, J. K. Parent behavior toward first and second children. *Genetic Psychology Monographs*, 1954, 49, 97-137.

Lawson, K., Daum, C., & Turkewitz, G. Environmental characteristics of a neonatal intensive care unit. *Child Development*, 1977, 48, 1633-1639.

Lazar, I., & Darlington, R. R. (Eds.), *Lasting Effects After Preschool*. Final Report, HEW Grant 90c-1311, to the Education Commission of the States, 1978.

Lazar, I., Hubble, V. R., Murray, H., Rosche, M., & Royce, J. *The Persistence of Preschool Effects*. Final Report, Grant No. 18-16-07843. Washington, D. C.; U.S. Government Printing Office, 1977.

Lebaiqz, K. Editorial correspondence: Mongoloid children and the burden of the family. *The Hastings Center Report*, Institute of Society, Ethics and the Life Sciences, 1972, 2, 12.

Lee, A. H. Relationship between birth weight and perceptual motor performance in children. *Perceptual and Motor Skills*, 1977, 45, 119-122.

Van Leeuwen, G. The nurse in prevention and intervention in the neonatal period. *Nursing Clinics of North America*, 1972, 8, 509-520.

Leiderman, P. H. The critical period hypothesis revisited: Mother to infant social bonding in the neonatal period. In F. D. Horowitz (Ed.), *Early Developmental Hazards: Predictors and Precautions*. Boulder, CO: Westview Press, 1978.

Leiderman, P. H., Leifer, A. D., Seashore, M. J., Barnett, C. R., & Grobstein, R. Mother-infant interaction: Effects of early deprivation, prior experience and sex of infant. *Research Publication of the Association for Research in Nervous and Mental Disease*, 1973, 51, 154-175.

Leiderman, P. H., & Seashore, M. J. Mother-infant separation: Some delayed consequences. In R. H. Porter & M. O'Connor (Eds.), *Parent-Infant Interaction* (Ciba Foundation Symposium 33). Amsterdam, The Netherlands: Associated Scientific Publishers, 1975.

Leiderman, P. H., Tulkin, S. R., & Rosenfeld, A. (Eds.), *Culture and Infancy*. New York: Academic Press, 1977.

Leifer, M. Psychological changes accompanying pregnancy and motherhood. *Genetic Psychology Monographs*, 1977, 95, 55-96.

Leifer, A. D., Liederman, P. H., Barnett, C. R., & Williams, J. A. Effects of mother-infant separation on mental attachment behavior. *Child Development,* 1972, 43, 1203-1218.

LeMasters, E. E. Parenthood as crisis. In H. J. Parad (Ed.), *Crisis Intervention: Selected Readings.* New York: Family Service Association of America, 1965.

Leonard, M. F., Rhymes, J. P., & Solnit, A. J. Failure to thrive in infants. *American Journal of Diseases of Children,* 1966, 8, 600-612.

Lester, B. M. Cardiac habituation of the orienting response to an auditory signal in infants of varying nutritional status. *Developmental Psychology,* 1975, 11, 430-442.

Lester, B. M., Emory, E. K., Huffman, S. L., & Eitzman, D. V. A multivariate study of the effects of high-risk factors on performance on the Brazelton neonatal assessment scale. *Child Development,* 1976, 47, 515-517.

Levenstein, P. The Mother-Child Home Program. In M. C. Day & R. K. Parker (Eds.), *The Preschool in Action* (2nd Ed.). Boston: Allyn and Bacon, 1976.

Levine, S. Infantile stimulation: A perspective. In A. Ambrose (Ed.), *Stimulation in Early Infancy.* New York: Academic Press, 1969.

Levinson, D., & Huffman, P. The traditional family ideology and its relation to personality. *Journal of Personality,* 1955. 23, 251- 273.

Levy, D. M. *Maternal Overprotection.* New York: W. W. Norton & Co., Inc., 1966.

Lewis, E. The management of stillbirth: Coping with an unreality. *Lancet,* 1976, 2, 619-620.

Lewis, M. State as an infant environment interaction: An analysis of mother-infant interaction. *Merrill-Palmer Quarterly,* 1972, 18, 95-122.

Lewis, M. Infant intelligence tests: Their use and misuse. *Human Development,* 1973, 16, 108-118.

Lewis, M. (Ed.), *Origins of Intelligence: Infancy and Early Childhood.* New York: Plenum Press, 1976 (a).

Lewis, M. What do we mean when we say "infant intelligence scores"? A sociopolitical question. In M. Lewis (Ed.), *Origins of Intelligence: Infancy and Early Childhood.* New York: Plenum Press, 1976 (b).

Lewis, M., & Goldberg, S. Perceptual-cognitive development in infancy: A generalized expectancy model as a function of the mother-infant interaction. *Merrill-Palmer Quarterly,* 1969, 15, 81-100.

Lewis, M., Johnson, N. What's thrown out with the bath water: A baby? *Child Development,* 1971, 42, 1053-1055.

Lewis, M., & Lee-Painter, S. An interactional approach to the mother-infant dyad. In M. Lewis & L. A. Rosenblum (Eds.), *The Effect of the Infant on Its Caregiver.* New York: Wiley, 1974.

Lewis, M., & Rosenblum, L. A. (Eds.), *The Effect of the Infant on Its Caregiver.* New York: Wiley, 1974.

Lewis, M., & Weintraub, M. The father's role in the child's social network. In M. E. Lamb (Ed.), *The Role of the Father in Child Development.* New York: Wiley, 1976.

Lewis, M., & Wilson, C. D. Infant development in lower class American families. *Human Development,* 1972, 15, 112-127.

Light, R. Abuse and neglected children in America: A study of alternative policies. *Harvard Educational Review,* 1973, 43, 556-598.

Lipsitt, L. P. Perinatal indicators and psychophysiological precursors of crib death. In F. D. Horowitz (Ed.), *Early Developmental Hazards: Predictors and Precautions.* Boulder, CO: Westview Press, 1978.

Liptak, G. S., Hulka, B. S., & Cassell, J. C. Effectiveness of physician-mother interactions during infancy. *Pediatrics,* 1977, 60, 186-192.

Liska, A. E. (Ed.), Introduction. In A. E. Liska (Ed.), *The Consistency Controversy.* Cambridge, MA: Schenkman, 1975, 1-20.

de Lissovoy, V. Child care by adolescent parents. *Children Today,* 1973, 2, 22-25.

Little, R. E., Schultz, F., & Mandell, W. Drinking during pregnancy. *Journal of Studies on Alcohol,* 1976, 37, 375-379.

Little, R. E., & Streissguth, A. P. Drinking during pregnancy in alcoholic women. *Alcoholism,* 1978, 2, 179-183.

Littman, B., et al. Caring for families of high-risk infants. *Western Journal of Medicine,* 1976, 124, 429-433.

Loesch, J. G., & Greenberg, N. H. Some specific areas of conflict observed during pregnancy: A comparative study of married and unmarried pregnant women. *American Journal of Orthopsychiatry,* 1962, 32, 624-636.

Lopata, H. Z. *Occupation: Housewife.* New York: The Oxford University Press, 1971.

Lorber, J. Results of treatment of myelomeningocele: An analysis of 524 unselected cases, with special reference to possible selection for treatment. *Developmental Medicine and Child Neurology,* 1971, 13, 279-303.

Lorber, J. Spina bifada cystics: Results of treatment of 270 consecutive cases with criteria for selection for the future. *Archives of Disorders of Childhood,* 1972, 47, 854-873.

Lorber, J. Early results of selective treatment of spina bifada cystica. *British Medical Journal,* 1973, 4, 201.

Lubchenco, L. O., Horner, F. A., Reed, L. H., Hix, L. E. Jr., Metcalf, D. R., Cohig, R., Elliot, N. C., & Bours, M. Sequelae of premature birth: Evaluation of premature infants of low birth weights of 10 years of age. *American Journal of Diseases of Children,* 1963, 106, 101.

Lubs, H. A., & de la Cruz, F. *Genetic Counseling.* New York: Raven Press, 1977.

Lumsdaine, A. A., & Glaser, R. (Eds.), *Teaching Machines and Programmed Learning.* Washington, DC: National Education Association, 1960.

Lynch, A. An MMPI scale for identifying at risk abusive parents. *Journal of Clinical Child Psychology,* 1975, 4, 22-24.

Lynch, M. A., & Roberts, J. Predicting child abuse: Signs of bonding failure in the maternity hospital. *British Medical Journal,* 1977, 60, 624-626.

Lynch, M. A., Roberts, J., & Gordon, M. Child abuse: Early warning in the maternity hospital. *Developmental Medicine and Child Neurology,* 1976, 18, 759-766.

Lytton, H. Observational studies of parent-child interaction: A methodological review. *Child Development,* 1971, 42, 651-683.

Maccoby, E. E., & Masters, J. Attachment and dependency. In P. Mussen (Ed.), *Manual of Child Psychology,* (3rd ed., Vol. 2). New York: Wiley, 1970.

Macfarlane, A. *The Psychology of Childbirth.* Cambridge: Harvard University Press, 1977.

Mack, R. W., & Johnston, F. E. The relationship between growth in infancy and growth in adolescence: Report of a longitudinal study among urban black adolescents. *Human Biology,* 1976, 48, 693-711.

Mack, R. W., & Kleinhenz, M. E. Growth, caloric intake, and activity levels in early infancy: A preliminary report. *Human Biology,* 1974, 46, 345-354.

Magrab, P. R. Psychosocial function: Normal development—infantile autism. In R. B. Johnston & P. R. Magrab (Eds.), *Developmental Disorders: Assessment, Treatment, Intervention.* Baltimore: University Park Press, 1976.

Mahler, M. S. Symbiosis and individuation: The psychological birth of the human infant. *Psychoanalytic Study of the Child,* 1974, 29, 89.

Maltzman, I., & Raskin, D. C. Effects of individual differences in the orienting reflex on conditioning and complex processes. *Journal of Experimental Research in Personality,* 1965, 1, 1-16.

Mameny, A. P., Jr., Dolan, A. B., & Wilson, R. S. Bayley's infant behavior record:

Relations between behaviors and mental test scores. *Developmental Psychology,* 1974, 16 ,696-702.

Mannino, F. V. Family structure, aftercare, and post-hospital adjustment. *American Journal of Orthopsychiatry,* 1974, 44, 61-69.

Marjonibanks, K. Birth order, family environment, and mental abilities: A regression surface analysis. *Psychological Reports,* 1976, 39, 759-765.

Martin, B. Parent-child relations. In F. B. Harowitz, (Ed.), *Review of Child Development Research,* Vol. 4. Chicago: University of Chicago Press, 1975.

Martin, J., Martin, D., Lund, C., & Streissguth, A. Maternal ingestion and cigarette smoking and their effects on newborn conditioning. *Alcoholism: Clinical Experimental Research,* 1977, 1, 243-247.

Martini, M. Interactions between caretakers and infants on the Marquesan Island of Ua Pou. In T. Field, A. Sostek & P. Vietze (Eds.), *Culture and Early Interactions.* Hillsdale, NJ: Lawrence Erlbaum, 1980.

Massie, H. N. The early natural history of childhood psychosis. *Journal of the American Academy of Child Psychiatry,* 1975, 14, 683-707.

Massie, H. N. Patterns of mother-infant behavior and subsequent childhood psychosis. A research and case report. *Child Psychiatry and Human Development,* 1977, 7, 211-230.

Massie, H. N. The early natural history of childhood psychosis: Ten cases studied by analysis of family home movies of the infancies of the children. *Journal of the American Academy of Child Psychiatry,* 1978, 17, 29-45.

Matas, L., Arend, R. A., & Sroufe, L. A. Continuity of adaptation in the second year: The relationship between quality of attachment and later competence. *Child Development,* 1978, 49, 547-556 .

Mayer, J. *Overweight: Causes, Cost, and Control.* Englewood Cliffs, NJ: Prentice-Hall, 1968.

Mayr, E. *Animal Species and Evolution.* Cambridge: Harvard University Press, 1963.

McAndrew, L. Children with a handicap and their families. *Child: Care, Health and Development,* 1976, 2, 213-237.

McArthur, C. Personalities of first and second children. *Psychiatry,* 1956, 19, 47-54.

McCall, R. B. Toward an epigenetic conception of mental development in the first three years of life. In M. Lewis (Ed.), *Origins of Intelligence: Infancy and Early Childhood.* New York: Plenum Press, 1976.

McCall, R. B. Challenges to a science of developmental psychology. *Child Deveolpment,* 1977, 48, 333-334.

McCall, R. B., Eichorn, D. H., & Hogarty, P. S. Transitions in early mental development. *Monographs of the Society for Research in Child Development,* 1977, 42, No. 171.

McCall, R. B., Hogarty, P. S., & Hurlburt, N. Transitions in infant sensorimotor development and the prediction of childhood IQ. *American Psychologist,* 1972, 27, 728-748.

McGowan, M. N. Post partum disturbance. *Journal of Nurse-Midwifery,* 1977, 22, 27-34.

McGuire, W. J. The nature of attitudes and attitude change. In G. Lindzey & E. Aronson (Eds.), *Handbook of Social Psychology.* (Vol. 3) Reading: Addison-Wesley, 1968.

Mcintyre, M. N. Need for supportive therapy for members of a family with a defective child. In H. A. Lubs & F. de la Cruz (Eds.), *Genetic Counseling.* New York: Raven Press, 1977.

McLaughlin, J., Sandler, H. M., Sherrod, K., Vietze, P. H., & O'Connor, S. Social-psychological characteristics of adolescent mothers and behavioral characteristics of their first-born infants. Unpublished manuscript, George Peabody, 1978.

McMillan, M. *The Nursery School.* London: J. M. Dent & Sons, 1919, Revised Edition, 1930.

McNemar, Q. *Psychological Statistics.* New York: Wiley, 1955.

Mead, G. H. *Mind, Self, and Society.* Chicago: University of Chicago Press, 1934.

Mech, E. V. Adoption: A policy perspective. In B. M. Caldwell & H. N. Ricciuti (Eds.), *Review of Child Development Research.* Chicago: University of Chicago Press, 1973.

Mednick, B. R. Breakdown in high-risk subjects: Familial and early environmental factors. *Journal of Abnormal Psychology,* 1973, 82, 469-475.

Mednick, S. A., & Schulsinger, F. A. Learning theory of schizophrenia. In Hammer et al. (Eds.), *Psychopathology: Contributions from the Social, Behavioral, and Biological Sciences.* New York: Wiley, 1973.

Mednick, S. A., Schulsinger, R., & Garfinkel, R. Children at high risk for schizophrenia: Predisposing factors and intervention. In M. L. Kietzman, S. Sutton, & J. Zubin (Eds.), *Experimental Approaches to Psychopathology.* New York: Academic Press, 1975.

Meier, J. H. Screening, assessment, and intervention for young children at developmental risk. In B. Z. Friedlander, G. M. Sterritt, & G. E. Kirk (Eds.), *Exceptional Infant* (Vol. 3), *Assessment and Intervention.* New York: Brunner/Mazel, 1975.

Melber, R. S. An approach for evaluating and improving maternity nursing care. *ANA Clinical Sessions,* 1968. New York: Appleton-Century-Crofts, 1969.

Mellbin, T., & Vuille, J. C. Relationship of weight gain in infancy to subcutaneous fat and relative weight at 10½ years of age. *British Journal of Preventive and Social Medicine,* 1976, 30, 239-243.

Mercer, R. T. Mothers' responses to their infants with defects. *Nursing Research,* 1974, 23, 133-137.

Mercer, R. T. Postpartum: Illness and acquaintance-attachment process. *American Journal of Nursing,* 1977, 77, 1174-1178.

Metropolitan Life Insurance Company. New weight standards for men and women. *Statistical Bulletin,* 1959, 40, 1-4.

Miller, D. B. Roles of naturalistic observation in comparative psychology. *American Psychologist,* 1977, 32, 211-219.

Miller, H. C. Fetal malnutrition in white newborn infants: Maternal factors. *Pediatrics,* 1973, 52, 504-512.

Miller, H. C. Maternal factors in "fetally malnourished" black newborn infants. *American Journal of Obstetrics and Gynecology,* 1974, 118, 62-67.

Miller, J. O. *Diffusion of Intervention Effects in Disadvantaged Families.* Occasional Paper, Urbana: University of Illinois, Coordination Center, National Laboratory of Early Childhood Education, 1968.

Milner, J., & Williams, P. Child abuse and neglect: A bibliography. *JSAS Catalog of Selected Documents in Psychology,* 1978, 8, 42.

Minde, K., Trehub, S., Corter, C., Boukydis, C., Celhoffer, B., & Marton, P. Mother-child relationships in the premature nursery: An observational study. Unpublished manuscript, Department of Psychiatry, The Hospital for Sick Children, Toronto, Canada, 1977.

Minturn, L., & Lambert, W. *Mothers of Six Cultures.* New York: Wiley, 1964.

Mitchell, R. The incidence and nature of child abuse. *Developmental Medicine and Child Neurology,* 1975, 17, 641-644.

Montessori, M. 1909. *The Montessori Method: Scientific Pedagogy as Applied to Child Education in "The Children's Houses"* (Revised edition). New York: Schocken Books, 1964.

Moore, A. U. Effects of modified maternal care in the sheep and goat. In G. Newton & S. Levene (Eds.), *Early Experience and Behavior.* Springfield, IL: Thomas, 1968.

Moss, H. A. Sex, age, and state as determinants of mother-infant interaction. *Merrill-Palmer Quarterly,* 1967, 13, 19-36.

Moss, H. A. Early sex differences in mother infant interaction. In R. C. Friedman, R. M. Richant, & R. L. Vandewiele (Eds.), *Sex Differences in Behavior.* New York: Wiley, 1974.

Moss, H. A., & Jones, S. J. Relations between maternal attitudes and maternal behavior as a function of social class. In P. H. Leiderman, S. R. Tulkin, & A. Rosenfeld (Eds.), *Culture and Infancy: Variations in the Human Experience.* New York: Academic Press, 1977.

Moss, H. A. An analysis of mother-infant interactions. Unpublished manuscript, NIMH, Bethesda, Maryland, 1977.

Mulvihill, J., Klimas, J., Stokes, D., & Risenberg, H. Fetal alcoholism: Seven new cases. *American Journal of Obstetrics and Gynecology,* 1976, 122, 937-941.

Nadelson, C. C. The pregnant teenager: Problems of choice in a developmental framework. *Psychiatric Opinion,* 1975, 12, 6-12.

Naeye, R. L., Blane, W., & Blane, P. C. Effects of maternal nutrition on the human fetus. *Pediatrics,* 1973, 52, 494-503.

Neale, J. M., & Weintraub, S. Children vulnerable to psychopathology: The Story Book High Risk Project. *Journal of Abnormal Child Psychology,* 1975, 3, 95-113.

Neel, J. V. On some pitfalls in developing an adequate genetic hypothesis. *American Journal of Human Genetics,* 1955, 7, 1-14.

Neuman, C. G., & Alpaugh, M. Birthweight doubling time: A fresh look. *Pediatrics,* 1976, 56, 469-473.

Newberger, E. H., Reed, R. B., Daniel, J. H., Hyde, J. N., Jr., & Kotelchuck, M. Pediatric social illness: Toward an etiologic classification. *Pediatrics,* 1977, 60, 178-185.

Newton, N. Emotions of pregnancy. *Clinical Obstetrics and Gynecology,* 1963, 6, 639-668.

Newton, N. R., & Newton, M. Relationship of ability to breast feed and maternal attitudes toward breast feeding. *Pediatrics,* 1950, 5, 869-875.

Nielsen, G., Collins, S., Meisel, J., Lowry, M., Engh, H., & Johnson, D. An intervention program for atypical infants. In B. Z. Friedlander, G. M. Sterritt, & G. E. Kirk (Eds.), *Exceptional Infant,* (Vol. 3), *Assessment and Intervention.* New York: Brunner/Mazel, 1975.

Nolan-Haley, J. H. Defective children, their parents, and the death decision. *Journal of Legal Medicine,* 1976, 4, 9-14.

Nuckholls, K. B., Cassell, J., & Kaplan, B. H. Psychological assets, life crises and the prognosis of pregnancy. *American Journal of Epidemiology,* 1972, 95, 431-441.

Nunnally, D., & Aguiar, M. Patients' evaluation of their prenatal and delivery care. *Nursing Research,* 1974, 23, 469-474.

Nunnally, J. *Psychometric Theory.* New York: McGraw-Hill, 1967.

Orthner, D., Brown, T., & Ferguson, D. Single-parent fatherhood: An emerging life style. *Family Coordinator,* 1976, 25, 429-438.

Oppe, T. E. Speculations on the relevance of developmental psychology to pediatrics. In R. Porter & M. O'Connor (Eds.), *Parent-Infant Interaction* (Ciba Foundation Symposium 33). Amsterdam, The Netherlands: Associated Scientific Publishers, 1975.

Osgood, C. E., Suci, G. J., & Tannenbaum, P. H. *The Measurement of Meaning.* Urbana, IL: University of Illinois Press, 1957.

Osofsky, H. J. Poverty, pregnancy outcome and child development. *Birth Defects: Infants at Risk,* 1974, 10, 37-49.

Osofsky, H. J. Relationship between nutrition during pregnancy and subsequent infant and child development. *Obstetrics, Gynecology Survey,* 1975 (a), 30, 227.

Osofsky, H. J. Relationships between prenatal medical and nutritional measures, pregnancy outcome, and early infant development in an urban poverty setting. *American Journal of Obstetrics and Gynecology*, 1975 (b), 12, 682-690.

Osofsky, H. J., & Kendall, N. Poverty as a criterion of risk. *Clinical Obstetrics and Gynecology*, 1974, 16, 103-119.

Osofsky, J. D. Neonatal characteristics and mother-infant interactions in two observational situations. *Child Development*, 1976, 47, 1138-1147.

Osofsky, J. D., & Danzger, B. Relationships between neonatal characteristics and mother-infant interaction. *Developmental Psychology*, 1974, 10, 124-130.

Ounsted, C., Oppenheimer, R., & Lindsay, J. Aspects of bonding failure: The psychopathology and psychotherapeutic treatment of families of battered children. *Developmental Medicine & Child Neurology*, 1974, 16, 447-456.

Ounsted, C., Oppenheimer, R., & Lindsay, J. The psychopathology and psychotherapy of the families: Aspects of bonding failure. In A. W. Franklin (Ed.), *Concerning Child Abuse*. Edinburgh, Scottland: Churchill Livingstone, 1975.

Overton, W. P. On the assumptive basis of the nature-nurture controversy: Additive versus interactive components. *Human Development*, 1973, 16, 74-89.

Page, E. B. Miracle in Milwaukee: Raising the IQ. In B. Z. Friedlander, G. M. Sterritt, & R. E. Kirk (Eds.), *Exceptional Infant*, (Vol. 3), *Assessment and Intervention*. New York: Brunner/Mazel, 1975.

Pakizegi, B. The interaction of mothers and fathers with their sons. *Child Development*, 1978, 49, 479-482.

Palani, P. E. Chromosomal and other genetic influences on birth weight variation. *Size at Birth*, (Ciba Foundation Symposium). Amsterdam, The Netherlands: Associated Scientific Publishers, 1974.

Palmer, F. H. Inferences to the socialization of the child from animal studies: A view from the bridge. In D. A. Goslin (Ed.), *Handbook of Socialization Theory and Research*. Chicago: Rand McNally, 1969.

Papajohn, J., & Spiegel, J. *Transactions in Families*. San Francisco: Jossey-Bass, 1975.

Pape, K. E., Buncic, R. J., Ashby, S., Fitzhardinge, P. M. The status at two years of low birth weight infants born in 1974 with birthweights of less than 1001 gm. *Journal of Pediatrics*, 1978, 92, 253.

Papousek, H., & Bernstein, P. The functions of conditioning stimulation in human neonates and infants. In A. Ambrose (Ed.), *Stimulation in Early Infancy*. New York: Academic Press, 1969.

Papousek, H., & Papousek, M. Cognitive aspects of preverbal social interactions between human infants and adults. In R. H. Porter & M. O'Connor (Eds.), *Parent-Infant Interaction* (Ciba Foundation Symposium). Amsterdam, The Netherlands: Associated Scientific Publishers, 1975.

Papousek, H., & Papousek, M. Mothering and the cognitive head start: Psychobiological considerations. In H. R. Schaffer (Ed.), *Studies in Mother-Infant Interaction*. New York: Academic Press, 1977.

Paraskevopoulos, J. & Hunt, J. McV. Object construction and imitation under differing conditions of rearing. *Journal of Genetic Psychology*, 1971, 119, 301-321.

Parke, R. D. Family interaction in the newborn period: Some findings, some observations, and some unresolved issues. In K. Riegal & J. Meacham (Eds.), *Proceedings of the International Society of Behavior Development*, 1974.

Parke, R. D. Perspectives on father-infant interaction. In J. D. Osofsky (Ed.), *Handbook of Infant Development*. New York: Wiley, 1979.

Parke, R. D., & Collmer, C. W. Child abuse: An interdisciplinary analysis. In E. M. Hetherington (Ed.), *Review of Child Development Research*, (Vol. 4) Chicago: University of Chicago Press, 1975.

Parke, R. D., & O'Leary, S. E. Father-mother-infant interaction in the newborn period: Some findings, some observations and some unresolved issues. In K. Riegel and J.

Meacham (Eds.), *The Developing Individual in a Changing World*, (Vol. 2), *Social and Environmental Issues*. The Hague: Mouton, 1976.

Parke, R. D., O'Leary, S., & West, S. Mother-father-newborn interaction: Effects of maternal medication between labor and sex of infant. Paper presented at a convention of the American Psychological Association, 1972.

Parke, R. D., Power, T. G., & Gottman, J. Conceptualizing and quantifying influence patterns in the family triad. In M. E. Lamb, S. J. Suomi, & G. R. Stephenson (Eds.), *The Study of Social Interaction: Methodological Issues*. Madison: University of Wisconsin Press, 1978.

Parke, R. D., & Sawin, D. B. Infant characteristics and behavior as elicitors of maternal and paternal responsibility in the newborn period. Paper presented at the Biennal Meeting of the Society for Research in Child Development, Denver, April 1975.

Parke, R. D., & Sawin, D. B. The father's role in infancy: A re-evaluation. *The Family Coordinator*, 1976, 25, 365-371.

Parke, R. D., & Sawin, D. B. Father-infant interaction in the newborn period: A re-evaluation of some current myths. In E. M. Hetherington & R. D. Parke (Eds.), *Contemporary Readings in Child Psychology*. New York: McGraw-Hill, 1977 (a).

Parke, R. D., & Sawin, D. B. The family in early infancy: Social interactional and attitudinal analyses. In F. A. Pederson (Ed.), *The Father-Infant Relationship: Observational Studies in a Family Context*. New York: Holt, Rinehart & Winston, 1980.

Parmelee, A. H., Kopp, C. B., & Sigman, M. Selection of developmental assessment techniques for infants at risk. *Merrill-Palmer Quarterly*, 1976, 22, 177-199.

Pasamanick, B., & Knobloch, H. Epidemiologic studies on the complications of pregnancy and the birth process. In G. Caplan (Ed.), *Prevention of Mental Disorders in Children*. New York: Basic Books, 1961.

Pasamanick, B., & Knobloch, H. Retrospective studies on the epidemiology of reproductive causality: Old and new. *Merrill-Palmer Quarterly*, 1966, 12, 7-26.

Patterson, G. R. Reprogramming the families of aggressive boys. In C. Thoresen (Ed.), *Behavior Modification in Education*. 72nd Yearbook, National Society for the Study of Education, 1973.

Paulson, M. Child trauma intervention: A community response to family violence, *Journal of Child Psychology*, 1975, 4, 26-29.

Pawlby, S. Imitative interaction. In H. R. Schaffer (Ed.), *Studies in Mother-Infant Interaction*. London: Academic Press, 1977.

Pawlby, S., & Hall, F. Interaction of infants whose mothers come from disrupted families. In T. Field, S. Goldberg, D. Stern, & A. Sostek (Eds.), *Interactions of High-Risk Infants and Children*. New York: Academic Press, 1979.

Payne, J. S., Mercer, C. D., Payne, R. A., & Davison, R. G. *Head Start: A Tragicomedy with Epilogue*. New York: Behavioral Publications, 1973.

Pedersen, F. A., Anderson, B. J., & Cain, R. L. An approach to understanding linkages between the parent-infant and spouse relationship. Paper presented at the Biennial Meeting of the Society for Research in Child Development, New Orleans, March 1977.

Perry, J. H., & Freedman, D. A. Massive neonatal environment deprivation: A clinical and neuroanatomical study. *Research Publication of the Association for Research on Nervous Mental Disease*, 1973, 51, 44-268.

Perry, J. C., & Stern, D. N. Mother-infant gazing during play, bottle feeding and spoon feeding. *Journal of Psychology*, 1975, 91, 207-213.

Philipps, C., & Johnson, N. E. The impact of quality of diet and other factors on birth weight of infants. *American Journal of Clinical Nutrition*, 1977, 30, 215-225.

Piaget, J. 1936. *The Origins of Intelligence in Children*. (M. Cooke, Transl.) New York: International Universities Press, 1952.

Piaget, J. 1937. *The Construction of Reality in the Child.* (M. Cooke, Transl.) New York: Basic Books, 1954.

Piaget, J. 1945. *Play, Dreams, and Imitation in Children.* (C. Gattegno & F. M. Hodgson, Transls.) New York: Norton, 1951.

Piaget, J. *Psychology of Intelligence.* New York: Harcourt, Brace, & World, 1950.

Piaget, J. 1947. *The Psychology of Intelligence.* (M. Piercy & D. E. Berlyne, Transls.) Paterson, NJ: Littlefield, Adams & Co., 1960.

Piaget, J. Problems of equilibration. In M. H. Appel & L. S. Goldberg (Eds.), *Topics in Cognitive Development* (Vol. 1), *Equilibration: Theory, Research and Application.* New York: Plenum Press, 1977.

Pines, D. Pregnancy and motherhood: Interaction between fantasy and reality. *British Journal of Medical Psychology,* 1972, 45, 333-343.

Pitt, B. Psychological aspects of pregnancy. *Midwife Health Visitor and Community Nurse,* 1977, 13, 140-142.

Pollitt, E., & Eichler, A. Behavioral disturbances among failure-to-thrive children. *Archives of American Journal of Diseases of Children,* 1976, 130, 24-29.

Pollitt, E., Eichler, A. W., & Chan, C. K. Psychosocial development and behavior of mothers of failure-to-thrive children. *American Journal of Orthopsychiatry,* 1975, 45, 525-537.

Porter, R., & O'Conner, M. (Eds.), *Parent-Infant Interaction* (Ciba Foundation Symposium 33). Amsterdam, The Netherlands: Associated Scientific Publishers, 1975.

Poskitt, E. M. E. Overfeeding and overweight in infancy and their relation to body size in early childhood. *Nutrition and Metabolism,* 1977, 21, 54-55.

Poskitt, E. M. E., & Cole, T. J. Nature, nurture, and childhood overweight. *British Medical Journal,* 1978, 1, 603-605.

Potter, H. W., & Klein, H. R. On nursing behavior. *Psychiatry,* 1957, 20, 39-46.

Powell, L. F. The effect of extra stimulation and maternal involvement on the development of low-birth-weight infants and on maternal behavior. *Child Development,* 1974, 45, 106-113.

Prechtl, H. F. R. The behavioral states of the newborn. *Brain Research,* 1974, 6, 185-212.

Prechtl, H., & Beintema, D. *The Neurological Examination of the Full Term Newborn Infant.* Clinics in Developmental Medicine, No. 12, London, Spastics Society with Heinemann Medical, 1964.

Provence, S., Naylor, A., & Patterson, J. *The Challenge of Daycare.* Yale University Press, 1977.

Pruette, L. G. *Stanley Hall: A Biography of a Mind.* New York: Appleton, 1926.

Prugh, D. Emotional problems of premature infants' parents. *Nursing Outlook,* 1953, 1, 461-464.

Rachels, J. Active and passive euthanasia. *New England Journal of Medicine,* 1975, 292, 78-80.

Raguis, N., Schachter, J., Elmer, E., Preismare, R., Bower, A. E., & Harway, V. Infants and children at risk for schizophrenia: Environmental and developmental observations. *Journal of the American Academy of Child Psychiatry,* 1975, 14, 150-177.

Ramey, C., Mills, P., Campbell, F., & O'Brien, C. Infants' home environments: A comparison of high-risk families and families from the general population. *American Journal of Mental Deficiency,* 1975, 80, 40-42.

Rapoport, J., Pandoni, C., Renfield, M., Lake, C. R., & Ziegler, M. G. Newborn dopamine-B-Hydroxylase, minor physical anomalies, and infant temperament. *American Journal of Psychiatry,* 1977, 134, 676-679.

Rau, J. H., & Kaye, H. Joint hospitalization of mother and child. Evaluation in vivo. *Bulletin of the Menninger Clinic,* 1977, 41, 385-394.

Reed, E. Genetic anomalies in development. In F. D. Horowitz (Ed.), *Review of*

Child Development Research (Vol. 4). Chicago: University of Chicago Press, 1975.

Rebelsky, F., & Hanks, C. Fathers' verbal interaction with infants in the first three months of life. *Child Development,* 1971, 42, 63-88.

Reich, W. T., & Smith, H. On the birth of a severely handicapped infant. *Hastings Center Report,* 1973, 3, 10-12.

Rendina, I., & Dickerscheid, J. D. Father involvement with first-born infants. *Family Coordinator,* 1976, 25, 373-379.

Rexford, E. N., Sander, L. W., & Shapiro. T. (Eds.), *Infant Psychiatry: A New Synthesis.* New Haven, CT: Yale University Press, 1976.

Reynolds, E. O. R., & Stewart, A. L. Intensive care and follow-up of infants of very low birth weight. In J. Dancer (Ed.), *Proceedings of the NIH Conference on Perinatal Intensive Care,* Bethesda, 1974. Bethesda, MD: National Institutes of Health, 1977.

Richards, M. P. H. (Ed.), *The Integration of a Child into a Social World.* London: Cambridge University Press, 1974.

Richards, M. P. M., & Bernal, J. F. Social interaction in the first days of life. In H. R. Schaffer (Ed.), *The Origins of Human Social Relations.* London: Academic Press, 1971.

Richards, M. P., & Bernal, J. F. An observational study of mother-infant interaction. In N. B. Jones (Ed.), *Ethological Studies of Child Behavior.* Cambridge, England: Cambridge University Press, 1972.

Richardson, S. A., Birch, H. G., & Hertzig, M. E. School performance of children who were severely malnourished in infancy. *American Journal of Mental Deficiency,* 1973, 77, 623-632.

Riegel, K. F. The influence of economic and political ideologies upon the development of developmental psychology. *Psychological Bulletin,* 1972, 78, 129-144.

Rimm, I. J., & Rimm, A. A. Association between juvenile onset obesity and severe obesity in 15,532 women. *American Journal of Public Health,* 1976, 66, 479-481.

Ringler, N. M., Kennell, J. H., Jarvella, R., Navojosky, B. J., & Klaus, M. H. Mother-to-child speech at two years: Effects of early postnatal contact. *Journal of Pediatrics,* 1975, 86, 141-144.

Rising, S. S. The fourth stage of labor: Family integration. *American Journal of Nursing,* 1974, 74, 870-874.

Roberts, J. A. F. The genetics of mental deficiency. *Eugenics Review,* 1952. 44, 71-83.

Robertson, J. A., & Fost, N. Passive euthanasia of defective newborn infants: Legal considerations. *The Journal of Pediatrics,* 1976, 88, 883-889.

Robson, K. S. The role of eye-to-eye contact in maternal-infant attachment. *Journal of Child Psychology and Psychiatry,* 1967, 8, 13-25.

Robson, K. S., & Moss, H. A. Maternal influences in early social visual behavior. *American Journal of Orthopsychiatry,* 1967, 37, 394-395.

Robson, K. S., & Moss, H. A. Patterns and determinants of maternal attachment. *Journal of Pediatrics,* 1970, 77, 976-985.

Roe, K. V. Infants' mother-stranger discrimination at 3 months as a predictor of cognitive development at 3 and 5 years. *Developmental Psychology,* 1978, 14, 191-192.

Rokeach, M. *Beliefs, Attitudes, and Values.* San Francisco: Jossey-Bass, 1968.

Rose, H. E., & Mayer, J. Activity, calorie intake, and the energy balance of infants. *Pediatrics,* 1968, 41, 18.

Rosen, B. C. Family structure and achievement motivation. *American Sociological Review,* 1961, 26, 574-585.

Rosenblith, J. F. Prognostic value of neonatal behavioral tests. *Early Child Development and Care,* 1973, 3, 31-50. Also in B. Z. Friedlander, G. M. Sterritt, & R. E. Kirk (Eds.), *Execeptional Infant,* (Vol. 3), *Assessment and Intervention.* New York: Brunner/Mazel, 1975.

Rosenblith, J. F. Relations between neonatal behaviors and those at 8 months. *Developmental Psychology*, 1974, 10, 779-792.

Rosenblum, L. A. Sex differences, environmental complexity, and mother-infant relations. *Archives of Sexual Behavior*, 1974, 3, 117-128.

Rosenthal, M. Attachment in mother-infant interaction. *Journal of Child Psychology and Psychiatry*, 1973, 14, 201-207.

Rosenzweig, M. R., & Bennett, E. L. Enriched environments: Facts, factors, and fantasies. In L. Petrinovich & J. L. McGauch (Eds.), *Knowing, Thinking, and Believing*. New York: Plenum, 1977.

Rosett, H., Ouellette, E., & Weiner, L. Fetal alcohol syndrome. *Annals of the New York Academy of Sciences*, 1976, 273, 123-129.

Roskies, E. *Abnormality and Normality: The Mothering of Thalidomide Children.* Ithaca, NY: Cornell University Press, 1972.

Ross, H. S., & Goldman, B. D. Infants' sociability towards strangers. *Child Development*, 1977, 48, 638-642.

Rossi, A. Transition to parenthood. *Journal of Marriage and the Family*, 1968, 30, 26-39.

Rowe. J., Clyman, R., Green, C., Mikkelsen, C., Haight, J., & Ataide, L. Follow-up of families who experience a perinatal death. *Pediatrics*, 1978, 62, 166-170.

Rubenstein, J. Maternal attentiveness and subsequent exploratory behavior in the infant. *Child Development*, 1967, 38, 1089.

Rubenstein, J. L., Pederson, F. A., & Yarrow, L. L. What happens when mother is away: A comparison of mothers and substitute caregivers. *Developmental Psychology*, 1977, 13, 529-530.

Rubin, J. Z., Provenzano, F. J., & Luria, Z. The eye of the beholder: Parents' view on sex of newborns. *American Journal of Orthopsychiatry*, 1974, 44, 512-519.

Rubin, R. Basic maternal behavior. *Nursing Outlook*, 1961, 9, 683-686.

Rubin, R. Puerperal change. *Nursing Outlook*, 1961, 9, 753-755.

Rubin, R. Maternal touch. *Nursing Outlook*, 1963, 11, 828-831.

Rubin, R. Attainment and the maternal role. *Nursing Research*, 1967, 16, 342-346.

Rubin, R. The neomaternal period. In B. Bergerson et al., (Eds.), *Current Concepts in Clinical Nursing* (Vol. 1). St. Louis: Mosby, 1967.

Rubin, R. Cognitive style in pregnancy. *American Journal of Nursing*, 1970, 70, 502-508.

Rubin, R. Fantasy and object constancy in maternal relationships. *Maternal Child Nursing Journal*, 1972, 1, 101-111.

Rubin, R. Maternal tasks in pregnancy. *Maternal Child Nursing Journal*, 1975, 4, 143-153.

Rubin, R. Binding-in in the post-partum period. *Maternal Child Nursing Journal*, 1977, 6, 67-75.

Rubin, R., Rosenblatt, C., & Balow, B. Psychological and educational sequelae of prematurity. *Pediatrics*, 1973, 52, 352-363.

Russell, M. Intrauterine growth in infants born to women with alcohol-related psychiatric diagnosis. *Alcoholism: Clinical Experimental Research*, 1977, 1, 225-231.

Rutter, M. *The Qualities of Mothering: Maternal Deprivation Reassessed.* New York: Aronson, 1974.

Ryan, J. Early language development: Towards a communicational analysis. In P. M. Richards (Ed.), *The Integration of a Child into a Social World*. Cambridge: Cambridge University Press, 1974.

Rynders, J. E., & Horrobin, J. M. Project EDGE: The University of Minnesota's communication stimulation program for Down's Syndrome infants. In B. Z. Friedlander, G. M. Sterritt, & G. E. Kirk (Eds.), *Exceptional Infant* (Vol. 3), *Assessment and Intervention*. New York: Brunner/Mazel, 1975.

Sackett, G. P. The lag sequential analysis of contingency and cyclicity in behavioral interaction research. In J. Osofsky (Ed.), *Handbook of Infant Development*. New York: Wiley, 1979.

Sackett, G. P., Stephenson, E. A., & Ruppenthal, G. C. Digital data acquisition systems for observing behavior in laboratory and field settings. *Behavioral Research Methods and Instrumentation*, 1973, 5, 334-348.

Salamy, A., & McKean, C. M. Postnatal development of human brainstem potentials during the first year of life. *Electroencephalography and Clinical Neurophysiology*, 1976, 40, 418-426.

Salans, L. B., Cushman, S. W., & Weissman, R. E. Studies of human adipose tissue. Adipose cell size and number in non-obese and obese patients. *Journal of Clinical Investigation*, 1973, 52, 929.

Salk, L. The role of the heartbeat in the relations between mother and infant. *Scientific American*, 1973, 228, 24-29.

Salk, L. The critical nature of the post-partum period in the human for the establishment of the mother-infant bond: A controlled study. In J. L. Schwartz & L. H. Schwartz (Eds.), *Vulnerable Infants: A Psychosocial Dilemma*. New York: McGraw-Hill, 1977.

Salo, K. E. Maternal employment and children's behavior: A review of literature. JSAS *Catalog of Selected Documents in Psychology*, 1975, 5, 277.

Sameroff, A. J. Learning and adaptation in infancy: A comparison of models. In H. W. Reese (Ed.), *Advances in Child Development and Behavior: VII*. New York: Academic Press, 1972.

Sameroff, A. J., Early influences on development: Fact or fancy? *Merrill-Palmer Quarterly*, 1975 (a), 21, 267-294.

Sameroff, A. J. Psychological needs of the mother in early mother-infant interactions. In G. Avery (Ed.), *Neonatology*. New York: Lippincott, 1975 (b).

Sameroff, A. J. The mother's construction on the child. Paper presented at the meeting of the International Society for the Study of Behavioral Development, Guilford, England, July 1975 (c).

Sameroff, A. J. Caretaking or reproductive causality? Determinants in developmental deviancy. In F. D. Horowitz (Ed.), *Early Developmental Hazards: Predictors and Precautions*. Boulder, CO: Westview Press, 1978.

Sameroff, A. J., Cashmore, T. P., & Dykes, A. C. Heartrate deceleration during visual fixation in human newborns. *Developmental Psychology*, 1973, 8, 117-119.

Sameroff, A. J., & Chandler, M. J. Reproductive risk and the continuum of caretaking casualty. In F. D. Horowitz, M. Hetherington, S. Scarr-Salapatek, & G. Spiegel (Eds.), *Review of Child Development Research* (Vol. 4). Chicago: University of Chicago Press, 1975.

Sameroff, A. J., & Feil, L. English and American parents' understanding of child development, 1980.

Sameroff, A. J., & Harris, A. Dialectical approaches to early thought and language. In M. H. Bornstein & W. Kessen (Eds.), *Psychological Development from Infancy*. New York: Erlbaum, 1979.

Sameroff, A. J., & Zax, M. Perinatal characteristics of the offspring of schizophrenic women. *Journal of Nervous and Mental Diseases*, 1973, 157, 191-199.

Sameroff, A. J. & Zax, M. In search of schizophrenia: Young offspring of schizophrenic women. In W. C. Wynne, R. L. Cromwell & S. Mathysse (Eds.), *The Nature of Schizophrenia: New Approaches to Research and Treatment*. New York: Wiley, 1978.

Sampson, E. E. Birth order, need achievement, and conformity. *Journal of Abnormal and Social Psychology*, 1962, 65, 155-159.

Sander, L. W. Issues in early mother-child interaction. *Journal of the American Academy of Child Psychiatry*, 1962, 1, 141-166.

Sander, L. W. Adaptive relationships in early mother-child interaction. *Journal of the American Academy of Child Psychiatry,* 1964, 3, 231-264.

Sander, L. W. The longitudinal course of early mother-child interaction: Cross-case comparison in a sample of mother-child pairs. In B. M. Foss (Ed.), *Determinants of Infant Behavior* (Vol. 4). London: Methuen, 1969.

Sander, L., Snyder, P., Rosett, H., Lee, A., Gould, J., & Ouellette, E. Effects of alcohol intake during pregnancy on newborn state regulation: A progress report. *Alcoholism: Clinical Experimental Research,* 1977, 1, 233-241.

Sander, L. W., Stechler, G., Burns, P., & Julia, H. Early mother-infant interaction and 24 hour patterns of activity and sleep. *American Journal of Orthopsychiatry,* 1970, 9, 102-103.

Sander, L. W., Stechler, G., Burns, P., & Lee, A. Changes in infant and caregiver variables over first 2 months. In E. B. Thoman (Ed.), *Origins of the Infant's Social Responsiveness.* Hillsdale, NJ: Erlbaum Associates, Inc., 1979.

Sander, L. W., Stechler, G., Julia, H., & Burns, P. Primary prevention and some aspects of temporal organization in early infant-caretaker interaction. In E. Rexford, L. Sander, & T. Shapiro (Eds.), *Infant Psychiatry: A New Synthesis.* New Haven: Yale University Press, 1976.

Sandgrund, A., Gaines, R., & Green, A. Child abuse and mental retardation: A problem of cause and effect. *American Journal of Mental Deficiency,* 1974 (a), 79, 327-333.

Sandgrund, A., Gaines, R., & Green, A. Child abuse: Pathological syndrome of family interaction. *American Journal of Psychiatry,* 1974 (b), 131, 882-886.

Sandgrund, A., Gaines, R., & Green, A. Aspects of bonding failure: The psychopathology and psychotherapeutic treatment of families of battered children. *Developmental Medicine and Child Neurology,* 1974 (c), 16, 447-456.

Sawin, D. B., Langlois, J. H., & Leitner, E. F. What do you do after you say hello? Observing, coding, and analyzing parent-infant interactions. *Behavior Research Methods and Instrumentation,* 1977, 9, 425-428.

Sawin, D. B., & Parke, R. D. Adolescent fathers: Some implications from recent research on paternal roles. *Educational Horizons,* 1976, 55, 38-43.

Scanlon, J. W. Address to the First Biennial Clinical Conference, National Perinatal Association, St. Louis, MO:, November, 1978.

Scanlon, J. W., & Alper, M. H. *Perinatal Pharmacology and Evaluation of the Newborn.* Boston: Little, Brown, 1974.

Scarr, S., & Weinberg, R. A. IQ test performance of Black children adopted by White families. *American Psychologist,* 1976, 31, 726-739.

Scarr-Salapatek, S. Genetics and the development of intelligence. In F. D. Horowitz (Ed.), *Review of Child Development Research* (Vol. 4). Chicago: University of Chicago Press, 1975.

Scarr-Salapatek, S., & Williams, M. L. The effects of early stimulation on low-birth-weight infants. *Child Development,* 1973, 44, 94-101.

Schacter, J., Elmer, E., Ragins, N., Wimberly, F., & Lachin, J. M. Assessment of mother-infant interaction: schizophrenic and non-schizophrenic mothers. *Merrill-Palmer Quarterly,* 1977, 23, 193-206.

Schaefer, E. S., & Bell, R. Q. Development of a parent attitude research instrument. *Child Development,* 1958, 29, 339-361.

Schaffer, H. R. (Ed.), *The Origins of Human Social Relations.* New York: Academic Press, 1971.

Schaffer, H. R. Cognitive components of the infant's responses to strangeness. In M. Lewis & L. Rosenblum (Eds.), *The Origins of Fear.* New York: Wiley, 1974.

Schaffer, H. R. (Ed.). *Studies in Mother-Infant Interaction.* (Proceedings of the Loch Lomond Symposium). London: Academic Press, 1977.

Schaffer, H. R., & Emerson, P. E. Patterns of response to physical contact in early human development. *Journal of Child Psychology and Psychiatry*, 1964, 5, 1-13.

Schaffer, R. *Mothering*. Harvard University Press, 1977.

Schaie, K. W. A general mold for the study of developmental problems. *Psychological Bulletin*, 1965, 64, 94-107.

Schiff, M., Duyme, M., Dumaret, A., Tomkiewicz, S., & Feingold, J. IQ and school failures of working-class adopted early into upper-middle-class families. Unpublished manuscript, 1978.

Schlesinger, E. R. Neonatal intensive care: Planning for services and outcomes following care. *Journal of Pediatrics*, 1973, 82, 916-920.

Schneider, C., Hoffmeister, J. K., & Helfer, R. E. A predictive screening questionnaire for potential problems in mother-child interaction. In R. E. Helper & C. H. Kempe (Eds.), *Child Abuse and Neglect*. Cambridge, MA: Ballinger, 1976.

Schwartz, B. K. Easing the adaptation to parenthood. *Journal of Family Counseling*, 1974, 2, 32-39.

Schwartz, J. C., Strickland, R. G., & Krolick, G. Infant day care: Behavioral effects at preschool age. *Developmental Psychology*, 1974, 10, 502-506.

Scott, J. P. *Early Experience and the Organization of Behavior*. Belmont, CA: Wadsworth Publishing, 1968.

Scott, N. T. Letter: Are there social differences in mothering? *Journal of Pediatrics*, 1974, 159, 145-146.

Sears, R. R., Maccoby, E. E., & Levine, H. *Patterns of Child Rearing*. Evanston, IL: Row, Peterson, 1957.

Seashore, M. J., Leifer, A. D., Barnett, C. R., & Leiderman, P. H. The effects of denial of early mother-infant interaction on maternal self-confidence. *Journal of Personality and Social Psychology*, 1973, 26, 369-378.

Seegmiller, B. R., & King, W. L. Relations between behavioral characteristics of infants, their mothers' behaviors, and performance on the Baylor Mental and Motor Scales. *Journal of Psychology*, 1975, 90, 99-111.

Semmens, J. P., & Lamers, W. M., Jr. *Teenage Pregnancy*. Springfield, IL: Charles C Thomas, 1968.

Senn, M. J. E., & Hartford, C. *The Firstborn: Experience of Eight American Families*. Cambridge, MA: Harvard University Press, 1968.

Serafica, F. C. The development of attachment behavior: An organism-developmental perspective. *Human Development*, 1978, 21, 119-140.

Serrano, C. V., & Puffer, R. R. Utilization of hospital birth weights and mortality as indicators of health problems in infancy. *Bulletin of the Pan American Health Organization*, 1975, 9, 325-345.

Shaffer, D., Pettigrew, A., Wolking, S., & Zajicek, E. Psychiatric aspects of pregnancy in schoolgirls: A review. *Psychological Medicine*, 1978, 8, 119-130.

Shaheen, E., Alexander, D., Truskowsky, M., & Barbero, G. Failure to thrive—A retrospective profile. *Clinical Pediatrics*, 1968, 7, 255.

Shapiro, V., Fraiberg, S., & Adelson, E. Infant-parent psychotherapy on behalf of a child in a critical nutritional state. *Psychoanalytic Study of the Child*, 1976, 31, 461-491.

Shaver, B. A. Maternal personality and early adaptation as related to infantile colic. In P. M. Shereshefsky & L. J. Yarrow (Eds.), *Psychological Aspects of a First Pregnancy and Early Postnatal Adaptation*. New York: Raven Press, 1973.

Shaw, C. A comparison of the patterns of mother-baby interaction for a group of crying, irritable babies and a group of more amenable babies. *Child Care Health Development*, 1977, 3, 1-12.

Shaw, M. W. Review of published studies of genetic counseling: A critique. In H. A. Lubs & F. de la Cruz (Eds.), *Genetic Counseling*. New York: Raven Press, 1977.

Shearman, R. P., Shutt, D. A., & Smith, T. G. The assessment and control of human fetal growth. *Size at Birth*, (Ciba Foundation Symposium). Amsterdam, The Netherlands: Associated Scientific Publishers, 1974.

Shereshefky, P. M., & Yarrow, L. J. (Eds.). *Psychological Aspects of a First Pregnancy and Early Postnatal Adaptation.* New York: Raven Press, 1974.

Sherrod, K. B., Friedman, S., Crawley, S., Drake, D., & Devieux, J. Maternal language to prelinguistic infants. Syntactic aspects. *Child Development,* 1977, 48, 1662-1665.

Sigman, M. The influence of medical neurological and environmental factors on the development of the preterm infant. Paper presented at NIH Conference on Pre- and Post-Term Birth: Relevance to optimal psychological development. Bethesda, Maryland, October, 1978.

Singer, A. Mothering practices and heroin addiction. *American Journal of Nursing,* 1974, 74, 77-82.

Singer, G., Stern, Y., & van der Spery, H. I. J. Emotional disturbance in unplanned versus planned children. *Social Biology,* 1976, 23, 254-259.

Skarin, K. Cognitive and contextual determinants of stranger fear in six- and eleven-month-old infants. *Child Development,* 1977, 48, 537-544.

Skeels, H. M. Adult status of children with contrasting early life experiences. *Monographs of the Society for Research in Child Development,* 1966, 31, (3), Serial No. 105, 1-65.

Skeels, H. M., & Dye, H. B. A study of the effects of differential stimulation on mentally retarded children. *Proceedings of the American Association of Mental Deficiency,* 1939, 44, 114-136.

Skinner, B. F. *Contingencies of Reinforcement.* New York: Appleton-Century-Crofts, 1969.

Skodak, M., & Skeels, H. M. A final follow-up study of 100 adopted children. *Journal of Genetic Psychology,* 1949, 75, 85-125.

Slade, C. I., Redl, O. J., & Manguten, H. H. Working with parents of high-risk newborns. *Journal of Obstetric and Gynecologic Nursing,* 1977, 6, 21-26.

Smart, M. S., & Smart, R. C. *Infants: Development and Relationships.* New York: The Macmillan Co., 1973.

Smilansky, M. Systems development-planning in education: An Israeli perspective. In D. A. Wilkerson (Ed.), *Educating all our Children: Thrust Toward Democracy.* Westport, CT: Mediax Associates, Inc., 1979.

Smith, D. W. *Recognizable Patterns of Human Malformations.* Philadelphia: Saunders, 1976.

Smith, H. T. A comparison of interview and observation measures of mother behavior. *Journal of Abnormal and Social Psychology,* 1958, 57, 278-282.

Solkoff, N., & Colten, C. Contingency awareness in premature infants. *Perceptual & Motor Skills,* 1975, 41, 709-710.

Solkoff, N., & Matuszak, D. Tactile stimulation and behavioral development among low-birthweight infants. *Child Psychiatry & Human Development,* 1975, 6, 33-37.

Solomon, R., & Decaire, T. Fear of strangers: A developmental milestone or an over-studied phenomenon? *Canadian Journal of Behavioral Science,* 1976, 8, 351-362.

Sosa, R., Kennell, J. H., Klaus, M., & Urrutia, J. J. The effect of early mother-infant contact on breast feeding. Infection and growth. *Ciba Foundation Symposium,* 1976, 45, 179-193.

Sostek, A. M., & Anders, T. F. Relationships among the Brazelton Neonatal Scale, Bayley Infant Scales, and early temperament. *Child Development,* 1977, 48, 320-323.

Sostek, A., Zaslow, M., Vietze, P., Kreiss, L., & Rubinstein, D. Contribution of context to interactions with infants in Fais and the U.S.A. In T. Field, A. Sostek & P. Vietze (Eds.) *Culture and Early Interactions.* Hillsdale, NJ: Erlbaum, 1980.

Spelke, E., Zelazo, P., Kager, J., & Kotelchuck, M. Father interaction and separation protest. *Developmental Psychology*, 1973, 9 ,83-90.

Spelt, D. The conditioning of the human fetus in utero. *Journal of Experimental Psychology*, 1948, 38, 338-346.

Sperber, Z., & Weiland, I. H. Anxiety as a determinant of parent-infant contact patterns. *Psychosomatic Medicine*, 1973, 35, 472-483.

Spielberger, C. D. (Ed.), *Anxiety and Behavior*. New York: Academic Press, 1966.

Sroufe, L. A. Wariness of strangers and the study of infant development. *Child Development*, 1977, 48, 731-746.

Sroufe, J. A., & Wunsch, J. P. The development of laughter in the first year of life. *Child Development*, 1972, 43, 1326-1344.

Sroufe, L. A., & Waters, E. Attachment as an organizational construct. *Child Development*, 1977, 48, 1184-1189.

Standley, K., Soule, A. B. III, Copans, S. A., & Duchowny, M. S. Local-regional anesthesia during childbirth: Effect on newborn behaviors. *Science*, 1974, 634-635.

Starr, R. (Ed.), *Prediction of Abuse*, 1978, in press.

Stein, S. C., Schut, L., & Ames, M. D. Selection for early treatment in myelomeningocele: A retrospective analysis of various selection procedures. *Pediatrics*, 1974, 54, 553-557.

Stein, Z., & Susser, M. Maternal starvation and birth defects. In S. Kelly et al. (Ed.), *Birth Defects: Risks and Consequences*. New York: Academic Press, 1976.

Steiner, G. *The Children's Cause*. Washington, D. C.: The Brookings Institute, 1976.

Stephenson, G. R., Smith, D. P. B., & Roberts, T. W. The SSR system: An open format event recording system with computerized transcription. *Behavior Research Methods & Instrumentation*, 1975, 7, 497-515.

Stern, D. N. A microanalysis of mother-infant interaction: Behavior regulating social contact between a mother and her 3½ month old twins. *Journal of the American Academy of Child Psychiatry*, 1971, 10, 501-517.

Stern, D. N. The goal and structure of mother-infant play. *Journal of the American Academy of Child Psychiatry*, 1974 (a), 13, 402-421.

Stern, D. N. Mother and infant at play: The dyadic interaction involving facial, vocal and gaze behaviors. In M. Lewis & L. Rosenblum (Eds.), *The Effect of the Infant on Its Caregiver*. New York: Wiley, 1974 (b).

Stern, D. N. *The First Relationship: Mother and Infant*. Cambridge: Harvard University Press, 1977.

Stern, D. N., & Gibbon, J. Temporal expectancies of social behavior in mother-infant play. In E. B. Thoman (Ed.), *Origins of the Infant's Social Responsiveness*. New York: Lawrence Erlbaum (Halsted Press), 1979.

Stern, L. Prematurity as a factor in child abuse. *Hospital Practice*, 1973, 8, 117-123.

Stevens, J. H., Jr., & Mathews, M. (Eds.). *Mother/Child-Father/Child Relationships*. Washington, DC: National Association for the Education of Young Children, 1978.

Stewart, K. R. *Adolescent Sexuality and Teenage Pregnancy: A Selected, Annotated Bibliography with Summary Forewords*. Chapel Hill, NC: Carolina Publishing Center, 1976.

Stewart, S. L., & Reynolds, E. O. R. Improved prognosis for infants of very low birth-weight. *Pediatrics*, 1974, 54, 724.

Stone, L. J., Smith, H. T., & Murphy, L. B. (Eds.). *The Competent Infant: Research and Commentary*. New York: Basic Books, 1973.

Stout, A. M. Parent behavior toward children of differing ordinal position and sibling status. Unpublished doctoral dissertation, University of California, 1960.

Streissguth, A. P. Psychologic handicaps in children with the fetal alcohol syndrome. *Annals of New York Academy of Science*, 1976, 273, 140-145.

Streissguth, A. P. Fetal alcohol syndrome. An epidemiologic perspective. *American Journal of Epidemiology*, 1978, 107, 467-478.

Streissguth, A. P. Maternal drinking and the outcome of pregnancy: Implications for child mental health. *American Journal of Orthopsychiatry*, 1977, 47, 422-431.

Streissguth, A. P., Herman, C. S., & Smith, D. W. Stability of intelligence in the fetal alcohol syndrome. A preliminary report. *Alcoholism*, 1978 (a), 2, 165-170.

Streissguth, A. P., Herman, C. S., & Smith, D. W. Intelligence, behavior, and dysmorphogenesis in the fetal alcohol syndrome. A report on 20 patients. *Journal of Pediatrics*, 1978 (b), 92, 363-367.

Strom, R., & Greathouse, B. Psychosocial development and behavior of mother of failure-to-thrive children. *American Journal of Orthopsychiatry*, 1975, 45, 525-537.

Stunkard, A. J. Behavioral treatments of obesity: Failure to maintain weight loss. In R. B. Stuart (Ed.), *Behavioral Self-Management*. New York: Brunner/Mazel, 1977.

Stunkard, A. J., D'Aquili, E., & Filion, R. D. L. Influence of social class on obesity and thinness in children. *Journal of the American Medical Association*, 1972, 221, 579-584.

Stunkard, A. J., & McLaren-Hume, E. M. The results of obesity: A review of the literature and report of a series. *Archives of Internal Medicine*, 1959, 103, 79-85.

Stunkard, A. J., & Mendelson, M. Obesity and the body image: I. Characteristics of disturbances in the body image of some obese persons. *American Journal of Psychiatry*, 1967, 123, 1296-1300.

Sugar, M. At risk factors for the adolescent mother and her infant. *Journal of Youth and Adolescence*, 1976, 5, 251-270.

Sugarman, M. Perinatal influences on maternal-infant attachment. *American Journal of Orthopsychiatry*, 1977, 47, 407-421.

Suran, B. G., & Rizzo, J. V. *Special Children: An Integrative Approach*. Glenview, IL: Scott, Foresman, and Company, 1979.

Sutton-Smith, B., Roberts, J. M., & Rosenberg, B. G. Sibling associations and role involvement. *Merrill-Palmer Quarterly*, 1964, 10, 25-38.

Sveger, T., Lindberg, T., Weilbull, B., & Ollson, V. L. Nutrition, overnutrition, and obesity in the first year of life in Malmo, Sweden. *Acta Paediatrica Scandinavica*, 1975, 64, 635.

Swanson, J. Nursing intervention to facilitate maternal-infant attachment. *Journal of Obstetric and Gynecologic Nursing*, 1978, 7, 35-38.

Taitz, T. S. Infantile overnutrition among artificially fed infants in the Sheffield region. *British Medical Journal*, 1971, 1, 315-316.

Tanguay, P. E. A pediatrician's guide to the recognition and initial management of early infantile autism. *Pediatrics*, 1973, 51, 903-910.

Tanner, J. M. Variability of growth and maturity in newborn infants. In M. Lewis & L. A. Rosenblum (Eds.), *The Effects of the Infant on Its Caregiver*. New York: Wiley, 1974.

Tanzer, C., & Block, J. *Why Natural Childbirth?* New York: Doubleday, 1972.

Taub, H. B., Goldstein, K. M., & Caputo, D. V. Indices of neonatal prematurity as discriminators of development in middle childhood. *Child Development*, 1977, 48, 797-805.

Tennes, K., & Carter, D. Plasma control levels and behavioral states in early infancy. *Psychosomatic Medicine*, 1973, 352, 121-128.

Thoman, E. B. Some consequences of early mother-infant interaction. *Early Child Development and Care*, 1974, 3, 249-261.

Thoman, E. B. Early development of sleeping behaviors in infants. In N. R. Ellis (Ed.), *Aberrant Development in Infant: Human and Animal Studies*. New York: Wiley, 1975 (a).

Thoman, E. B. How a rejecting baby may affect mother-infant synchrony. *Parent-Infant Interaction*, (Ciba Foundation Symposium 33). Amsterdam, The Netherlands: Associated Scientific Publishers, 1975 (b).

Thoman, E. B. Sleep and wake behaviors in neonates: Consistencies and consequences. *Merrill-Palmer Quarterly,* 1975 (c), 211, 295-314.

Thoman, E. B. Infant development viewed within the mother-infant relationship. In E. Quilligan & N. Kretchmer (Eds.), *Perinatal Medicine.* New York: Wiley, 1978.

Thoman, E. B., Acebo, C., Dreyer, C. A., Becker, P. T., & Freese, M. P. Individuality in the interactive process. In E. B. Thoman (Ed.), *Origins of the Infant's Social Responsiveness.* Hillsdale, NJ: Lawrence Erlbaum Associates, Inc., 1978.

Thoman, E. B., Barnett, C. R., & Leiderman, P. H. Feeding behaviors of newborn infants as a function of parity of the mother. *Child Development,* 1971, 42, 1471-1483.

Thoman, E. B., & Becker, P. T. Issues in assessment and prediction for the infant born at risk. In T. Field, A. Sostek, S. Goldberg, & H. H. Shuman (Eds.), *Infants Born at Risk.* New York: Spectrum, 1979.

Thoman, E. B., Becker, P. T., & Freese, M. P. Individual patterns of mother-infant interaction. In G. P. Sackett (Ed.), *Application of Observational/Etiological Methods to the Study of Mental Retardation.* Baltimore: University Park Press, 1979.

Thoman, E. B., Korner, A. F., & Beason-Williams, L. Modification of responsiveness to maternal vocalization in the neonate. *Child Development,* 1977, 48, 563-569.

Thoman, E. B., Korner, A. F., & Kraemer, H. C. Individual consistency in behavioral states in neonates. *Developmental Psychobiology,* 1976, 9, 271-283.

Thoman, E. B., Leiderman, P. H., & Olson, J. P. Neonate-mother interaction during breast feeding. *Developmental Psychology,* 1972, 6, 110-118.

Thoman, E. B., Miano, V. N., & Freese, M. P. The role of respiratory instability in the sudden infant death syndrome. *Developmental Medicine and Child Neurology,* 1977, 19, 729-738.

Thoman, E. B., Turner, A. M., Leiderman, P. H., & Barnett, C. R. Neonate-mother interaction: Effects of parity on feeding behavior. *Child Development,* 1970, 41, 1103-1111.

Thomas, A., & Chess, S. *Temperament and Development.* New York: Brunner/Mazel, 1977.

Thomas, A., Chess, S., Birch, H. G., Hertzig, M. E., & Korn, S. *Behavioral Individuality in Early Childhood.* New York: New York University Press, 1963.

Thomas, E. A. C., & Martin, J. A. Analyses of parent-infant interaction. *Psychological Review,* 1976, 83, 141-156.

Thomas, H. Psychological assessment instruments for use with human infants. *Merrill-Palmer Quarterly,* 1970, 16, 179-223.

Thompson, W. R. Development and biophysical bases of personality. In E. F. Borgotta & W. W. Lambert (Eds.), *Handbook of Personality Theory and Research.* Chicago: Rand McNally, 1968.

Thompson, W. R., & Grusec, J. Studies of early experience. In P. H. Mussen (Ed.), *Carmichael's Manual of Child Psychology* (3rd ed., Vol. 1). New York: Wiley, 1970.

Thorndike, E. L. Measurement of twins. *The Journal of Philosophy, Psychology and Scientific Method,* 1905, 2, 547-553.

Thurstone, L. L. The measurement of social attitudes. *Journal of Abnormal and Social Psychology,* 1931, 26, 244-269.

Tizard, J. Early malnutrition, growth and mental development in man. *British Medical Bulletin,* 1974, 30, 169-174.

Tizard, B., & Rees, J. A comparison of the effects of adoption, restoration to the natural mother, and continued institutionalization on the cognitive development of four-year old children. *Child Development,* 1974, 45, 92-99.

Tizard, J., & Tizard, B. The institution as an environment for development. In M.

Richards (Ed.), *The Integration of a Child into a Social World.* London: Cambridge University Press, 1974.

Tjossen, T. D. (Ed.), *Intervention Strategies for High Risk Infants and Young Children.* NICHD Mental Retardation Research Centers Series. Baltimore: University Park Press, 1976.

Trause, M. A. Stranger responses: Effects of familiarity, stranger's approach and sex of infant. *Child Development,* 1977, 48, 1657-1661.

Trevarthen, C. B. Conversations with a two-month-old. *New Scientist,* 1974, 62, 230-235.

Trevarthen, C. B. The nature of an infant's play. Paper presented at the International Society for the Study of Behavioral Development, Guilford, CT, 1975.

Trnavsky, P. A., Brown, J. V., & Bakeman, R. Sociological characteristics: Differences between mothers of preterms and mothers of fullterms from a low-income population (Tech. Rep. 6). Atlanta: Georgia State University, Infancy Laboratory, April, 1978.

Tronick, E., Adamson, L., Wise, S., Als, H., & Brazelton, T. B. Mother-infant face to face interaction. In Gosh, S. (Ed.), *Biology and Language.* New York: Academic Press, 1975.

Tronick, E., Als, H., & Adamson, L. The communicative structure of face to face interaction. In M. Bullowa (Ed.), *Before Speech: The Beginnings of Human Communication.* Cambridge: Cambridge University Press, 1979.

Tronick, E., Als, H., Adamson, L., Wise, S., & Brazelton, B. The infant's response to entrapment between contradictory messages in face-to-face interactions. *Journal of the American Academy of Child Psychiatry,* 1978, 17, 1-13.

Tronick, E., Als, H., & Brazelton, T. B. The infant's capacity to regulate mutuality in face-to-face interaction. *Journal of Communication,* 1977 (a) 27.

Tronick, E., Als, H., & Brazelton, T. B. Mutuality in mother-infant interaction. *Journal of Communication,* 1977 (b), 27, 74-79.

Tronick, E., Als, H., & Brazelton, T. B. Monadic phases: A structural descriptive analysis of infant mother face-to-face interaction. *Merrill-Palmer Quarterly,* 1980, 26, 1, 3-24.

Tronick, E., & Brazelton, T. B. Clinical uses of the Brazelton Neonatal Behavioral Assessment. In B. Friedlander, G. Sterritt, & G. Kirk (Eds.), *Exceptional Infant* (Vol. 3). New York: Brunner/Mazel, 1975.

Tronick, E., & Brazelton, T. B. A structural descriptive analysis of infant-mother face to face interaction. *Child Development,* 1978.

Tulkin, S. R. Social class differences in maternal and infant behavior. In P. H. Leiderman, S. R. Tulkin, & A. Rosenfield (Eds.), *Culture and Infancy: Variations in the Human Experience.* New York: Academic Press, 1977.

Tulkin, S. R., & Cohler, B. J. Childrearing attitudes and mother-child interaction in the first year of life. *Merrill-Palmer Quarterly,* 1973, 19, 95-106.

Tulkin, S. R., & Kagan, J. Mother-child interaction in the first year of life. *Child Development,* 1972, 43, 31-41.

United States Commission on Civil Rights. *Racial Isolation in the Public Schools* (Vol. 1). Washington, DC: U.S. Government Printing Office, 1967.

Uzgiris, I. C., & Hunt, J. McV. *Assessment in Infancy: Ordinal Scales of Psychological Development.* Urbana: University of Illinois Press, 1975.

Vandenberg, S. G. The nature and nurture of intelligence. In D. C. Glass (Ed.), *Genetics.* New York: Rockefeller University Press and The Russell Sage Foundation, 1968.

Veevers, J. E. The social meanings of parenthood. *Psychiatry,* 1973, 36, 291-310.

deVries, M. W., & deVries, M. R. Cultural relativity of toilet training readiness: A perspective from East Africa. *Pediatrics,* 1977, 60, 170-177.

Wachs, T. D. Utilization of a Piagetian approach in the investigation of early-experience effects: A research strategy and some illustrative data. *Merrill-Palmer Quarterly*, 1976, 22, 11-30.

Wachs, T. D. Relationship of infants' physical environment to their Binet performance at 2.5 years. *International Journal of Behavioral Development*, 1979.

Wachs, T. D., Uzgiris, I. C., & Hunt, J. McV. Cognitive development in infants of different age levels and from different environmental backgrounds: An exploratory investigation. *Merrill-Palmer Quarterly*, 1971, 17, 283-317.

Waechter, E. H. Bonding problems of infants with congenital anomalies. *Nursing Forum*, 1977, 16, 298-318.

Walberg, H., & Marjoribanks, K. Differential mental abilities and home environment: A canonical analysis. *Developmental Psychology*, 1973, 9, 363-368.

Waleko, K. Manipulation of a multigravida's feelings of vulnerability. *Maternal-Child Nursing Journal*, 1974, 3, 103-131.

Wallace, H. M., Gold, E. M., Goldstein, H., & Oglesby, A. C. A study of services and needs of teenage pregnant girls in the large cities of the United States. *American Journal of Public Health*, 1973, 63, 5-16.

Wallin, J. E. W. Intelligence irregularity as measured by scattering in the Binet scale. *Journal of Educational Psychology*, 1922, 13, 140-151.

Walker, H. Placebo versus social learning effects in parent training procedures designed to alter the behaviors of aggressive boys. Unpublished doctoral dissertation, University of Oregon, 1971.

Walker, L. Investigating the semantic properties of two concepts. Available from the author at The University of Texas, School of Nursing, 1700 Red River St., Austin, Texas 78701.

Walters, C. E. Prediction of postnatal development from fetal activity. *Child Development*, 1965, 36, 801-808.

Walters, C. E. *Mother-Infant Interaction*. New York: Human Sciences Press, 1975.

Ward, J. H., & Jennings, E. *Introduction to Linear Models*. Englewood Cliffs, NJ: Prentice-Hall, 1973.

Warner, R. H., & Rosett, H. L. The effects of drinking on offspring. *Journal of Studies of Alcohol*, 1975, 36, 1345-1420.

Warren, N. Malnutrition and mental development. *Psychological Bulletin*, 1973, 80, 324-328.

Waters, E. The reliability and stability of individual differences in infant-mother attachment. *Child Development*, 1978, 49, 483-494.

Watson, J. S. Memory and contingency analysis in infant learning. *Merrill-Palmer Quarterly*, 1967, 13, 55-76.

Weber, C. U., Foster, P. W., & Weikart, D. P. *An Economic Analysis of the Ypsilanti Perry Preschool Project*. Ypsilanti, Michigan: High/Scope Educational Research Foundation, 1978.

Weikart, D. P., Epstein, A. S., Schweinhart, L., & Bond, J. T. *The Ypsilanti Preschool Curriculum Demonstration Project*. Ypsilanti, MI: High/Scope Educational Research Foundation, 1978.

Weikart D. P., & Lambie, D. Preschool intervention through a home-teaching program. In J. Hellmuth (Ed.), *The Disadvantaged Child* (Vol. 2). Seattle Wash.: Special Child Publication, 1967.

Weintraub, M. Fatherhood: The myth of the second-class parent. In J. H. Stevens & M. Matthews (Eds.), *Mother/Child, Father/Child Relationships*. Washington, DC: NAEYC, 1978.

Weintraub, M., & Frankel, J. Sex differences in parent-infant interaction during free play, departure, and separation. *Child Development*, 1977, 48, 1240-1249.

Wente, A. S., & Crockenberg, S. B. Transition to parenthood: Lamaze preparation, adjustment difficulty, and the husband-wife relationship. *Family Coordinator*, 1976, 25, 351-357.

Westman, J. C. (Ed.), *Individual Differences in Children.* New York: Wiley, 1973.

White, B. L. *Human Infants: Experience and Psychological Development.* Englewood Cliffs, NJ: Prentice-Hall, 1971.

White, B. L. *The First Three Years of Life.* Englewood Cliffs, NJ: Prentice-Hall, 1975.

White, B. L. *Experience and Environment: Major Influences on the Development of the Young Child,* (Vol. 2). Englewood Cliffs, NJ: Prentice-Hall, 1978.

White, B. L., Kaban, B., Shapiro, B., & Attanucci, J. Competence and experience. In I. C. Uzgiris & F. Weitzmann (Eds.), *The Structuring of Experience.* New York: Plenum Press, 1977.

White, B. L., & Watts, J. C. *Experience and Environment: Major Influences on the Development of the Young Child.* Englewood Cliffs, NJ: Prentice-Hall, 1973.

Whitelaw, A. G. L. Influence of maternal obesity on subcutaneous fat in the newborn. *British Medical Journal,* 1976, 1, 985-986.

Whitelaw, A. G. L. Infant feeding and subcutaneous fat at birth and at one year. *The Lancet,* 1977, 2, 1098-1099.

Whiten, A. Postnatal separation and mother-infant interaction. Paper presented at the Conference of the International Society for the Study of Behavioral Development, University of Surrey, 1975.

Whiten, A. Assessing the effects of perinatal events on the success of the mother-infant relationship. In H. R. Schaffer (Ed.), *Studies in Mother-Infant Interaction.* New York: Academic Press, 1977.

Wicker, A. W. Attitudes versus actions: The relationship of verbal and overt behavioral responses to attitude objects. *Journal of Social Issues,* 1969, 25, 41-78.

Widdowson, E. M. Immediate and long-term consequences of being large or small at birth: A comparative approach. *Size at Birth,* (Ciba Foundation Symposium). Amsterdam, The Netherlands: Associated Scientific Publishers, 1974.

Wiel, A. Infantile obesity. In M. Winick (Ed.), *Childhood Obesity.* New York: Wiley, 1975.

Wiener, G., Rider, R. V., Oppel, W. C., Fischer, L., & Harper, P. A. Correlates of low birth weight: Psychological status at six to seven years of age. *Pediatrics,* 1965, 35, Part 1.

Wiesenfeld, A. R., & Klorman, R. The mother's psychophysiological reactions to contrasting affective expressions by her own and an unfamiliar infant. *Developmental Psychology,* 1978, 14, 294-304.

Wilkinson, P. W., Pearlson, J., Parku, J. M., Phillips, P. R., & Sykes, P. Obesity in childhood: A community study in Newcastle upon Tyne. *The Lancet,* 1977, 1, 350-352.

Will, J. A., Self, P. A., & Datan, N. Maternal behavior and perceived sex of infants. *American Journal of Orthopsychiatry,* 1976, 46, 123-134.

Willerman, L. Activity level and hyperactivity in twins. *Child Development,* 1973, 44, 288-293.

Willerman, L. *The Psychology of Individual and Group Differences.* San Francisco: Freeman, 1979.

Willerman, L., Broman, S. H., & Fiedler, M. Infant development, preschool IQ, and social class. *Child Development,* 1970, 41, 69-77.

Willerman, L., & Fiedler, M. F. Intellectually precocious preschool children: Early development and later intellectual accomplishments. *Journal of Genetic Psychology,* 1977, 131, 13-20.

Williams, C. C., Williams, R. A., Griswold, M. J., & Holmes, T. H. Pregnancy and life change. *Journal of Psychosomatic Research,* 1975, 19, 123-129.

Williams, T. H. Childrearing practices of young mothers: What we know, how it matters. *American Journal of Orthopsychiatry*, 1974, 44, 70-75.

Willmuth, R. Prepared childbirth and the concept of control. *Journal of Obstetric and Gynecological Nursing*, 1975, 4, 38-41.

Wilson, E. O. *Sociobiology: The New Synthesis.* Cambridge: Harvard University Press, 1975.

Winer, B. J. *Statistical Principles in Experimental Design.* New York: McGraw-Hill, 1971.

Winick, M. (Ed.), *Childhood Obesity.* New York: Wiley, 1975.

Withers, R. F. J. Problems in the genetics of human obesity. *Eugenics Review*, 1964, 56, 81-89.

Wohlwill, J. F. Methodology and research strategy in the study of developmental change. In L. R. Goulet & P. B. Baltes (Eds.), *Life-Span Developmental Psychology: Research and Theory.* New York: Academic Press, 1970.

Wohlwill, J. F. *The Study of Behavioral Development.* New York: Academic Press, 1973.

Wolff, P. H. Observations on newborn infants. *Psychosomatic Medicine*, 1959, 21, 110-118.

Wolff, P. H. The causes, controls, and organization of behavior in the neonate. *Psychological Issues*, (Vol. 5, Monograph 17). New York: International Universities Press, 1966.

Wolff, P. H. The natural history of crying and other vocalizations in early infancy. In B. M. Foss (Ed.), *Determinants of Infant Behavior*, (Vol. 4). London: Methuen, 1969.

Wolff, P. H. Mother-infant relations at birth. In J. G. Howells (Ed.), *Modern Perspectives in International Child Psychiatry.* New York: Brunner/Mazel, 1971.

Wolff, P. H. Organization of behavior in the first three months of life. *Early Development*, 1973, 51, 132-153.

Wolff, P. H. Current concepts: Mother-infant interactions in the first year. *New England Journal of Medicine*, 1976, 295, 999-1001.

Woodrow, H. The relation between abilities and improvement with practice. *Journal of Educational Psychology*, 1938, 29, 215-230.

Woodrow, H. Factors in improvement with practice. *Journal of Psychology*, 1939, 7, 55-70.

Wright, L. The theoretical and research base for a program of early stimulation care and training of premature infants. In J. Hellmuth (Ed.), *Exceptional Infant* (Vol. 2). *Studies in Abnormalities.* New York: Brunner/Mazel, 1971.

Wulbert, M., Ingles, S., Kriegermann, E., & Mills, B. Language delay and associated mother-child interactions. *Developmental Psychology*, 1975, 11, 61-70.

Yando, R., Zigler, E., & Litzinger, S. A further investigation of the effects of birth order and number of siblings in determining children's responsiveness to social reinforcement. *Journal of Psychology*, 1975, 89, 95-111.

Yang, R. K., & Bell, R. Q. Assessment of infants. In P. McReynolds (Ed.), *Advances in Psychological Assessment* (Vol. 3). San Francisco: Jossey-Bass, Inc., 1975.

Yang, R. K., Federman, E. J., & Douthitt, T. C. The characterization of neonatal behavior: A dimensional analysis. *Developmental Psychology*, 1976, 12, 204-210.

Yang, R. K., & Halverson, C. F., Jr. A study of the "inversion of intensity" between newborn and preschool-age behavior. *Child Development*, 1976, 47, 350-359.

Yang, R., Zweig, A. R., Douthit, T. C., & Federman, E. J. Successive relationships between maternal attitudes during pregnancy, analgesic medication during labor and delivery, and newborn behavior. *Developmental Psychology*, 1976, 12, 6-14.

Yarrow, L. J. The development of focused relationships during infancy. In J. Hellmuth

(Ed.), *Exceptional Infant* (Vol. 1), *The Normal Infant.* New York: Brunner/ Mazel, 1967.

Yarrow, L. J., & Goodwin, M. Some conceptual issues in the study of mother-infant interactions. *American Journal of Orthopsychiatry,* 1965, 35, 473-481.

Yarrow, L. J., Pedersen, F. A., & Rubenstein, J. Mother-infant interaction and development in infancy. In R. H. Leiderman, S. R. Tulkin, & A. Rosenfeld, (Eds.), *Culture and Infancy: Variations in the Human Experience.* New York: Academic Press, 1977.

Yarrow, L. J., Rubenstein, J. L., & Pedersen, F. A. *Infant and Environment: Early Cognitive and Motivational Development.* New York: John Wiley & Sons, 1975.

Yarrow, M. R., Campbell, T. D., & Burton, R. V. Recollections of childhood: A study of the retrospective method. *Monographs of the Society for Research in Child Development,* 1970, 35, (5), Serial No. 138.

Zaslow, R. W., & Breger, L. A theory and treatment of autism. In L. Breger (Ed.), *Clinical Cognitive Psychology.* Englewood Cliffs, NJ: Prentice-Hall, 1969.

Zax, M., Sameroff, A. J., & Babigian, H. M. Birth outcomes in the offspring of mentally disordered women. *American Journal of Orthopsychiatry,* 1977, 47, 218-230.

Zegiob, L., & Forehand, R. Maternal interactive behavior as a function of race, socioeconomic status, and sex of the child. *Child Development,* 1975, 46, 564-568.

Zemlick, M. J., & Watson, R. I. Maternal attitudes of acceptance and rejection during and after pregnancy. *American Journal of Orthopsychiatry,* 1953, 23, 570-584.

Zigler, E., & Child, I. L. Socialization. In G. Lindzey & E. Aronson (Eds.), *Handbook of Social Psychology* (2nd ed., Vol. 3). Reading, MA: Addison-Wesley, 1969.

Zigler, E., & Trickett, P. K. IQ, social competence, and evaluation of early childhood intervention programs. *American Psychologist,* 1978, 33, 789-798.

Zuk, G. H., Miller, R. L., Bartram, J. B., & Kling, F. Maternal acceptance of retarded children: A questionnaire study of attitudes and religious background. *Child Development,* 1961, 32, 525-540.

NAME INDEX

Abramowicz, H. K., 60, 397n.
Acebo, C., 104, 111, 114, 440n.
Adams, D. K., 163, 421n.
Adamson, 46, 97, 150, 151, 156, 214, 398n., 402n., 441n.
Ahern, F. M., 60, 419n.
Ainsworth, M. D. S., 78, 79, 82, 96, 142, 397n., 401n.
Ajzen, I., 236, 237, 237n., 238n., 241, 242, 243, 348, 410n.
Alpaugh, M., 79, 428n.
Als, H., 46, 97, 147-51, 156, 214, 398n., 402n., 441n.
Altmann, S. A. 301, 398n.
Ames, M. D., 201, 398n.
Anderson, B. J., 179, 189, 398n., 430n.
Arend, R. A., 5, 426n.
Ashby, W. R., 156, 398n.
Ashton, R., 97, 98, 398n.
Altaide, L., 208, 433n.
Atkin, R., 47, 398n.
Attanucci, J., 44, 443n.

Babigian, H. M., 344, 445n.
Badger, E., 43, 50, 51, 52, 398n., 399n., 420n.
Bakeman, R., 120, 121, 123, 124, 142, 215, 271-99, 272, 273, 274, 277, 280, 282, 284, 287, 291, 294, 297, 298, 307, 313, 331, 352, 354, 359, 399n., 403n., 413n., 441n.
Bakow, H., 259, 399n.
Baldwin, A., 270, 399n.
Baldwin, B., 72, 415n.
Baltes, P. B., 263, 399n.

Barnard, K. E., 172, 399n.
Barnett, C. R., 94. 162, 163, 239, 244, 399n., 436n., 440n.
Bartram, J. B., 209, 445n.
Bateson, P. P. G., 300, 400n.
Bayley, N., 227, 400n.
Becker, P. T., 99, 100, 101, 104, 111, 114, 440n.
Becker, W., 241, 242, 348, 400n.
Beckwith, L., 97, 120, 121, 123, 127, 142, 400n., 406n.
Bee, H. L., 127, 400n.
Bell, R. Q., 241, 255, 256, 257, 258, 258n., 260-65, 268, 269, 355, 400n., 435n., 444n.
Bell, S., 78, 79, 82, 397n.
Benfield, D. G., 198, 200, 208, 400n.
Bennett, E. I., 58, 433n.
Bereiter, C., 49, 356, 401n.
Bernal, J., 79, 183, 274, 432n.
Bessman, S. P., 68, 401n.
Binet, A., 37, 40, 401n.
Birch, H., 344, 401n.
Biron, P., 74, 401n.
Blehar, M. C., 142, 401n.
Block, J., 178, 439n.
Blomin, R., 71, 404n.
Bloom, B., 8, 401n.
Bobbitt, R. A., 323, 401n.
Borjeson, M., 74, 83, 401n.
Bower, T. G. R. 161, 172, 402n.
Bowers, A., 11, 415n.
Bowlby, J., 154, 402n.
Brachfeld, S., 121, 123, 412n.
Bradley, R., 216, 402n., 408n.

447

Bray, R., 47, 398n.
Brazelton, T. B., 46, 71, 92, 97, 124, 133, 134, 137, 139, 147-51, 154, 171, 172, 214, 215, 238, 239, 241, 244, 256, 259, 398n., 402n., 420n., 441n.
Breger, L., 208, 445n.
Brody, S., 94, 402n.
Broman, S. H., 58, 65, 216, 403n., 443n.
Bronfenbrenner, U., 175, 176, 301, 403n.
Bronner, A., 11, 415n.
Brook, C. D. G., 73, 83, 83n., 84, 403n.
Brooks, J., 255, 403n.
Broussard, E. R., 226, 234, 239, 240, 244, 403n.
Brown, J. V., 80, 97, 120, 121, 123, 124, 252, 271-99, 271, 272, 273, 274, 277, 280, 282, 284, 287, 297, 298, 354, 359, 399n., 403n., 441n.
Brown, T., 175, 428n.
Bruch, H., 72, 77, 78, 80, 403n.
Bruner, J., 157, 403n.
Bugen, L. A., 159, 160, 197-99, 211, 404n.
Burns, D., 51, 399n.
Burt, C., 17, 404n.
Burton, R. V., 348, 445n.
Buss, A. H., 71, 80, 404n.

Cain, R. L., 189, 430n.
Caldwell, B. M., 216, 217, 408n.
Call, J., 96, 404n.
Callaway, E., 59, 404n.
Campbell, A. G. M., 201, 408n.
Campbell, D. T., 243, 348, 404n., 445n.
Caplan, G., 171, 404n.
Caputo, D. V., 240, 413n.
Carey, W. B., 80, 95, 215, 404n.
Carmichael, L., 32, 404n.
Causey, R., 249, 404n.
Chandler, M. J., 120, 175, 344, 345, 356, 434n.
Chapple, E. D., 133, 135, 138, 404n.
Charney, E., 75, 79, 405n.
Chess, S., 77, 80, 215, 238, 405n., 440n.
Chomsky, N., 97, 405n.
Cicirelli, V. G., 9, 405n.
Clarke-Stewart, K. A., 120, 142, 177, 405n.
Clausen, J., 59, 405n.
Clifton, R. K., 131, 413n.
Clyman, R., 208, 433n.
Cochran, W. G., 323, 405n.
Cohen, D. B., 61, 405n.
Cohen, E. S., 121, 127, 142, 400n., 406n.
Cohen, L. B., 255, 406n.
Cohler, B. J., 239, 241, 242, 406n., 441n.

Cole, T. J., 75, 431n.
Coleman, R. W., 238, 406n.
Colen, B. D., 201, 406n.
Collipp, P. J., 72, 406n.
Collmer, C. W., 177, 193, 429n.
Condon, W. S., 97, 146, 147, 406n.
Cook, S. W., 238n., 406n.
Cooke, R., 8
Crawley, S. B., 136, 406n.
Cremin, L. A., 8, 406n.
Criticos, A., 136, 406n.
Crockenberg, S. B., 178, 442n.
Cronbach, L., 245, 406n.
Crook, J. H., 300, 407n.
Cushman, S. W., 84, 434n.

Dabba, Jr., J. M., 287, 399n.
Darlington, R. R., 10n., 423n.
Darwin, C., 14
David, M., 67
Davidson, R. G., 11, 430n.
Davis, A., 94, 407n.
Davison, M., 47, 398n.
De la Cruz, F., 210, 211, 425n.
Dennis, W., 17, 28, 407n.
Deutsch, C. P., 10, 235, 407n.
Deutsch, M., 10
Deutscher, I., 235, 407n.
DeVries, M. R., 348, 407n.
DeVries, M. W., 348, 407n.
Diamond, J. M., 159, 197, 204-207, 209, 407n.
Diamond, M. C., 58, 407n.
Dietrich, K. N., 128, 407n.
DiVitto, B., 121, 123, 124, 407n., 412n.
Dohrenwend, B., 199, 407n.
Dohrenwend, B., 199, 407n.
Donovan, W. L., 132, 411n.
Douthitt, T., 258, 258n., 259, 444n.
Dreyer, C. A., 104, 111, 114, 440n.
Drillien, C. M., 172, 408n.
Duff, R. S., 201, 408n.
Dugdale, A. E., 84, 408n.
Duncan, S., 133, 408n.
Dunn, J. B., 16, 80, 97, 142, 408n.
Dye, H. B., 28, 59n., 63, 67, 437n.

Eagly, A. H., 236, 416n.
Eichorn, D. H., 265, 408n.
Eid, E. K., 75, 408n.
Eimas, P., 147, 408n.
Elardo, R., 216, 408n., 409n.
Ellis, H. L., 204, 409n.
Elwer, E., 162, 409n.

Engelmann, S., 49, 356, 401n.
Epstein, H. T., 12, 84, 409n.
Erikson, E. H., 46, 409n.
Escalona, S.K., 256, 409n.

Fanaroff, A. A., 176, 409n.
Federman, E. J., 258, 259, 444n.
Feil, L., 352, 434n.
Feiring, C., 175, 409n.
Feldstein, S., 133, 418n.
Ferguson, C. A., 135, 409n.
Ferguson, D., 175, 428n.
Festinger, L. A., 22n., 409n.
Feuerstein, R., 43, 409n., 410n.
Fiedler, M., 65, 216, 443n.
Field, T. M., 87, 88, 89, 120-43, 152, 171,
    354, 355, 359, 410n.
Fisch, R. O., 75, 410n.
Fishbein, M., 156, 214, 236, 237n., 238n.,
    241, 242, 243, 249, 348, 410n.
Fiske, D. W., 122, 131, 243, 404n., 410n.
Fitzhardinge, P. M., 200, 410n.
Fletcher, A. B., 159, 197, 200-203
Fletcher, J., 205, 209, 411n.
Fomon, S. J., 77, 82, 411n.
Fost, N., 200, 411n.
Foster, P. W., 10n., 442n.
Fredrickson, W. T., 273, 403n.
Freeman, J. M., 204, 411n.
Freese, M. P., 99, 100, 104, 111, 114, 118,
    242, 411n., 440n.
Friedlander, B. Z., v-vi, 159, 160, 190-96,
    197, 203, 205, 206, 208, 209, 211, 358
Friedman, S., 136, 406n.
Frodi, A. M., 132, 411n.
Froebel, F., 10, 411n.
Frost, N., 201, 206, 432n.

Gajdusek, D. C., 99, 411n.
Galton, F., 14
Garland, M. J., 200, 201, 418n.
Garn, S. M., 72, 74, 75, 84, 411n., 412n.
Geiken, K., 175, 412n.
Gesell, A., 32, 412n.
Gewirtz, H. B., 140, 412n.
Gewirtz, J. L., 140, 412n.
Ghodssi, M., 19
Gibbon, J., 97, 438n.
Giefer, E., 74, 415n.
Glaser, R., 41, 425n.
Glidden, 59
Golani, I., 96, 412n.

Goldberg, S., 120, 121, 123, 124, 125, 134,
    140, 407n., 410n., 412n., 424n.
Golden, R. R., 59, 413n.
Goldstein, K. M., 240, 241, 413n.
Goldston, S., 198, 413n.
Goodman, 67
Goodrich, W., 257
Gorham, K. A., 208, 210-11, 413n.
Gottesman, I. I., 59, 413n.
Gottman, J., 175, 188, 287, 291, 294, 312,
    331, 430n., 431n.
Graham, F. K., 131, 256, 413n.
Gray, S. W., 10, 51, 188, 413n., 421n.
Green, C., 208, 433n.
Green, J. A., 136, 137, 414n.
Greenberg, N. H., 95, 413n.
Greenough, W. T., 33, 58, 414n.
Gregg, C. S., 162, 409n.
Grinker, J., 73, 414n.
Grunebaum, H. U., 242, 406n.
Gunther, M., 97, 414n.
Gussow, G. D., 344, 401n.
Gustafson, G. E., 136, 414n.

Habermas, J., 156, 414n.
Hager, A., 73, 414n.
Haight, J., 208, 433n.
Hall, F., 120, 142, 430n.
Hall, G. S., 10
Halverson, Jr., G. F., 258n., 262, 263, 264,
    265, 268, 414n.
Harlow, H. F., 163, 414n.
Harris, A., 358, 434n.
Harris, Z. J., 40, 415n.
Hartner, M. S. S., 226, 234, 239, 240, 244,
    403n.
Hartz, A., 74, 75, 415n.
Hawkins, II, R. C., vii-x, 5, 70-75, 72, 78,
    80, 81, 159, 160, 197, 208-11, 347, 359,
    415n.
Healy, W., 11, 415n.
Hebb, D. O., 36, 131, 133, 415n.
Heber, F. R., 64, 415n.
Hegmann, J. P., 58, 415n.
Helfer, R. E., 162, 234, 239, 415n., 436n.
Hepler, R., 273, 403n.
Herndon, 67
Herrnstein, R., 13, 416n.
Hersher, L., 163, 416n.
Herzberger, S., 47, 398n.
Hill, V., 170, 416n.
Hilton, I., 94, 416n.
Himmelfarb, S., 236, 416n.

Hinde, R. A., 300, 400n.
Hirsch, J., 13, 14, 73, 414n., 416n., 421n.
Hodgins, A. A., 49, 50, 51, 356, 420n.
Hoffman, L., 175, 416n.
Hoffmeister, J. K., 234, 239, 436n.
Hogarty, P. S., 91, 426n.
Holden, R. H., 66, 416n.
Hollenbeck, A. R., 216, 310, 417n.
Hollingshead, A. B., 220, 417n.
Holmes, T., 199, 417n.
Holzinger, K. J., 17, 417n.
Honzik, M. P., 91, 417n.
Hubble, I., 10n., 423n.
Huffman, P., 244, 424n.
Humphrey, 24
Humpreys, L., 47, 398n.
Hunt, E., 58, 417n.
Hunt, J. McV., 3, 4, 7-54, 13, 15, 15n., 17,
 18, 19, 22, 23, 24, 31, 34, 35, 38, 40,
 45, 45n., 46, 47, 52, 64, 65, 67, 84, 346,
 347, 356, 359, 399n., 417n., 418n., 421n.,
 429n., 441n., 442n.
Hunter, R. S., 162, 170, 171, 418n.
Hurlburt, N., 91, 426n.
Hymel, S., 174-89, 213

Jackson, J. C., 256, 413n.
Jacobs, B. A., 128, 418n.
Jacobsen, B., 66, 421n.
Jacobson, M., 136, 406n.
Jaffe, J., 133, 418n.
Jansen, A. R., 200, 201, 418n.
Jencks, C., 45, 418n.
Jenkins, G. M., 302, 418n.
Jennings, E., 248, 442n.
Jensen, A. R., 13, 14, 17, 56, 418n., 419n.
Johannsen, W., 16, 419n.
John, E. R., 47, 419n.
Johnson, C. A., 60, 419n.
Johnson, D. L., 121, 127, 421n.
Johnson, N., 256, 259, 424n.
Johnson, R. C., 60, 419n.
Johnston, F. E., 75, 425n.
Jones, 120, 121, 125
Jones, H. E., 39, 419n.
Jones, O., 137, 142, 419n.
Jones, S. J., 239, 428n.
Jones-Kearns, 258n., 268, 269, 414n.

Kaback, M. M., 210, 419n.
Kaban, B., 44, 443n.
Kagan, J., 122, 127, 239, 256n., 419n.,
 420n., 441n.

Kant, 36
Kaplan, D. M., 171, 404n.
Karnes, M. B., 49, 50, 51, 64, 356, 420n.
Kaye, K., 124, 154, 420n.
Keefer, C., 143, 420n.
Kendon, A., 133, 138, 420n.
Kennedy, J., 171, 172, 420n.
Kennedy, J. F., 8
Kennedy, W. A., 58, 403n.
Kennell, J. H., 165, 168, 173, 176, 200, 354,
 409n., 420n., 421n.
Kety, S. S., 66, 421n.
Kilbride, H. W., 121, 127, 128, 421n.
Kinney, D. K., 66, 421n.
Kirk, G. E., v, 38, 52, 418n., 421n.
Kitzinger, S., 178, 421n.
Klaus, M. H., 164, 165, 168, 169, 173, 176,
 188, 354, 409n., 421n.
Klaus, R., 51, 413n.
Klein, M., 162, 421n.
Kleinhenz, M. E., 76, 78, 80, 425n.
Kling, F., 209, 445n.
Klopfer, M. S., 163, 421n.
Klopfer, P. H., 163 421n.
Knittle, J. L., 73, 421n.
Knobloch, H., 120, 344, 355, 430n.
Koch, H. L., 94, 421n.
Koch, R., 68, 401n.
Kogan, K. L., 125, 142, 422n.
Kohn, M. L., 349, 422n.
Koluchová, J., 65, 422n.
Kopf, R. C., 171, 422n.
Kopp, C. B., 92, 142, 400n., 430n.
Korner, A. F., 101, 215, 238, 422n., 440n.
Koslowksi, B., 133, 151, 402n.
Kraemer, H. C., 101, 440n.
Krech, 58
Kreiss, L., 143, 437n.
Kris, E., 238, 406n.
Krug, R., 241, 242, 348, 400n.
Kubicek, L., 127, 422n.
Kuo, Z. Y., 32, 422n.

Lamb, M. E., 132, 175, 411n., 423n.
Lambie, D., 51, 442n.
Langman, J., 61, 423n.
LaPiere, R. T., 235, 423n.
Lashley, K. S., 157, 423n.
Lasko, J. K., 94, 423n.
Lazar, L., 10n., 423n.
Leavitt, M. E., 132, 411n.
Legaiqz, K., 201, 423n.
Leib, S. A., 208, 400n.

Leiderman, P. H., 94, 216, 239, 244, 423n., 436n., 440n.
Leifer, A. D., 239, 244, 436n.
Leifer, M., 238, 423n.
Leonard, M. F., 95, 424n.
Levenstein, P., 49, 50, 424n.
Levinson, D., 244, 424n.
Lewis, M., 91, 127, 140, 215, 238, 256, 259, 424n.
Lieb, S. A. 198, 400n.
Lieberman, A. F., 142, 401n.
Liska, A. E., 238n., 424n.
Lloyd, J. K., 73, 403n.
Locke, J., 36
Lockie, M. S., 127, 400n.
Lopata, H. Z., 176, 425n.
Lorber, J., 201, 204, 425n.
Lubchenco, L. O., 172, 425n.
Lumsdaine, A. A., 41, 425n.
Lynch, A. A., 162, 425n.

Macfarlane, A., 215, 425n.
Mack, R. W., 75, 76, 78, 80, 425n.
Maddi, S. R., 122, 131, 410n.
Main, M., 133, 151, 402n.
Malthus, P. T., 14
Maltzman, I., 47, 425n.
Manosevitz, M., 80, 213, 215-33, 349, 353
Marcy, T. G., 142, 400n.
Martini, M., 143, 426n.
Mason, E., 171, 404n.
Massie, H. N., 128, 151, 152, 154, 155, 426n.
Matas, L., 5, 426n.
Mayer, J., 74, 76, 426n., 432n.
Mayr, E., 156, 426n.
McCall, R. B., 65, 91, 265, 426n.
Mcintyre, M. N., 208, 211, 211n., 426n.
McKean, C. M., 58, 423n.
McLaren-Hume, E. M., 156, 427n.
Mead, G. H., 156, 427n.
Medel, G., 55
Mednick, S. A., 71, 427n.
Mellbin, T., 76, 427n.
Mendelson, M., 73, 439n.
Mercer, C. D., 11, 430n.
Miano, V. N., 118, 440n.
Mikkelsen, C., 208, 433n.
Mill, J., 18
Mill, J. S., 18
Miller, D. B., 300, 427n.
Miller, J. O., 51, 427n.
Miller, R. L., 209, 445n.
Minde, K., 176, 427n.
Montessori, M., 10, 427n.

Moore, A., 163, 416n., 427n.
Morgan, S. T., 273, 403n.
Moss, H. A., 128, 234, 239, 258n., 265, 268, 269, 354, 418n., 428n.
Murray, H., 10n., 423n.

Neel, J. V., 67, 428n.
Neuman, C. G., 79, 428n.
Nicholas, P. L., 58, 403n.
Nixon, R., 13
Notarius, C., 312, 413n.
Nunnally, D., 242, 428n.
Nyman, B. A., 127, 400n.

Ogston, W. D., 146, 406n.
O'Leary, S., 178, 430n.
Olson, J. P., 94, 440n.
Orthner, D., 175, 438n.
Osgood, C. E., 241, 244, 258n., 428n.
Osofsky, H. J., 215, 428n., 429n.

Papajohn, J., 209, 429n.
Pape, K. E., 200, 429n.
Papousek, H., 46, 429n.
Papousek, M., 46, 429n.
Paraskevopoulos, J., 15, 429n.
Parke, R. D., 93, 159, 174-89, 175, 177, 178, 181, 182, 183, 184, 186, 188, 193, 213, 301, 348, 429n., 430n.
Parmelee, A. H., 92, 142, 400n., 430n.
Pasamanick, B., 120, 344, 355, 430n.
Patterson, G. R., 347, 348, 352, 430n.
Pawlby, S., 120, 127, 136, 137, 142, 143, 410n., 419n., 430n.
Payne, J. S., 11, 430n.
Payne, R. A., 11, 430n.
Pedersen, F. A., 39, 46, 175, 176, 189, 430n., 445n.
Penticuff, J. H., vii-x, 159, 161-73, 354
Pestalozzi, 37
Pharis, M. E., 80, 213, 215-33, 349, 353
Piaget, J., 11, 19, 23, 33, 34, 36, 39, 48, 121, 136, 156, 349, 350, 352, 356, 430n., 431n.
Plato, 36
Plomin, R., 80, 404n.
Poskitt, E. M. E., 75, 76, 431n.
Power, T. G., 174-89, 175, 213, 430n.
Provence, S., 238, 406n.
Pruette, L. G., 11, 431n.
Prugh, D., 171, 431n.

Quinlin, K. A., 195, 202

Rachel, J., 205, 431n.
Rahe, R., 199, 417n.
Raskin, D. C., 47, 425n.
Rees, J., 67, 440n.
Reynolds, E. O. L., 200, 438n.
Rhymes, J. P., 95, 424n.
Richards, M. P. M., 79, 80, 97, 183, 274, 408n., 432n.
Richardson, L., 136, 406n.
Richardson, S. A., 60, 397n.
Richmond, G., 163, 416n.
Richmond, J., 9, 10
Riegel, K. F., 356, 432n.
Rimm, A. A., 73, 74, 415n., 432n.
Rimm, I. J., 73, 432n.
Rizzo, J. V., 208, 209, 211, 439n.
Roache, M., 10n., 423n.
Roberts, J. A. F., 59, 60, 162, 425n., 432n.
Roberts, T. W., 301, 438n.
Robertson, J. A,, 201, 206, 432n.
Robson, K. S., 96, 432n.
Rogers, P. P., 136, 406n.
Rokeach, M., 238n., 432n.
Rose, H. E., 76, 432n.
Rosen, B. C., 94, 432n.
Rosenblum, L. A., 215, 238, 424n.
Rosenfeld, A., 217, 423n.
Rosenzweig, M. R., 58, 433n.
Roskies, E., 358, 359, 433n.
Rowe, J., 200, 208, 433n.
Royce, J., 10n., 423n.
Rubin, R., 239, 433n.
Rubinstein, D., 143, 437n.
Rubinstein, J. L., 39, 46, 165, 175, 433n., 445n.
Ruppenthal, G. C., 274, 301, 434n.
Ryan, J., 156, 433n.
Ryder, R. G., 258n.

Sackett, G. P., 215, 253, 274, 291, 300-340, 301, 307, 355, 434n.
Salamy, A., 58, 434n.
Salans, L. B., 84, 434n.
Salapatek, P., 255, 406n.
Salzer, U., 47, 398n.
Sameroff, J., 5, 101, 120, 174, 175, 216, 301, 338, 341-59, 344, 345, 345n., 349, 350, 352, 355, 358, 434n.
Sampson, E. E., 94, 434n.
Sander, L. W., 77, 97, 98, 121, 126, 146, 147, 238, 406n., 434n., 435n.
Sawin, D. B., vii-x, 182, 183, 184, 430n.
Scanlon, J. W., 173, 435n.

Scarr, S., 30, 435n.
Schaefer, E. S., 241, 435n.
Schaffer, H. R., 122, 435n.
Schaie, K. W., 265, 399n.
Schiff, M., 31, 32, 436n.
Schneider, C., 234, 239, 436n.
Schulsinger, R., 71, 427n.
Schut, L., 201, 398n.
Schwartz, E. L., 47, 419n.
Sears, R. R., 94, 436n.
Seashore, M. J., 167, 168, 239, 244, 436n.
Selltiz, C., 238n., 406n.
Setty, R. M., 72, 415n.
Shakow, D., 40, 415n.
Shapiro, B., 44, 443n.
Shapiro, V., 162, 436n.
Shockley, W. B., 13
Shriver, E. K., 8
Shriver, R. S., 8
Sigman, M., 92, 142, 430n., 437n.
Silberstein, R. M., 240, 413n.
Simon, T., 40, 401n.
Skeels, H. M., 28, 29, 36, 56, 57, 57n., 59n., 63, 67, 437n.
Skinner, B. F., 347, 437n.
Skodak, M., 29, 56, 57, 57n., 437n.
Slade, C. I., 171, 437n.
Smilansky, M., 15, 15n., 437n.
Smith, D. P. B., 301, 438n.
Smith, D. W., 61, 437n.
Smith, H. T., 348, 437n.
Snyder, R. A., 273, 403n.
Solnit, A. J., 95, 424n.
Sostek, A., 120, 143, 410n., 437n.
Spelt, D., 257, 438n.
Spencer, H.. 8
Spiegel, J., 209, 429n.
Spielberger, C. D., 122, 438n.
Sroufe, J. A., 136, 438n.
Sroufe, L. A., 5, 426n.
Standley, K., 179, 398n.
Starr, R. H., 128, 407n.
Stein, S. C., 201, 204, 438n.
Steiner, G. Y., 8, 438n.
Stephenson, E. A., 274, 301, 434n.
Stephenson, G. R., 301, 438n.
Stern, D. N., 97, 98, 120, 127, 133, 135, 138, 151, 153, 158, 287, 410n., 438n.
Stern, L., 162, 421n.
Stern, W., 40
Sterritt, G., v
Stewart, S. L., 200, 438n.
Stout, A. M., 94, 438n.

Streissguth, A. P., 121, 127, 400n., 421n.
Stunkard, A. J., 72, 73, 80, 439n.
Suci, G. J., 241, 244, 428n.
Suran, B. G., 208, 209, 211, 439n.
Sutton-Smith, B., 94, 439n.
Sveger, T., 76, 439n.

Taitz, T. S., 75, 439n.
Tannenbaum, P. H., 241, 244, 428n.
Tanzer, C., 178, 439n.
Taub, H. B., 240, 413n.
Taylor, J., 175, 409n.
Teska, J. A., 49, 50, 51, 356, 420n.
Thoman, E. B., 87, 88, 89, 91-119, 94, 99, 100, 101, 104, 111, 114, 118, 215, 225, 238, 242, 354, 359, 411n., 439n., 440n.
Thomas, A., 77, 80, 215, 440n.
Thompson, M. A., 136, 406n.
Thorndike, E. L., 14, 440n.
Thurstone, L. L., 236, 440n.
Tinsley, B. R., 174-89, 213
Tizard, B., 67, 440n.
Trevarthen, C. B., 46, 128, 135, 441n.
Trickett, P. K., 10, 445n.
Trnavsky, P. A., 272, 441n.
Tronick, E., 46, 87, 89, 91, 98, 129, 131, 133, 134, 144-58, 147-51, 156, 214, 215, 298n., 354, 402n., 441n.
Tulkin, S. R., 127, 216, 239, 241, 423n., 441n.
Turner, A. M., 94, 440n.

Uzgiris, I. C., 15, 19, 47, 441n., 442n.

Vandenberg, S. G., 63, 441n.
VanEgeren, L. F., 127, 400n.
Vietze, P., 121, 126, 143, 437n.
Volkmar, F., 52, 421n.
Vollman, J. H., 198, 208, 400n.
Vuille, J. C., 76, 427n.

Wachs, T. D., 47, 442n.
Waldrop, M. F., 258, 258n., 355, 400n.
Walker, H., 348, 442n.
Walker, L. O., vii-x, 80, 234-50, 214, 244

Wallin, J. E. W., 40, 442n.
Walters, C. E., 257, 442n.
Ward, J. H., 248, 442n.
Watson, J. S., 140, 442n.
Watts, D. G., 302, 418n.
Watts, J. C., 44, 48, 443n.
Weber, C. U., 10n., 442n.
Weikart, D. P., 10n., 49, 51, 442n.
Weinberg, R. A., 30, 435n.
Weinraub, M., 255, 403n.
Weiss, J. L., 242, 406n.
Weissman, R. E., 84, 434n.
Weller, G. M., 258, 355, 400n.
Wente, A. S., 178, 442n.
West, S., 178, 430n.
White, B. L., 44, 48, 443n.
Whitelaw, A. G. L., 75, 82, 83, 443n.
Whiten, A., 166, 443n.
Wicker, A. W., 235, 238n., 443n.
Wiel, A., 79, 443n.
Wilkinson, P. W., 83, 443n.
Willerman, L., 4, 55-69, 57n., 65, 66, **216,** 346, 356, 359, 416n., 443n.
Williamson, M. L., 68, 401n.
Wilson, C. D., 127, 140, 424n.
Wilson, E. O., 300, 444n.
Winer, B. J., 318
Winick, M., 72, 444n.
Wise, S., 46, 97, 150, 402n., 441n.
Withers, R. F. J., 74, 444n.
Wohlwill, J. F., 92, 265, 269, 356, **444n.**
Wolff, O. H., 73, 403n.
Woltereck, R., 16
Woodrow, H., 38, 444n.
Wunsch, J. P., 136, 438n.

Yang, R. K., 252, 255-70, 258, 259, 260-65, 355, 444n.
Yarrow, L. J., 39, 46, 175, 445n.
Yarrow, M. R., 348, 445n.

Zaslow, M., 143, 437n.
Zaslow, R. W., 208, 445n.
Zax, M., 344, 434n., 445n.
Zigler, E., **10**
Zuk, G. H., 209, 445n.

SUBJECT INDEX

All page numbers for tables and figures appear in italics.

Achievement tests, 41
Adolescence, compensatory education in, 43
Adoption:
  and genetic studies of intelligence, 56
  and obesity, 74, 79
Alcohol and biophysical risks, *viii*
American Medical Association (AMA), 205
Amniocentesis, 210
Anencephalics, 202
Anoxia, 91, 344
Apgar score, 240
Approach-withdrawal, maternal-twins and, *153*, 154
Attachment disturbances, 142
Attentiveness of infants, 131
Attitudes, parental, and parent-infant relationships, 234-49, 348
  conclusion on, 249
  methodological considerations on, 240-43
  preliminary research design on, 244-49
  discussion of, 247-49
  method of, 244-45
  results on, 245-47, *246, 247*
  theoretical considerations on, 236-40
    dimensionality, 236-37
    neonatal perception, 238-40
Attribution theory in social psychology, 348

Badger instrument, 43-44
Badger's Teaching Guides for Infants/ Toddlers, 20
Bayley Scales of Infant Development, 65, 117, 165, 216, *230*
  DEVN-AVG, 227, 229, 231
  DEVN-OWN, 227, 229, 231
Behavior codes, 274
Behaviorism:
  on reflexes, 36
  for weight control, 72
Bethesda Longitudinal Study, 255-70
  basic considerations on, 256-58
  conclusion on, 269-70
  length of time, 265-69, *266, 267*
  longitudinal relations, 261-65, *264*
  maturity in, 259-60
  reactivity-irritability in, 259, 260
  reflexive/discriminative sucking in, 260
Biophysical risks, *viii*
  conceptualization framework on, ix-x
  and obesity, 70
Birth order:
  and feeding practices, 94-95
  and maternal activity, 127-28
  and obesity, 79
Birth weight as biophysical risk, *viii*, 344
Bonding, maternal-infant, 46, 161, 165
Brain development and environmental factors, 33, 58
Brazelton Neonatal Behavioral Assessment Scale, 92, 241, 244, 256

455

Breast feeding and obesity, 79. *See also* Feeding patterns

Caretaking:
  casualty in, 120, 121
  environment of, 347-52
Categorical level, 350-51, 358
Cell assemblies concept, 36
Central nervous system, conduction, selective breeding for, 58-59
Cerebral palsy, 142
Child abuse, 162, 176
  literature on, 170
Childbirth, preparation for, 178
Child guidance movement, 11
Child-rearing and heritability, 14
Children of the Creche (Dennis), 28
Children's Cause, The (Steiner), 8
Chromosomes and retardation, 61. *See also* Genes
Cipher language, 99-100
Cloning, 16
Cognition, achievement/demands in, 11
Collaborative Perinatal Research Project, 216
Communicative behaviors, mother-infant, *284, 285*
Compensating level, 350, 351
Compensatory education, 11-12, 44, 49
  in adolescence, 43
  failure of, 13
Competence, 44-45
  self-ratings in, 229
Compulsiveness, 11
Computers and direct observation, 301
Concrete operations stage of development, 350
Context of development, 356-57
Criterion-referenced approach, 4
  tests, 41-42, 53
Critical periods in obesity development, 84
Cue-exchange, mother-infant, 96-97
Culture:
  and decision-making, 209-210
  retardation and, 64
Custody cases, fathers in, 175-76
Cybernetic systems of communication, 145-46, 157

Daily Infant Feeding/Sleeping Record, 80n.
Damaged newborns, nontreatment of, 204-207
Damtamyte, 274

Deaf, supportive environment for, 345-46
Decision-making and culture, 209-10
Dendritic aborizations, 58
Depression and psychosocial risks, *ix*
Developmental model, 353
Diagnosis, tests for, 39-42
Diapering, paternal participation in, 184, *185, 187*
Diathesis-stress model on obesity. *See* Obesity, infantile, diathesis-stress model for
Digital recording system, 274
Digo tribe, 349
Direct observation techniques, 300-301
Divorce and fathers, 175
Down's syndrome, 18, 59, 125, 142, 201

Early separation/reproductive casualty. *See* Reproductive casualty/early separation, disruption of attachment formation due to
Educability, goal of,
  and early experience, 10
  indices of, 15
  and potential, 14
EEG, 59
Electro-General Corporation, 274
Emory University School of Medicine, 272
Emotional deprivation and developmental failure, 95-96
Empathy and personal disability, 193
Environmental enrichment and intelligence, 65
Environment and heredity, relative importance of, 14-15, 55-59
Equilibration (equilibrium), 11, 33
Equilibrium (equilibration), 11, 33
Essay on the Principles of Population (Malthus), 14
Ethics, medical, treatment of newborns, 204-207
Euthanasia:
  alternatives to, 208-11
  ethics of, 204-207
  passive, 201
Extinction, 47
Eye pigment, inheritance of, 61
Face-to-face interactions, disturbance in, 150-54, *151, 153*
Family support system, 43
Fat cell hypothesis on obesity, 73
Fathers and risk, hospital-based intervention model on, 174-89
  discussion of, 188-89

fathers as caretakers, 175-77
hospital-based intervention program, 179-87, *185, 187*
intervention as father support system, 177-79
and childbirth, 178-79
Feedback and psychosocial risks, *viii*
Feeding patterns, 124
and birth order, 94-95
behavior scored, *280*
and bonding, 165
and obesity, 71-85, 347
and paternal behavior, 181, 184
and reproductive casualty, 164-65
Fertilizer effects, 4, 63
Fetal development:
of brain, 68-69
research on, vii
Formal operational stage of development, 350
Funding and public awareness, vi

Games, infant-parent, 136-37
G.A.P. Committee on Child Psychiatry, 239
Gaze of infant:
aversion of, 172
and maternal behavior, 129-30, *130*
Gender prediction, *225*
General systems perspective, 88, 216
Genes. See also Genetics of psychosocial risk: Genotypes; Heritability
counseling on, 210-11, 211n.
and environment, relative importance of, 14-15, 55-59
Genetics of psychosocial risk, 44, 55-69
conceptual framework on, ix-x
genetic perspective, 4, 67-68
inherited characteristics, 57-59
and mental retardation, 59-67, *62*
neurological damage, 63-67
prevention of, 63-67
operational definition of, vii
in pregnancy/early infancy, *viii-ix*
Genotypes. See also Genes; Genetics of psychosocial risk
and environment, 55, 346
and phenotypes, 3, 16, 18, 347
Gestural imitation, 20, *21*, 22
Grady Memorial Hospital, 272
Great Britain, treatment of infants in, 204-205
Great Society of the 1960s, v

Habituation, 47
Hair color, inheritance of, 61
Harvard Preschool Project, 44, 45
Heart rates of infants, 131-32, *132*
Hereditary Genius (Galton), 14
Heredity. *See also* Genes
and environment, 14-15, 55-59
and intelligence, 13, 55-59
Heritability:
approach to, 346
defined, 57n.
hypothesis on, 12-13
indices of, 15, 16-17
of intelligence, 53, 55-59
on range of reactions, 13-18
and retardation, 13-18
Heterozygote fetuses, 68
High-risk infants:
early interactions and later development, 141-43
interactions of, 120-43
qualitative differences, 133-41
phases of interaction, 134-41
quantitative differences, 121-33
inverted U, 121-33, *130, 132*
Hippocratic Oath, 202
Home Observation for Measurement of the Environment (HOME), 216
Hormone levels:
antepartum/postpartum, 163
and biophysical risks, *viii*
Hospitals, 162, 170, 171. *See also* Fathers and risk, hospital-based intervention model on
Hot house effects, 4, 63
"How Much Can We Boost IQ and Scholastic Achievement?" (Jensen), 13
Hunter's syndrome, 68
Hyaline membrane disease, 200
Hyperactivity:
of mothers, 121-24, 135, 138, 140
and physical risks, *ix*
Hypoactivity:
of infants, 126
of mothers, 121-24, 126, 129
Hyporesponsive infants, 126, 135

Impact of Head Start, The (Cicirelli et al.), 9
Individual differences, perspectives on, 3, 4, 41
Infanticide, 197, 201

Infants Ideals (II), attitudes on, 245, *246, 247,* 248
Infantized imitative behaviors, 135-36
Inheritability. *See* Heritability
Intelligence. *See also* IQ; Mental retardation
  inheritance of, 13, 55-59
  and neural conduction, 58-59
  and obesity, 56
  polygenic continuum for, 60
  and poverty, 52
  and socio-economic status, 16, 23, 30-32, 65
  tests on, prediction by, 37-39
Intelligence and Experience (Hunt), 8
Interactional model, 353
Introversion, 264-65
IQ. *See also* Intelligence; Stanford-Binet test
  genetic basis of, 56-57, 57n.
  and heredity, 13
  longitudinal testing of, 12
  and maternal speech, 142
  mental age/chronological age in, 40
  and obesity, 84
  and orphanage rearing, 28-30
  and plasticity, 53
  as predictor, 37-39
  in retardation, 59-60, 64-68
  scores of, 356
  and social class, 16, 23
  and socio-economic status, 16, 23, 30-32
  in twins, 17-18
  variance in, 13-14
Israel, migration to, 16

Kennedy Awards, 29
Kibbutzim, intelligence of, 16
Kikuyn tribe, 349

Labor, prolonged, 91-92
Lag sequential analysis, observational study, 300-41
  analysis of sequential significance, 331-33, *332*
  autocontingency effects, 328-30, *329*
  autolags, 315-21, *316, 317, 320*
  conclusion on, 340
  criterion on, 310-11
  crosslags, 321-23, *322*
  definition/procedures on, 307-10
  greater than 1 lags, 312-13
  lag contingencies, 323-28, *324, 327*

lag model, 301-306
  probability computation, 302-307, *303, 304, 306*
  research paradigm on, 338-40, *339*
  statistical significance of, 313-15, *314*
  and vectors, 333-37, *334, 336*
Lamaze training, 178
Language:
  delays in, 142
  development of, 24-25
  isomorphic relations in, 157
  and mother-infant nonlinguistic communication, 97-98
  phonological component of, 40
  skills for, 45, 45n., 52
  training in, 4
Learning and psychosocial risks, *viii*
Likert technique, 242
Lip-reading, 345
Locomotive abilities, 48
Longitudinal study of mother-infant interaction, 75-76, 83, 98-99, 120, 142, 239, 255-70

Malnourishment and infant gestation, 239
Maternal deprivation, 163
Maternal Ideals (MI), attitudes on, 245, *246,* 246-48, *247*
Maternal Ideals-Maternal Security-Maturity (MI-MSM) complex, 246-48, *246, 247*
Maternal self-confidence paired comparisons (MSC), 244-48, *246, 247*
Means development, 20, *21*
Meningitis, 204
Meningomyeloceles, 201
Mental retardation, plasticity and hierarchical achievements, 3, 5, 9-54
  evidence of plasticity, 18-32
    non-metrical effects of interventions, 24-28, *25, 26*
  heritability or range of reactions, 13-18
  and incompetence/poverty, 49-54
  and psychological development theory, 32-42
    and diagnostic tests, 39-40
    and learning-teaching goals, 40-49
    and predictive tests, 37-39
    and psychosocial risk, 59-67, *62*
  risk assessment, 42-48
Metera Center, Athens, 15, 20
Models of development, 345-46
Mother-Child Home Program, 49

Morphogenesis, 61
  timing of, *62*
Multitrait-multimethod approach in parental attitudes, 243, 247-48
Municipal Orphanage of Athens, 22, 23
Municipal Orphanage of Tehran, 19, 28
Myelination, timing of, *62*
Myelomeningocele child, 204

National Institute of Child Health and Human Development, 8
National Institute of Mental Health, 198
  International Research Program, 257
National Perinatal Association, 173
Neonatal Behavioral Assessment Scale, 259
Neonatal Perception Inventories (NPI), 239-41, 245-49, *246, 247*
Neural conduction and intelligence, 58-59
Neurotic inhibitions, 11
Nilo-Hamitic genetic origins, 349
Norm-referenced tests, 38, 41, 42, 53
Norms:
  attitudinal, 237
  social/personal, 348-49
Nurseries, high-risk, 161-62
Nursery schools, compensatory goals in, 10

Obesity, infantile, diathesis-stress model for, 5, 70-85, 87-89
  and adoption, 74, 79
  and birth order, 79
  case study of, 82
  and feeding/sleepng patterns, 71-85, 347
  genetic studies, 74-75
  hypothesis on, 81-82
  implications of, 82-85
  longitudinal studies on, 75-76, 83
  methodology for, 79-80
  and overnutrition, 76-82
  prediction of, 73-74
  risk factors in environment, 70-71, 79-80
  and sleep, 71-73
Object construction, 23
Object permanence, 20, *21*, 22, 23
Object relations, 20, *21*
Observation procedures, 275-76
Office of Child Development, 10
Office of Economic Opportunity, 13
Ontogenesis and environmental factors, 32
Operational causality, 20, *21*
Origin of Species (Darwin), 14
Orphanage of the Queen Farah Pahlavi Charity Society, 15, 17, 18

Overnutrition, 76, 347
Overprotectiveness, 126, 142

Parent and Child Center of Mt. Carmel, 22, 23
Parent Attitude Research Institute (PARI), 240, 241
Parent-infant interactions, asynchrony/disruption in, 91-119, 178
  behaviors recorded, 101, 103, *103*
  case studies, 104-17, *105, 106, 108, 112-16*
  code-recording behaviors, 99-101
  communication model, 96-98
  discussion of, 117-19
  earliest patterns of interaction, 93-95
  emphasis upon, 92-93
  longitudinal study strategies for, 98-99
  mother-infant interaction and development dysfunction, 95-96
Pediatric News, 201
Personal model, 353
Phenotypes/genotypes in research, 3, 16, 18, 347. *See also* Genes; Genetics of psychosocial risk
Phenylalanine, 68
Phenylketonuria (PKU), 68
Phrenoblysis, 12
Plasticity in psychological development, 3-4
Play:
  and development, 10
  and parent-infant interaction, 182-83
Postpartum period and parental attitudes, 238-39
Poverty and mental retardation, 49-54
Prediction, reliability in, 91
Premature infants, 95, 118, 166, 344. *See also* Prenatal contexts, parental models for; Preterm/full-term infant-mother dyads
  and activity, 354-55
  intensive care for, 200-201
  neurological immaturity of, 171-72
  and parental attitudes, 239
  risk in, 88
  vocalizations of, 279
Prenatal contexts, parental models for, 215-53. *See also* Premature infants
  contextual differences, 231-32
  and developmental continuity, 216
  evaluating contexts, 217-18
  models research, 218-31

development pace, *230*
difficulty ratings, *228*
gender prediction, *225*
sample change items, *221*
sample characteristics, *219*
sex preferences, *224*
prospectus on, 232-33
Preoperational stage of development, 350, 358
Pregnancy:
confirmation of, 220
preparation for, 178-79
psychosocial risks in, *viii-ix*
Preterm/full-term infant-mother dyads, 271-99. *See also* Premature infants
behavioral dialogues, 282-86, *284-85*
flow analysis, 286-91, *286, 288*
pattern analysis, 291-96, *292, 293, 295*
method on, 272-76
observations, 273-74
procedure/apparatus, 274-76, *276*
subjects, 272-73
results on, 276-82, *277, 278, 280, 281*
summary on, 298-99
variable stability, 96-98, *297*
Project Head Start, 9, 10, 11, 12, 13, 14, 27, 49, 53, 359
Prospectivistic level, 350, 352
Psychoanalysis:
on attitudes, 235
and child guidance movement, 11
Psychosis:
natural history of, 152
and psychosocial risks, *ix*
Psychosocial risk, genetics of. *See* Genetics of psychosocial risks; Obesity, infantile, diathesis-stress model for
Psychotherapy, adjunctive, 210-11, 211n.

Questionnaires on prenatal contexts, 218-20

Racial Isolation in the Public Schools (U.S. Commission on Civil Rights), 9
Radiation and genome, 61
Range of reaction concept, 16
Recapitulation theory, 10-11
Reciprocal obligations, *viii*, 156
REM sleep, 100
Reproductive casualty/early separation:
conclusions on, 169-73

disruption of attachment formation due to, 120, 121, 161-73
and feeding, 164-65
interactional deprivation, 163-64
Retardation, mental. *See* Mental retardation
Risk factors, psychosocial, taxonomy on, 361-95
environmental, 363-76
infant developmental status of birth, 376-82
infant and environmental interaction, 382-85
outcomes, 385-95
outline on, 362
RNA/DNA ratios, 58. *See also* Genes
Ross Conference on Pediatric Research, 200

Sampling techniques, 79-80
Sanctity of life, 190-203
physician's perspective on, 200-203
Schemes for relating to objects, 20, *21, 22*
Schizophrenia, 66, 344, 353
Self-actualization, family, 191
Self-appraisals of mothers, 229, 239
Semantic differential technique, 241-42, 244
Sensorimotor organization, 34-35, 142
stage of development, 36, 39, 350, 357
Separation of psychosocial risks, *viii*. *See also* Reproductive casualty/early separation
Serial ordering, 34
Sex differences, 354-55
attitudes on, 182
Sex preferences on children, 224
Sleep:
of infants, characteristics of, 110-12
and obesity, 71-73
Social competence, defined, 10
Social Darwinism, 8
Social Readjustment Rating Scale, 199
Social skills in infancy, 144-58
consequences of developmental disruption, 154-58, *155*
face-to-face interactions, disturbance in, 150-54, *151, 153*
mother-infant interaction, joint regulation of, 145-50, *148, 149*
Socio-cultural model, 353
Socio-economic class:
and development, 8
and hypoactivity, 121

and intelligence, 16, 23, 30-32, 65
and parental expectations, 231-32
and prenatal contexts, 220
and psychological development, 28
and psychosocial risks, *viii*
and values, 349
and verbal stimulation, 127
Stability and Change in Human Characteristics (Bloom), 8
Stanford-Binet test, 65, 142, 216. *See also* IQ
Stereotypes, enculturated role, 197
Stimulus/response, 33
Stress and psychosocial risks, *viii*
Sucking:
  behavior, 100-101
  reflexive/discriminative, 260
Superego development, 11
Symbiosis, 350
Symbiotic level, 350, 357
Synchronization, interactive, 146-47
Systems theory, 88, 216

Tay-Sachs disease, 210
Teaching machines, 41
Teenage mothers, 50-52, 126
Tehran Orphanage, 46
Time-lapse photography, 97
Tobacco and biophysical risks, *viii*
Toy Demonstrators Visit Handbook, 50
Toys for learning, 50
Traditional Family Ideology Scale, 245, *246*

Parent-Child Relationships Subscale, 244, 245
Transactional process and individual adaptation, 5
Turntaking, infant-parent, 137-38
Twins, monozygotic/dizygotic, 16-18
  birth order and maternal activity, 127
  maternal interaction with, 152-54
  and obesity, 74, 83, 83n.
Tyrosine, 68

United Services for Effective Parenting (USEP), 52
University of Cincinnati Medical School, 43, 50, 52
University of Minnesota, 29
University of Texas, vii, 217
  Student Health Center, 70n.
U.S. Commission on Civil Rights, 9
Uzgiris-Hunt Scales, *21*

Videotape:
  for maternal-infant transactions, 81-82
  for paternal-infant interactions, 179-89
Vocalizations:
  games in, 46-47
  imitation in, 20, *21*, 40
  infant, 142
  maternal, 122-24, *123*
  and preterm infants, 279

Westinghouse Learning Corporation, 9
WISC, 64. *See also* IQ